KINESIOLOGY

Application to Pathological Motion

KINESIOLOGY

Application to Pathological Motion

Gary L. Soderberg, LPT, PhD

Associate Professor
Physical Therapy Education
College of Medicine
The University of Iowa
Iowa City, Iowa

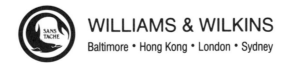

WILLIAMS & WILKINS
Baltimore • Hong Kong • London • Sydney

Senior Editor: John Butler
Associate Editor: Carol Eckhart
Copy Editor: Stephen Siegforth
Design: Bob Och
Illustration Planning: Reginald R. Stanley
Production: Raymond E. Reter

Copyright ©, 1986
Williams & Wilkins
428 East Preston Street
Baltimore, MD 21202, U.S.A.

Printed in the United States of America

Library of Congress Cataloging in Publication Data

Main entry under title:

Soderberg, Gary L.
  Kinesiology—application to pathological motion.

  Includes bibliographies and index.
  1. Physical therapy. 2. Human mechanics. 3. Kinesiology. I. Title. [DNLM: 1. Biomechanics. 2. Movement. 3. Movement Disorders. WE 103 S679k]
RM701.S64 1986   612'.7   85-6247
ISBN 0-683-07857-7

90 91 92 93 94
10 9 8 7 6 5 4 3

Dedicated to Susie, Kendra, Curt, Kristine
and colleagues and students who
offered challenge and influence

Preface

This volume has evolved from numerous years of teaching, clinical observation, and researching phenomena associated with normal and pathological motion. The work assimilates materials fundamental to both kinesiology and pathokinesiology so that professional program entry level students in health or related fields may achieve an understanding of principles applied to normal and pathological movement. The work is primarily intended for physical therapists but has broad application across any discipline that incorporates movement science.

The primary objective of this volume is to present knowledge in sufficient depth so as to provide a true understanding of factors which predispose abnormal motion. This text assumes prerequisite knowledge in physics, pathology, gross and applied anatomy, and physiology. No intention exists of reviewing fundamentals, for example, the physiology of muscle contraction as related to human movement. Serious attempts have been made to include applications of basic principles and sciences to movement dysfunction. The reader and student will also find an abundance of resource material that may be utilized to further enhance the understanding of kinesiology and pathokinesiology.

The content of the work is broken into three major sections. The first includes fundamentals of evaluating movement; muscle mechanics and applied neurology; articular function; and material properties of biological tissues. The second and major section deals with articular kinesiology and pathokinesiology, while the third section discusses posture, gait, and ergonomics. Included with each of the latter two sections will be reiterations of the principles established in the first section. Numerous examples will be provided for the application of the fundamentals attended to in the early sections of the volume. The material in this volume is intended to foster the establishment of adequate competencies for provision of patient care and to serve as a precursor for further study and a greater understanding of pathological motion.

Gary L. Soderberg

Acknowledgment

The preparation of this work would not have been possible without the diligent assistance of many others. Particular thanks is expressed to all students who graciously critiqued the work during and after the development of the manuscript. Don Neumann, a therapist and doctoral candidate, provided invaluable feedback as the volume evolved. Similar thanks is expressed to graduate student Dave Johnson, a therapist held in high regard because of his knowledge of the clinical management of musculoskeletal dysfunction. Chapter reviewers also contributed significantly to the quality and inclusiveness of the content. Among them were Bob Lamb of the Medical College of Virginia, and Bruce Miller, Supervisor of the Musculoskeletal Division of the Physical Therapy Department of the University of Iowa Hospitals and Clinics. Other chapter reviewers included Jim Andrews, Tom Cook, Don Shurr, and Carolyn Wadsworth. Thanks is also expressed to Chanatip Suksang for the illustrative work. My special appreciation is extended to Judy Biderman for her splendid organization and attention to the required detail. Finally, recognition needs to be given to the remainder of the faculty of the University of Iowa Educational Programs in Physical Therapy for their tolerance while the preparation of this manuscript was pursued.

Contents

1

Principles Applied to Movement

Fundamental to the study of kinesiology and pathological motion are the terms and associated units used to describe motion and the forces producing or resulting from motion. Also essential is an overview of factors that influence motion. Then, relating these factors to movement is essential to understanding normal and abnormal movement. This chapter focuses on an overview of the factors pertinent to the description of motion. The information presented in each of the topics will be referred to and elaborated upon in later chapters, primarily those discussing the individual joints.

TERMINOLOGY
Systems and Units

Much of the information directly related to kinesiology and the description of pathological motion is presented with units and/or terminologies that use different systems of measurement. The student of normal and disturbed motion must have a working understanding of the meaning of the fundamental units as well as the ability to make conversion between the different quantities of the various measurement systems. Further, without this level of comprehension the student and practitioner will have difficulty reading and effectively comparing results presented in the literature. For these and other purposes this section will present the fundamental units of measurement systems as they relate to kinesiology and pathological motion.

Recently the International System of Units, known as SI, has become rather widely accepted. The SI, a modern version of MKSA (meter, kilogram, second, ampere), is based on seven fundamental units which by convention are regarded as dimensionally independent. Of most importance to the study of movement are length (meter), mass (kilograms), and time (seconds) because they are base units in the system (Fig. 1.1) (5). From these units other quantities are derived. Note that with few exceptions, such as joules per second for power, the units are all derived from the base units. Of frequent interest is force, defined as the action or effect of one body on another. This quantity, derived from the product of mass (kilograms) and acceleration (meters per square second), is in newtons. Other systems of measurement in use but to be avoided are:

 English absolute (foot, pound mass, second, and poundal)
 Metric gravitational (meter, metric slug, second, kilogram force)
 English gravitational (foot, slug, second, pound force)

From the systems and units described above note that the principal departure of SI from the gravimetric system of metric engineering units is the use of

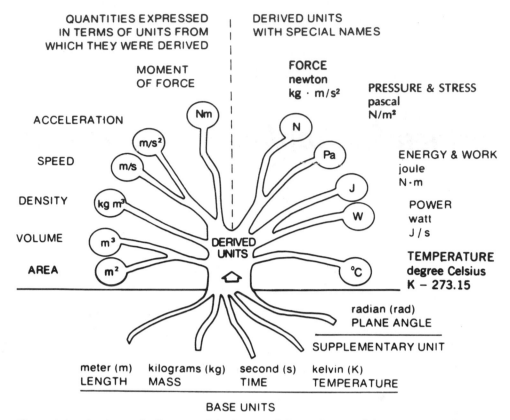

Figure 1.1.   A schematic diagram of the base and derived units of the International System of Units. (From Frankel VH, Nordin M: *Basic Biomechanics of the Skeletal System.* Philadelphia, Lea & Febiger, 1980, p 4.

explicitly distinct units for mass and force. In SI, the name kilogram is restricted to the unit of mass. The kilogram-force, from which the suffix "force" was in practice often erroneously dropped, should not be used. In its place the SI unit of force, the newton, defined as force which applied to mass of 1 kg gives it an acceleration of 1 m/s² (1 kgm/s²), is used. Likewise, the newton rather than the kilogram-force is used to form derived units which include force. For example, pressure or stress (newtons per square meter = pascals), energy and work (newtons × meters = joules), and power (newtons × meters per second = watts) are all commonly used (15).

Considerable confusion exists from use of the term weight as a quantity to mean either force or mass. In commercial and everyday use, the term weight often means mass. Thus, when one speaks of a person's weight, the quantity often referred to is mass. This technically incorrect use of the term weight in everyday life will probably persist. In science and technology, the term weight of a body means the force that if applied to the body would give it an acceleration equal to the local acceleration of a free falling body. The adjective "local" in the phrase "local acceleration of a freely falling body" means at that particular location on the surface of the earth. In this context the local acceleration of gravity is designated by the symbol g, with observed values of g differing by over 0.5% at various points on the earth's surface. The use of "gravity force" (mass times acceleration of gravity) instead of weight with this meaning is recommended. Because of the dual use of the term weight as a quantity, this term should be avoided in technical practice except under circumstances in which its meaning is completely clear. When the term is used, it is important to know whether mass or force is intended and to use SI units properly by using kilograms for mass or newtons for force (1; J. Andrews, University of Iowa, personal communication, 1982.)

The use of the same name for units of force and mass causes confusion. When the non-SI units are used, a distinction should be made between force and mass, for example, lbf to denote force in gravimetric engineering units and lbm for mass (1). Table 1.1, modified from White and Panjabi (13), gives conversion factors for entities specified in the presently used inch, pound system and the new SI system proposed for use in the United States. To obtain the measurement unit when the SI unit is given, multiply the SI quantity by the numerator factor X. Use the denominator factor Y as the multiplier to convert from the right-hand column to the SI system. The latter is much preferred (13).

Another unit frequently encountered in the literature is the kilopond (kp). It is a gravimetric measure of force equal to 1 kg of mass at the earth's surface. Conversions are kp or kg(f) times 2.205 to arrive at lb(f). Conversely, lb(f) times 0.4536 equals kps. To convert newtons to kiloponds multiply by 0.1020. To change kiloponds to newtons multiply by 9.81.

An example of using conversions occurs if one uses the foot-pound output of the Cybex (Division of Lumex, Ronkonkoma, NY), an electromechanical device frequently used in clinical settings. Assume that the patient generates 80 lbf-ft (same as foot-pounds) of torque during isometric knee extension. To convert to SI multiply by 1.3558 (see Table 1.1). The newton meters of torque should = 108.46. Other conversion tables exist and the student/practitioner should either select one or generate commonly used measures that are most consistent with their needs (5, 13).

Movement Description

In addition to the entities described and quantified above there are other terms to which a specific meaning is attached. Each is basic to understanding kinesiology, and each will be used later in this volume. The discussion that ensues presents the most important and useful concepts. A complete list of terms can be found in White and Panjabi (13).

Reference Frames

In order to adequately describe motion a reference frame is required. This reference frame, often arbitrarily located, is used so that displacement data adequately represent the motion or motions occurring. Often, human motion is described relative to the location of the body in a given room or location. Clinically, however, therapists will register motion with respect to the perceived axis of a given joint. Although clinical technique is prone to inaccuracies the method is not likely, because of practicalities, to be significantly altered.

Degrees of Freedom

An additional general concept that should be understood is degrees of freedom. By definition this is the number of independent coordinates in a system that are necessary to accurately specify the position of an object in space. For example, a pure hinge joint would have 1° of freedom because only one

Table 1.1.   Conversions

Entity	SI	→X→ ←Y←	Misc. units
Acceleration	m/sec²	3.2808 0.3048	ft/sec²
Angle	rad	57.296 0.0175	degree
Area	m²	10.763 0.0929	ft²
	m²	1550.0 0.000645	inch²
Density	kg/m³	0.0624 16.018	lbm/ft³
	kg/m³	0.0000361 27680.	lbm/inch³
Energy, work	N·m = J[a]	0.7376 1.3558	ft lbf
Force	N	0.2248 4.4482	lbf
	N	$\dfrac{X}{9.81}$	kgf
Length	m	3.2808 0.3048	ft
	m	39.370 0.0254	inch
Mass	kg	2.2046 0.4536	lbm
Mass moment of inertia	kg m²	23.730 0.0421	lbm ft²
Moment, torque	Nm	0.7376 1.3558	lbf ft
	Nm	$\dfrac{X}{9.81}$	kgf m
Pressure, stress	N/m² = Pa[a]	$\dfrac{X}{98,066}$	kgf/cm²
	N/m² = Pa[a]	0.000145 6895.6	lbf/inch²
Stiffness	N/m	5.667 0.177	lbf/inch
Velocity	m/sec	3.2808 0.3048	ft/sec
Volume	m³	35.313 0.0283	ft³
	m³	61023. 0.0000164	inch³

[a] Official recommended units of SI.

coordinate exists around which motion will take place. Anatomical joints are said to have 1 to 3° of freedom, depending upon the structure. However, later in this volume a case will be made for all joints having 6° of freedom.

Kinematics and Kinetics

Fundamental to the analysis and description of motion are the terms associated with the collection of information used in the description of human motion. For example, kinematics is used to mean the description of motion without regard to the forces. Systems commonly in use include filming techniques and goniometry, i.e., any method that collects displacement data. On the other hand, kinetics is the term applied to the study of force or forces applied to the body. These forces can be internally generated forces, such as muscular tensions or restraint forces produced by tensions in ligaments. External forces, such as gravity and segmental masses, must also be taken into account. The application and magnitude of all the forces determines whether motion does or does not take place, forming the basis for isometric and isotonic exercise forms. The forces, of both internal and external generation, produce the resultant effects at joints, determining the magnitude of the compression, shear, and rotation that occurs at these joints. It is these joint forces that are often of ultimate interest to the clinician. Discussion of these joint forces will occur in each of the subsequent chapters on the joints.

Other factors are common to the motion of the human body and the respective segments. Inertia, a well-known property of bodies, will be discussed in subsequent sections of this chapter. The topic of body segment parameters will also be discussed. How these and other quantities influence and interact during motion will be elucidated throughout the remainder of this volume.

REPRESENTATION OF MUSCLE FORCES
Vector Representation of Muscle

Typically, tensile forces as generated by muscles satisfy the criteria for and are subsequently vector quantities. You will recall from basic physics that vectors are represented by magnitude (length), a line of application (in this case, the action line of the muscle), a direction, and a point of application. Vectors can also be used to represent displacement, velocity, accelerations, and certainly muscle forces or tensions generated within muscles. On the other hand, scalar quantities have magnitude only. Temperature is an example.

Frequently, attempts are made to compose and resolve vectors in order to adequately represent the motion segment or segments of the human body. Composition is defined as combining two forces into one. Classical methods of solution are the parallelogram and the trigonometric method. A corollary occurs in muscle when we attempt to describe the line of action of the anterior and middle deltoid muscle segments in abduction of the glenohumeral joint. Conversely, resolution is replacing a single force by two or more forces. This will be emphasized in Chapter 2 by showing how the tensile force from muscle can be resolved into rotary and stabilizing components.

Torque

When discussing the rotary component of these tensile forces the term torque must be introduced. A synonym is moment, defined as the measure of the tendency of a force to produce rotation about a point or axis. Moments should be described in newton-meters, but they can also be described in any other units of force and distance (Table 1.1). They may also be described as positive or negative, clockwise or counterwise, or by other conventions. Specifically, the moment is determined by the force multiplied by the perpendicular distance from the line of application of the force to the axis around which the turning motion is occurring (Fig. 1.2). Further, note that any force that passes through

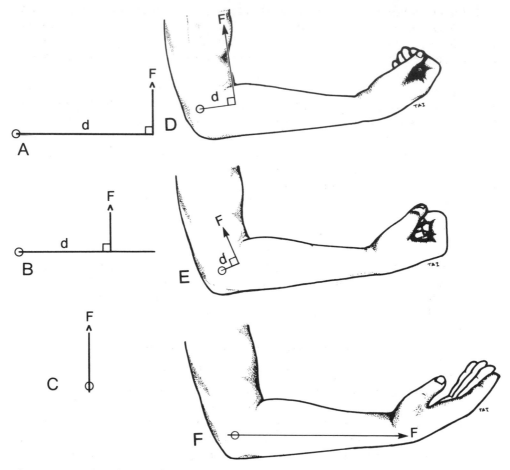

Figure 1.2. (A) In this graphical representation the muscle force (*F*) is applied perpendicularly to a segment at some distance (*d*). (B) A force of similar magnitude is now applied closer to the axis of rotation (O) and would have less of a turning effect because d is less. (C) In this case F passes through O; thus, there is no perpendicular distance. The result is zero moment. *D, E,* and *F* show the correlary situation at the elbow.

the center of rotation will have zero moment since the distance is zero (Fig. 1.2). Therefore, in all cases there are two ways to increase the effective moment; increase the force and/or increase the distance at which the force is applied.

Applications of Force Systems

In human motion the turning effect will be the result of the sum of the moments produced by the variety of forces and their point of attachment. Figure 1.3 shows one muscle force represented by F, the weight of the arm G, and the weight of the mass held in the hand, W (9). F, or the force in the muscle, would be multiplied by the distance a, since this is the appropriate perpendicular distance to the axis O. Likewise, b would be used for G and c would be used for W. The sum of these three respective moments would be represented in an equation by $(F)(a) - (G)(b) - (W)(c) = 0$. In such an equation if the sum of the three terms were zero, static equilibrium would be demonstrated. If not equal to zero the segment would rotate according to the direction of the greatest moment application. In the case shown in Figure 1.3 the mass of the weight in

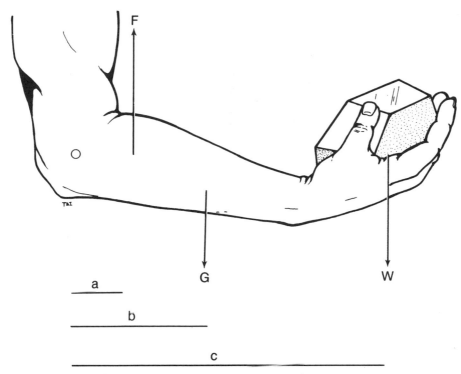

Figure 1.3.   A lateral view of the arm with a mass held in the hand. See text for description.

the hand (W) and the weight of the forearm (G) produce the tendency for a clockwise moment, while the muscle force F produces the opposite effect; thus, positive and negative signs are given to the respective terms. Thus, the direction that the arm will turn depends on the magnitudes of the forces and their respective distances from O. These moments may be called an external or resistive moment that is opposed or controlled by the internal or muscular moment.

A simple configuration for a single plane motion is shown as an example in Figure 1.4. Rarely, if ever, are forces applied to the segment perpendicularly. This is particularly true of muscle insertions. In cases where the forces are applied at an angle other than 90° trigonometric functions can be used to calculate the component of the force that will have a turning effect. Consider Figure 1.4 to analyze the effect of the application of the muscle force at an angle of insertion of 45°. Clearly not all of the tensile force generated in muscle can have a rotation (R) effect. Rather, significant force is shunted (S) into the joint itself. The magnitude of the force that will have a turning effect will vary with the magnitude of the trigonometric function associated with the angle of insertion of the muscle producing the moment. This example and Table 1.2 provide an index of the magnitude of the effect of the change in angle of insertion. Specifically, in this example, only 0.7071 of the force in the tendon will have a turning effect on any segment. Further discussion of this factor is provided in the next chapter, while a review of trigonometry and a complete table of functions are found in Appendix A.

For a practical example of a situation that uses moments assume the configuration in Figure 1.5. A therapist pushing against the patient's arm with a force F1

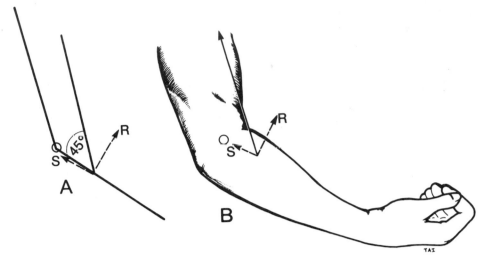

Figure 1.4. Diagrammatic mechanical (*A*) and anatomical (*B*) representation of two body segments with a musculotendinous unit spanning a joint with a specified axis of rotation (O). Muscle force is shown with the solid vector. The respective force into the joint (*S*) and the rotary effect (*R*) are shown as dashed vectors. See text for further description.

Table 1.2.   Angle of Insertion—Trigonometric Functions

Degrees	Cosine function
10	0.9848
20	0.9397
30	0.8660
40	0.7660
45	0.7071

will tend to move the patient sideways but will not cause rotation about the shoulder (S), since the line of force passes through S. A weight F2, held in the hand, however, would produce a clockwise moment equal to F2 × d (Fig. 1.5*A*). Now, after removing the weight, the therapist exerts an upward force F3 at an angle A with the vertical (Fig. 1.5*B*). It will create a counterclockwise moment equal to F3 × d or F3 × cos A × D (i.e., the component of the force through H perpendicular to S). Either solution, F3 × d or F3 cos A × D, yields the same answer. In the former method the force F3 remained the same, and the distance was modified. In the latter, note two things. One, that D remained constant but the force was modified, and two, that the other component of F3, (F3 sin A), has no moment about S because F3 × sin A × 0 = 0. Thus, the moment of a force can be represented by the sum of the moments of its two components.

Each of the examples provided thus far have been systems that are predominantly coplanar. For thorough analyses, however, there are usually coplanar force systems that require three-dimensional solutions. As a result, an understanding of the fundamentals of vector algebra is required. For those interested an overview of the topic is presented in Appendix B. Further discussion and applications of the topic, considered outside of the scope of this volume, can be found in Miller and Nelson (8) and Winter (15).

In analyzing various exercises and assessing their relative difficulty, consideration should be given to the point of rotation, the proportion of the body weight

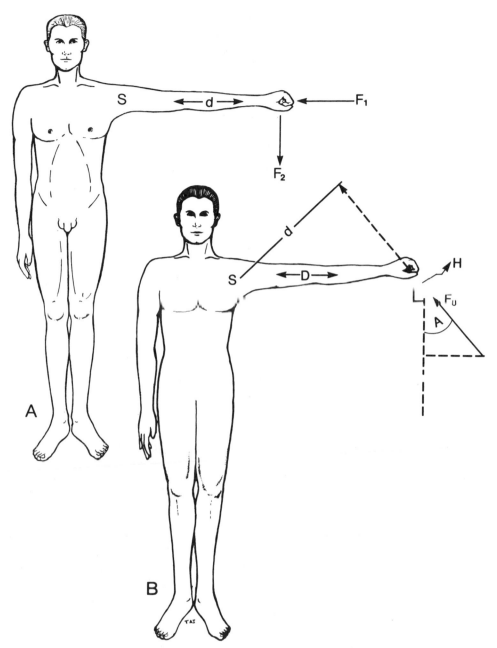

Figure 1.5. Diagrammatic representation of the effect of forces on the shoulder. See text for specific description.

being supported, raised, or lowered, and whether or not there are any external resistances. In addition, we need to consider what muscles are acting to produce the desired movement. More sophisticated analyses include the moments created by the nonmuscular forces about the point of rotation. In total, then, the muscles must create appropriate moments of force to produce the desired movements.

Finally, muscles within the human body are capable of acting by producing a

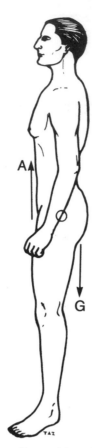

Figure 1.6. Lateral view of the standing subject. The anteriorly placed vector depicts force from the abdominal mucles (*A*), tilting the anterior rim of the pelvis superiorly. The posteriorly placed vector represents force from the gluteal musculature (*G*) that pulls the posterior pelvis inferiorly. Considered together the two forces act as a force couple to rotate around the axis noted in the pelvis as O.

force couple, defined as two parallel forces equal in magnitude but opposite in direction. Examples are countless, but one of import is shown in Figure 1.6. The implications for this mechanical system as occurring in the human body will be demonstrated during our study of each of the various segments of the body (14).

FRICTION

The role of frictional forces in kinesiological problems or in clinical practice is frequently ignored. However, in many instances the presence or lack of friction will determine the degree of success of the applied therapy. In gait, for example, friction is necessary between the foot and the supporting surface so that force can be transmitted up the leg in contact with the floor. The same is true for patients using crutches. Witness the potentially disastrous circumstances associated with use of extremely worn crutch tips. Exercise equipment also has frictional characteristics, whether they be in pulley devices or in the mechanical bearings of resistive equipment. Friction during administration of traction, usually considered as negligible, may be considerable. Further, frictions within the body are important to normal function. Primary examples are increased friction associated with degenerative joint diseases or in cases of inflammatory conditions of tendons, such as tenosynovitis.

Other examples are available from a study of joint motion. Because the bony surfaces are bathed in a fluid medium, friction between the surfaces is minimized. Further discussion of this factor will follow in Chapter 3. In addition, muscles contain fluids. Thus, in treatment, consideration must be given to the influence of high and low loads and the impact of velocity, particularly when viscosity of the fluid affects the friction present in joints. Other types of friction include dry, rolling, and internal friction.

Coefficient of Friction

Friction is described by means of a coefficient of friction. This coefficient is a ratio of forces, the force required for motion divided by the compressive (normal) force between the two bodies. The coefficient of friction is unitless, because it is the ratio of two forces. Consider the situation in Figure 1.7 where an object rests on a surface. In this free body diagram the N or normal force is equal to the load of 100 newtons. Now, if a push (P) of 5 newtons is applied to the load, a force parallel to the surface is developed that is called F, the frictional force. This value may be any value up to a maximum value, and, based on $F_{max} = \mu N$, will depend upon μ and the normal force. μ, as known from your practical experiences, depends upon the materials of the surfaces of the two objects as well as the degree of lubrication. Certainly two surfaces of sandpaper provide greater friction than two Teflon surfaces, given the same amount of compression between the two surfaces and the same pushing force. Returning to our example, assume that we push harder, so that 50 newtons of force are required to start the object moving. Substitution into the equation yields $50 = \mu 100$. Division shows that the coefficient of friction is 0.5. Conversely, if μ is known and N is known, the force needed to move the object can be calculated by simple multiplication. Note that the area of the surface is not a factor in considering the friction. Further, if frictional force is plotted against the pushing force we note that the static friction will always be greater than the kinetic friction. In other words, getting the object in motion will be more difficult than keeping the object in motion (8).

Clinical Relevance

Seldom will clinicians need to calculate the specific μ or be concerned with the amount of force required to produce motion. However, if a patient of large mass is supine on a table during pelvic traction the therapist must be cognizant

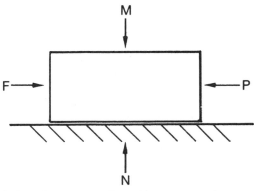

Figure 1.7. A mass (M) resting on a surface. N represents the normal force, P a pushing force, and F the frictional force. See text for further description.

that the force required to produce distraction is dependent on the mass (normal force) and the coefficient of friction.

Brand states that the coefficient of friction in joints is in the range of 0.005 to 0.01. Such a finding is interesting when considered in view of μ's of 0.005 to 0.1 in mechanical systems (2). Even skating on ice lubricated by water produces a μ of only 0.03. Walker has produced a table of values that shows coefficients that range from 0.142 to 0.163 for cobalt-chrome hip replacements sliding on themselves for different lubricants and different concentrations of albumin, globulin, and hyaluronic acid (12). That joint lubrication is superior to man-made systems points out the effectiveness of the human body in controlling factors critical to efficient performance. More specific discussion of lubrication in joints is included in Chapter 3 on articular mechanics and function.

FREE BODY DIAGRAMS

In many instances analytic or descriptive approaches will be based upon forces applied to a given body or segment of a body. An accurate representation of all the forces is called a free body diagram because an artificial boundary or limit of any structure or segment can be made at any location, depending on the problem that needs to be solved. In actuality the correct placement of the external forces acting on the body is essential for the correct interpretation or solution of any system on which forces are acting. The forces are represented by vectors and typically include muscle forces, gravity, friction, wind resistance, ground reaction forces, and fluid forces. They are graphically represented by the magnitude, direction, and angle at which the force is applied. Therefore, a correct quantitative graphical solution to the problem or configuration is implied (Fig. 1.8). Identification or use of incorrect free body diagrams results primarily from lack of inclusion of all the forces or from adding unnecessary forces. Application of the principles of free body diagrams will be stressed in several of the chapters on joints.

BODY SEGMENT PARAMETERS

In the process of analyzing normal and abnormal human motion, there are various measures that are pertinent when motion is quantified. Length, mass,

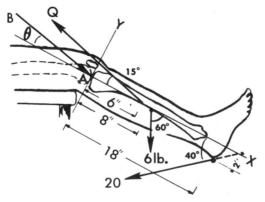

Figure 1.8. An example of a free body diagram. Each of the respective forces is shown with a vector. (From Williams M, Lissner HR: In LeVeau B (ed): *Biomechanics of Human Motion*. Philadelphia, WB Saunders, 1977.)

volume, density, center of mass, and moment of inertia are known as body segment parameters because they provide the data needed in kinematic analyses and in formulae required to complete kinetic analyses. Practically, these data have been used in comprehensive analyses of pathological motion, in the design of industrial tools and seating devices, and for development of prostheses. In actuality, little work has been completed on body segment parameters because the work is tedious and difficult. Accurate techniques are probably available, but frequently the expense or degree of complexity prevents the completion of comprehensive studies. The texts of Miller and Nelson (8) and Winter (15) provide discussions of these parameters. Williams and Lissner also thoroughly discuss their importance (14). Most using these measures will use the data from the work of Dempster (4). The following material will provide an overview of the parameters and stress their importance in the study of kinesiology and pathokinesiology.

Segment length, or link, data are important from the standpoint of allowing the determination of end points for each body part. Identification of these points, usually at specific anatomical landmarks, enables the definition of segment displacement, yielding the ultimate data of interest, the velocities and accelerations. Although identification of specific landmarks are difficult to accurately reproduce, these methods appear to produce reliable data.

Mass, defined as weight/gravity, is a function of two other parameters, the volume and the density of a particular segment. Keeping in mind the earlier discussion under the terminology section of this chapter, the concept becomes important because mass is distributed differently in each segment of the body. Further, each body segment, or link, has a specific mass and location of the center of mass (the location where mass is centered). Table 1.3 provides a compilation of the percentages of weights for each of the segments of the body (15).

Of particular relevance is the location of the center of mass, also shown in Table 1.3, of each of the body segments. This is because the location of the center of mass determines the relative ease, or difficulty, with which the segment will turn. Consider the free body diagram in Figure 1.9, an isolated link with an identified center of mass. If a force (F) is applied such that the force passes through the center of mass, no rotation will occur. Rather the segment would move linearly across the surface of the page. A more realistic view is shown in Figure 1.10. With no load the center of mass will be located more proximal to the axis of rotation (A) than in the instance when a 10-lb mass is held in the hand (B). Thus, if an attempt is being made to move the arm from this position, more difficulty will be encountered in the latter case because the mass moment of inertia is larger. This is due to the fact that both the mass and the distance from the axis of rotation to the center of the mass have increased. Note that this increased mass and the distribution of the mass are both factors because the moment of inertia (I) = mass × the radius of gyration. This "special" average of the distribution of all of the mass particles from the point of rotation (i.e., the radius of gyration) is necessary for the calculation of the mass moment of inertia (I). Additional discussion of this topic will be presented in Chapter 13, "Posture and Gait."

The factors of volume and density, mentioned as constituents of mass, are less important because they are accounted for in the mass quantity. Density is a

Table 1.3. Anthropometric Data[a]

Segment	Definition	Seg weight/tot body wt[b]	Center of mass/segment length[b]		Radius of gyration/segment length[b]			Density
			Prox-imal	Distal	C of G	Prox-imal	Distal	
Hand	Wrist axis/knuckle II middle finger	0.006	0.506	0.494	0.297	0.587	0.577	1.16
Forearm	Elbow axis/ulnar styloid	0.016	0.430	0.570	0.303	0.526	0.647	1.13
Upper arm	Glenohumeral axis/elbow axis	0.028	0.436	0.564	0.322	0.542	0.645	1.07
Total arm	Glenohumeral joint/ulnar styloid	0.050	0.530	0.470	0.368	0.645	0.596	1.11
Foot	Lateral malleolus/head metatarsal II	0.0145	0.50	0.50	0.475	0.690	0.690	1.10
Shank	Femoral condyles/medial malleolus	0.0465	0.433	0.567	0.302	0.528	0.643	1.09
Thigh	Greater trochanter/femoral condyles	0.100	0.433	0.567	0.323	0.540	0.653	1.05
Total leg	Greater trochanter/medial malleolus	0.161	0.447	0.553	0.326	0.560	0.650	1.06
Head and neck	C7-T1 and 1st rib/ear canal	0.081	1.000		0.495	1.116[c]		1.11
Thorax and abdomen	C7-T1/L4-L5[d]	0.355[c]	0.63	0.37				
Trunk head neck	Greater trochanter/glenohumeral joint[d]	0.578[c]	0.66	0.34	0.503	0.830	0.607	

[a] From Winter DA: *Biomechanics of Human Movement*. New York, Wiley, 1979.
[b] Data from Dempster W: Space Requirements of the Seated Operator. WADC Technical Report 55–159. Report released to the Office of Technical Services, Dept of Commerce, Washington, DC, July 1955.
[c] Calculations required.
[d] These segments are presented relative to the length between the greater trochanter and the glenohumeral joint.

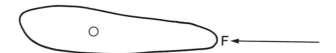

Figure 1.9. An isolated segment with an identified center of mass (O). *F* represents the application of a force.

function of the type of tissue(s) that make up the segment, and the volume is contingent upon the quantity of the tissue. Differences in body types result from the degree of each tissue present in the individual.

LAWS OF MECHANICS GOVERNING MOTION

To completely analyze human motion in a clinical sense or with sophisticated techniques both kinematics and kinetics are involved. The need for this information results in the necessity to collect information that will describe the motion and the forces producing the motion. Simon et al have suggested a clinical method to analyze four-dimensional motion (10), while Soderberg and Gabel

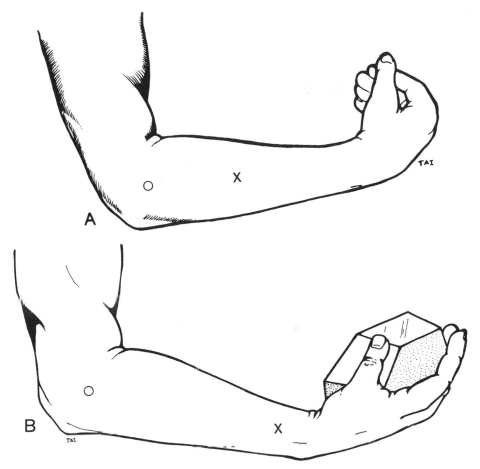

Figure 1.10. A forearm and hand segment with an axis of rotation O and a center of mass X. (A) When a mass (M) is added to the hand the mass moment of inertia is larger, making movement more difficult (B).

(11) have proposed a method for sagittal plane analysis. More sophisticated approaches have been used in many laboratories, a common example being that of Crowninshield et al in a study of the human hip (3).

Displacement, Velocity, and Acceleration

There are several concepts related to kinematics that are important to clarify. Although the basic constituents of the description of motion are the same, the derivation of the quantities differs, depending upon whether the motion is angular or linear. Table 1.4 shows the derivation of each of the three quantities and provides the symbol and terminology for each. Therapists will have interest in both. During gait, for example, the patient must move from one location to another and, considering the total body, a displacement per time period would enable the calculation of the patient's velocity. However, individual segment displacements, shown in Figure 1.11, are responsible for the walking. Once the displacement and time are known, velocities and accelerations can also be determined (Table 1.4, Fig. 1.11A). Note that high quality displacement data are essential because these quantities are also used in the velocity and acceleration

Table 1.4.   Displacement, Velocity, and Acceleration

Formulas	Units
Linear	
Displacement d-	Meters
Velocity d/t = v	Meters/sec
Acceleration $\dfrac{v_2 - v_1}{t_2 - t_1} = a$	Meters/sec/sec
Angular	
Displacement θ (angle)	Radians or degrees
Velocity $\dfrac{\theta}{t} = \omega$	Radians/sec
Acceleration $\dfrac{\omega_2 - \omega_1}{t_2 - t_1} = \alpha$	Radians Degrees/sec/sec

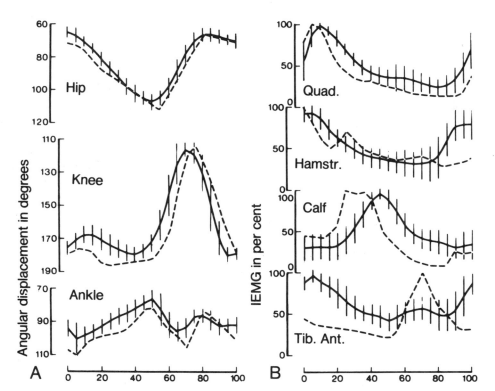

Figure 1.11.   Angular displacements for sagittal plane motion of the hip, knee, and ankle for normal subjects (———) and for patient (– – –) during a gait cycle. (A) The role and relationship of the electromyogram (IEMG) shown in B will be discussed in subsequent chapters. (From Richards C, Knutsson E: Evaluation of abnormal gait patterns by intermittent light photography and electromyography. Scand J Rehabil Med 3(Suppl):61–68, 1984.)

calculations. Average velocity may also be used by adding the appropriate quantities and dividing by the number of values included in the numerator. Instantaneous linear or angular velocity is calculated by division of the difference of two displacements by the difference in the time interval. The closer that time approximates zero the better the representation of instantaneous velocity.

Use of an example will clarify differences associated with the kinematics of linear and angular motion. Shown in Figure 1.12 is segment AC that has been

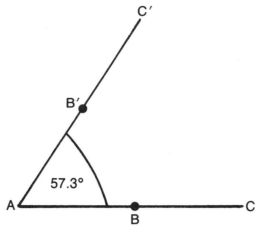

Figure 1.12. Segment AC with an intermediate point *B* identified. The segment is then displaced to a new location, indicated by *B'* and *C'*. See text for details.

displaced through one motion, 57.3°, to position AC'. Given that the segment moved through the range in 1 sec the angular velocity would be 57.3°/sec. However, the linear velocity of point B to B' on the segment would be considerably different than point C to C'. This can be clearly demonstrated by connecting B to B' and C to C', noting the length of the lines. Because both displacements were completed in the same amount of time due to the fixed location of the points, C would have a greater linear velocity because of the larger displacement. To generalize then, every part of a rigid body has the same angular displacement, velocity, and acceleration, but the linear values for any part are a function of the distance from the point of rotation. Maximum angular velocities for human performance are approximately 18 rad/sec, but in most functional activities the value is usually less than 1 rad.

There are a number of specific laws that govern motion. A complete treatise is not intended for incorporation into this volume. However, the fundamentals as applied to movement will be discussed so that some understanding of the limitations and applications presented in later chapters will be more readily understood.

Force, Mass, and Acceleration

Newton's law of $F = M \times a$ is of most importance. Applied to linear motion the mass portion is considered to be the segment mass previously described. The acceleration, determined by a number of available kinematic techniques, would be used in producing the appropriate product in newtons of force. However, for angular motion of the segment consider that the torque, or turning effect, results from the product of the moment of inertia and the angular acceleration ($T = I\alpha$). In turn, as noted above, moment of inertia is dependent on the product of the mass times the square of the radius of gyration (ρ). Therefore, the determining equation becomes moment = mass times ρ^2 times the angular acceleration ($T = m\rho^2\alpha$).

Impulse and Momentum

The $F = m \times a$ relationship is also of import in other applications to human motion. Substituting v/t for a yields $F = m \times v/t$. Multiplication of both sides by t produces F × t = m × v, or the impulse-momentum relationship. The implications will be specifically discussed in later chapters. Similarly, for angular motion M × t = I × angular acceleration. Note that momentum is dependent on velocity and that inertia always exists, regardless of velocity.

Work, Energy, and Power

Other laws are applied to work, energy, and power. Simply put, the amount of work is the product of the force in the direction of movement times the distance the body supplying the resistance is moved. For angular motion the work is equal to the moment times the angular displacement. Units are, therefore, newton-meters (not to be confused with torque), or the preferred term, joules (Table 1.1). When time becomes a consideration power is the preferred quantity. Power is the rate of doing work (force times distance divided by time). The measurement unit is watts. Energy, or the capacity to do work, occurs in many different forms. Of primary interest is mechanical energy, consisting in turn of potential energy or kinetic energy. Potential energy is equal to the product of mass, gravity, and height, yielding a quantity in joules. Kinetic energy is equal to ½ mass × velocity^2 for linear motion and ½ I^2 for angular motion. Since work and kinetic energy calculations produce the same units it can easily be shown that for a given kinetic energy so much work can be done. Clarification of these concepts has been presented by Knuttgen as they apply to exercise science (6). Laird and Rozier have discussed the implications of these mechanical principles as applied to exercise as a modality (7). An in-depth discussion of mechanical work, energy, and power is also presented in Chapter 5 of the Winter volume (15). Applications of these principles will be included in Chapter 13, "Posture and Gait."

Statics and Dynamics

Under any given set of circumstances it is possible for any given link or system of links to be stationary (static) or in motion (dynamic). Equations governing the system are equilibrium equations that will determine whether or not the system is in equilibrium or undergoing motion. Williams and Lissner thoroughly develop the rationale for these equations and apply them to a number of situations applicable to therapeutics (14).

Solution of Problems

In practical circumstances there is a reasonable protocol to follow in the solution of link segment problems. However, detailed descriptions of the necessary procedures are beyond the scope of this volume. In brief, first complete an accurate free body diagram. Then, kinematic data must be gathered so that velocities and accelerations of the various body parts are available for use in equations of motion. Data on body segment parameters are also necessary for inclusion into equations demanding either mass or the mass moment of inertia. Information on associated kinetics is also required and is usually obtained by a force-transducing device. These techniques range in sophistication from the multidimensional force plate to a simple hand-held dynamometer. Once all these data are available it would be possible to arrive at the joint reaction forces and the net muscle moments responsible for creating or controlling the motion. Problems analyzing three-dimensional motion become elaborate, and a true appreciation of the complexities requires study of engineering mechanics and the appropriate mathematics necessary for solution. Those that desire more complete information on this topic are referred to the texts by Miller and Nelson (8) and Winter (15).

SUMMARY

The information in this chapter presents concepts related to the description of human motion. The material is fundamental to the following chapters, and thorough understanding is recommended. However, the information presented in this chapter should be used as a reference if review is needed. Each of the concepts presented in this chapter will be reinforced in some subsequent chapter, so that specific applications are made to both normal and pathological human motion.

References

1. *ASTM Standard for Metric Practice (E 380-79).* Philadelphia, American Society for Testing and Materials, 1980.
2. Brand RA: Joint lubrication. In Albright JA, Brand RA (eds): *The Scientific Basis of Orthopedics.* New York, Appleton-Century-Crofts, 1979.
3. Crowninshield RD, Johnston RC, Andrews JG, et al: A biomechanical investigation of the human hip. *J Biomech* 11:75–85, 1978.
4. Dempster W: Space Requirements of the Seated Operator. WADC Technical Report 55-159. Report released to the Office of Technical Services, Dept of Commerce, Washington, DC, July 1955.
5. Frankel VH, Nordin M: *Basic Biomechanics of the Skeletal System.* Philadelphia, Lea & Febiger, 1980.
6. Knuttgen HG: Force, work, power, and exercise. *Med Sci Sports* 10.227–228, 1978.
7. Laird CE, Rozier CK: Toward understanding the terminology of exercise mechanics. *Phys Ther* 59:287–292, 1979.
8. Miller DI, Nelson RC: *Biomechanics of Sport.* Philadelphia, Lea & Febiger, 1973.
9. Schenck JM, Cordova FD: *Introductory Biomechanics,* ed 2, Philadelphia, FA Davis, 1980.
10. Simon SR, Nuzzo RM, Koskinen MM: A comprehensive clinical system for four dimensional motion analysis. *Bull Hosp Joint Dis* 38:41–44, 1977.
11. Soderberg GL, Gabel R: A light emitting diode system for the analysis of gait: a method and selected clinical examples. *Phys Ther* 58:426–432, 1978.
12. Walker PS: *Human Joints and Their Artificial Replacements.* Springfield, IL, Charles C Thomas, 1977.
13. White AA, Panjabi MM: *Clinical Biomechanics of the Spine.* Philadelphia, JB Lippincott, 1978.
14. Williams M, Lissner HR: In LeVeau B (ed): *Biomechanics of Human Motion.* Philadelphia, WB Saunders, 1977.
15. Winter DA: *Biomechanics of Human Movement.* New York, Wiley, 1979.

2

Muscle Mechanics and Neurology

MUSCLE MECHANICS

Diverse muscular function is required by the variety of conditions necessary for efficient and effective human motion. This chapter includes discussion of several physiologic aspects that allow for a wide range of muscular functions. For example, important relationships in muscle mechanics are the length-tension and force-velocity features. However, force-time characteristics and an understanding of tension resulting from eccentric and concentric contractions are also critical to the topic of muscle mechanics. Neural control will be discussed briefly, with the intention of stressing the role played by the muscle spindle and Golgi tendon organ in sensing muscle length and contributing to adjusting muscular tension.

Muscle Morphology

The obvious purpose of muscle is to contract so as to produce efficient and smooth movement of the body. In general, muscle form has been arranged accordingly, depending upon location and specific function. Although muscles have been identified as fusiform and pennate, some have taken triangular, cruciate, spiral, and other forms (36). That muscle displays great diversity of lengths is demonstrated by the 30-cm length of the sartorius when compared to the 1.4-cm length of the dorsal interossei. Similarly, fiber organization appears to be based on function.

If muscle is considered according to two pure forms, fusiform and pennate, the possibility exists for a number of comparisons to be made. Fusiform typically means spindle-shaped or spindle-like in form. An example is the sartorius muscle with parallel muscle fibers that extend from the anterior rim of the pelvis to the medial aspect of the knee. Pennate, meaning feather-shaped, is typified by the bipennate gastrocnemius muscle, while a multipennate muscle would be the deltoid. In considering function, if fusiform fibers can shorten by 30% of their initial length, then a relatively great range of motion could be achieved. In fact, fusiform muscles have been credited with the ability to contract through three times as great a distance as the pennate structure. In contrast, the configuration of the pennate muscle influences the actual distance through which the muscle can contract. For example, a pennate muscle whose fibers are quite parallel to a central tendon would come close to simulating the shortening ability of the fusiform muscle. Compare this to a pennate muscle whose fibers are more perpendicular to the central tendon and have a relatively limited ability to shorten and exert tension via the insertional tendon. A diagram from Tricker and Tricker provides a demonstration by use of the cosine of the angle of attachment (Fig. 2.1) (35). Note that as the angle between the central tendon approaches 45° the effective amount of force in the direction of muscle pull would be only 70.71% of the force generated by fiber contraction (Table 1.2). At 60° the effective force would be only 50% of the tension generated by muscle contraction. Thus, the fusiform muscle has been credited with the ability to contract through a great range of motion, while the pennate muscle generally shortens a much lesser total distance. The cross-sectional area of the pennate muscle is, however, usually much greater than that of the fusiform fiber. Therefore, muscles of pennate structure have the potential for creating the greatest amount of tension, since there is a rather direct relationship between cross-sectional area and muscular tension generated.

There are other differences if the purest form of fiber arrangement remains under consideration. Typically, the fusiform fibers attach at a distance closest to the joint, while the pennate fibers have a tendency to attach a greater distance from the axis of rotation of a particular joint. The importance of this will be

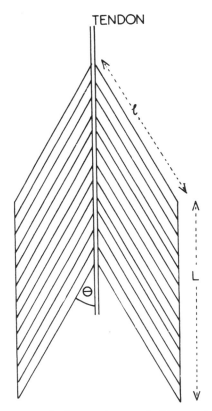

Figure 2.1. A typical arrangement of pennate muscle fibers relative to the central tendon of attachment. *L* is total muscle length and *l* is the length of a single fiber. The force exerted equals LAx/1 × f cos Θ, where A is the total cross sectional area and x is the number of fibers per unit area measured perpendicularly to the fibers. (From Tricker RAR, Tricker BJK: *The Science of Human Movement.* New York, Elsevier Publishing Co, 1967, p 266.)

brought out in a subsequent chapter. Before discussing other features of muscle, suffice it to say that in general mechanical terms, the fusiform muscle has the capability to lift a lesser load through a greater range of motion, therefore yielding generally less power at perhaps a greater velocity. Conversely, the pennate structure can typically lift a greater load through a lesser range of motion and, therefore, has generally high power capabilities but velocities that are significantly slower than the fusiform structure.

While this consideration of the morphology of muscle is of some significance, it should be pointed out that these considerations have been developed with the purest forms of fiber arrangement. In actuality, muscles in the human are a compromise between the fusiform and the pennate type of structure. According to the *Handbook of Physiology*, the angles of pennation are usually 30° or less (2). Because these attachment angles produce cosine function values of 0.866 or greater, the result may be that muscle length is far more important than angle of pennation in the production of muscle tension.

There are a host of other factors that play a role in muscle function. For example, consideration must be given to two joint muscles and their ability to maintain appropriate length during the course of a contraction. Another factor is that many muscles attach only after significant modification of the angle of insertion. One such change occurs as the quadriceps tendon uses the patella to increase the angle of insertion. Other examples include the volar carpal groove and the tendon of the flexor digitorum profundus lifting the superficialis tendon at the terminal digits of the fingers. The significance of these length and insertion factors will be detailed in the following chapters.

Fundamental Considerations

Before progressing to three-dimensional motion, evaluation of muscle function should be completed in one plane. Assume, for the sake of example, that we have one muscle that spans a pure hinge joint flexed to 45° (Fig. 2.2). A tension

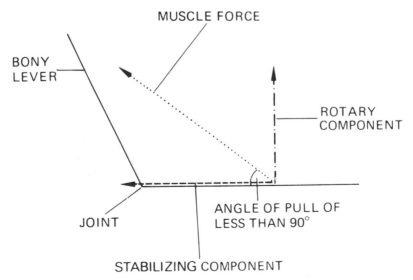

Figure 2.2. Schematic view of a pure hinge joint with the muscle force described by a vector. See text for description. (From Macdonald FA: *Mechanics for Movement: Notes for Physiotherapy Students.* London, G Bell and Sons, 1973, p 47.)

generated within the muscle will have two effects when the force is resolved. One component of the muscle tension will be transmitted into the joint, thus applying compression to the joint. The other component will be a rotary component or one that will create a moment or torque about the hinge axis. As the joint angle changes in position the various stabilization or rotary effects will be modified. Figure 2.3 demonstrates a joint angle of greater than 90°, under which conditions a contracting muscle would tend to distract the joint, thus producing a subluxing or dislocating force. From these examples it is clear that muscular angles of insertion that are 90° will provide a purely rotary force and thus exert the most effective torque.

In considering three-dimensional motion, there are two useful laws that have been cited by MacConaill and Basmajian (21). The first, the law of approximation, states that when a muscle contracts the muscle tends to bring its attachments together. This is a straightforward concept, but the point should be made that neither the muscle origin or insertion is identified as standardly done in textbooks of anatomy. Labeling of the origin and insertion should be disregarded since the motion created will depend upon which segment is stabilized. In many cases muscle will reverse origins and insertions in order to function effectively. For example, the gluteus medius muscle contracts during the stance phase of gait in order to effectively stabilize the pelvis on the weight-bearing femur. During standing posture the anterior tibialis muscle and triceps surae muscles alternately pull the lower leg forward and backward about the ankle joint axis. Other examples will be provided in subsequent chapters on each joint.

The second law is known as the law of detorsion. This law states that when a muscle contracts the tendency will be to bring the origin and insertion into one and the same plane. This law, demonstrated in Figure 2.4, particularly applies to

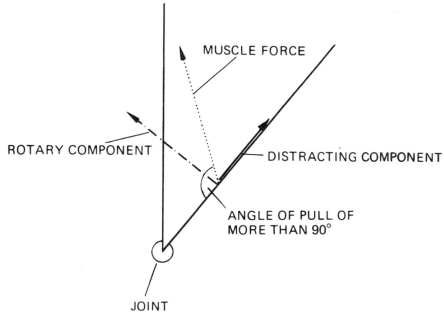

Figure 2.3.   Schematic view of the same joint in a different position. Note that the effects of the muscle force are different from those shown in Figure 2.2. (From Macdonald FA: *Mechanics for Movement: Notes for Physiotherapy Students.* London, G Bell and Sons, 1973, p 47.)

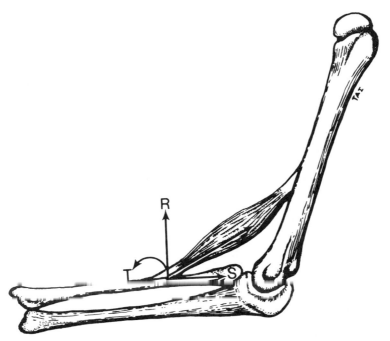

Figure 2.4. A schematic view of the law of detorsion. The muscle force vector, shown along the muscle, will tend to generate force into the joint (*S*) as well as create a moment (*R*). If the muscle attachment on the mobile segment is broad or not located in the midline of the segment a twisting (*T*) effect will also occur or tend to occur, depending on the degrees of freedom in the joint.

muscles that are twisted prior to contraction. Examples include the sternocleidomastoid, the hip adductors, and pectoralis major. This law is important because it stresses that motion is three-dimensional and that origin and insertion will in effect be brought into one and the same plane.

MacConaill, in 1949, proposed that muscles be labeled as "spurt" or "shunt," depending on the characteristics of the muscle location (20). For example, muscles that insert most distal in relationship to the joint on which they act tend to compress the joint rather than produce a turning effect. Therefore, this muscle would be labeled as a shunt muscle, since most of the generated tension is shunted into the joint. The most commonly cited example is the brachioradialis muscle. Another good example is the coracobrachialis muscle because glenohumeral joint compression tends to occur instead of flexion. Conversely, muscles such as the biceps with a great turning or moment effect would be identified as a spurt muscle. In this case attachments are close to the joint axis around which motion is occurring. Others have criticized the spurt and shunt classification system on the basis of mechanical principles (15). They point out that if in fact a muscle would be considered a shunt muscle according to MacConaill's criteria the muscle would have the opposite function if considered to act on the proximal rather than the distal segment. Consider, for example, the brachioradialis muscle. In the case where the hand and wrist were fixed and the upper arm allowed to move, the muscle would be a spurt muscle (elbow flexion) rather than a shunt muscle. So, in the common case where muscles act on the proximal segments, i.e., reverse functions, the muscle also changes classification.

Muscle Tension

As is well known, the type of muscle contraction varies. Definitions have not been commonly accepted. The student/clinician must use this as an observandum against indiscriminate use because the same term may be interpreted differently. The most common terminologic variations are described below.

The most consistently used term is isometric. In this contraction type, constant muscle length is implied because segments remain fixed. However, since there is considerable shortening at the protein filament level in any condition of tension generation, no contraction appears to satisfy isometric conditions (12).

Isotonic contractions, literally translated as same tension or force, are typically broken down into two subcategories. They have been defined by O'Connel and Gowitzke (24) as:

isotonic—sometimes called concentric or shortening contraction; a muscle contraction in which the internal force produced by the muscle exceeds the external force of the resistance; the muscle shortens and movement is produced.

eccentric—a muscle contraction in an already shortened muscle, to which an external force greater than the internal force is added, and the muscle lengthens while continuing to maintain tension.

Bouisset, in *New Developments in Electromyography and Clinical Neurophysiology*, provides another system for definitions (9):

isometric—external resistance is equal to the internal force developed by the muscle, and there is no external movement.

isotonic—a muscle contraction when the external force is constant.

anisotonic—a contraction during periods of increasing or decreasing external force.

anisometric—a muscle contraction resulting when external resistance is smaller or greater than the internal muscle force—if smaller, muscle shortens (concentric or positive work); if greater, muscle lengthens (eccentric or negative work).

It is readily recognized that there are some commonalities in definitions. Although Bouisset (9) may have more sensical forms of definitions, the most frequently used are those provided by O'Connel and Gowitzke (24), with the exception that concentric and eccentric contractions are both considered forms of isotonic exercise.

More recently isokinetic contractions have become a popular exercise mode. A literal interpretation of the term isokinetic means constant or same force. In actuality these electromechanical hydraulic systems enable exercise through a range of motion at a constant angular velocity. However, patients and/or normals will typically not have the constant force output implied in the definition. In reality the device allows individuals to perform at constant velocity, thus making constant force a possibility but not a requirement. In fact, as will be described in subsequent chapters, changes in the forces and resulting torques may be indicative of pathology. Finally, although concentric and eccentric forms of isokinetic exercise may be performed, the latter is limited by loading requirements and concerns for patient safety.

Functional Roles

Muscle function frequently will be classified by its functional role in movement. When a muscle is labeled as a prime mover, the intention is that the muscle is the single most important force creating a particular torque. An assistant mover is a servile muscle or one that can aid the prime mover to act as an "emergency" muscle either when great force is required or when paralysis has occurred. An agonist simply means a muscle that performs a similar action, while an antagonist means a muscle that has an opposite action. For example, the biceps brachii and brachialis muscles are agonists, while the triceps brachii muscle is an antagonist. A stabilizer is classically considered a muscle that will steady or support so that another muscle may act effectively. Wrist extensors commonly perform this function so that the hand can be used effectively. This contraction is generally an isometric. Finally, a muscle can assume the role of a synergist. In this case the muscle will control or neutralize undesired actions produced by other active muscles. Earlier editions of Brunnstrom's revised text, in fact, further defined two categories of synergists (19). The helping synergist is two muscles with a common joint action but each with an action antagonistic to each other. The anterior gluteus medius muscle internal rotation and abduction function compared to the posterior gluteus medius muscle external rotation and abduction function provides a useful example. Pure or true synergy is identified as the condition when a muscle contracts statically to prevent an action in one of the joints traversed by two or more joint muscles. An example at the hand and wrist can be used. To make an effective closure of the fingers, long flexors originating in the forearm will be active. Because during the grasp there would be a tendency for the wrist to flex, the wrist extensors become active for purposes of maintaining the wrist in a neutral position. Thus, the extensors have neutralized the tendency for flexion.

The student should note that there are many other classification systems and terms available; for example, postural, impulse, slow or rapid tension, ballistic, and cocontraction. In addition, the terms fast, slow, and intermediate are assuming a more precise definition and role in considerations applied to human movement. None of the classification systems enjoys any advantages over the others, and they should be considered only as descriptors of the functional ability or capability of muscle.

In summary, there are multiple factors that influence muscle function. Figure 2.5 is an attempt to demonstrate the interactive environment in which the musculotendinous unit functions. Some factors have now been discussed. the remainder will be included in subsequent sections.

Structural Models

Numerous models of the musculotendinous unit as a functional unit have been described and presented in the literature (Fig. 2.6) (25). Hill was among the most prolific original workers in this area, successfully describing the force-velocity relationship over 40 yr ago (14). More recently others have produced results that closely parallel in vivo responses of muscle (28, 34). Although the model used makes some difference, the relationship of the elements within the muscle, in addition to viscosity, is primarily responsible for the mechanical properties described in the following sections.

Length-Tension

The models in Fig. 2.6 show the basic elements responsible for producing the length-tension relationship. *CE* designates the contractile component or the overlap of actin and mysosin filaments. The *PE* or parallel elastic component is made up of the connective tissues surrounding the muscle filaments. The series

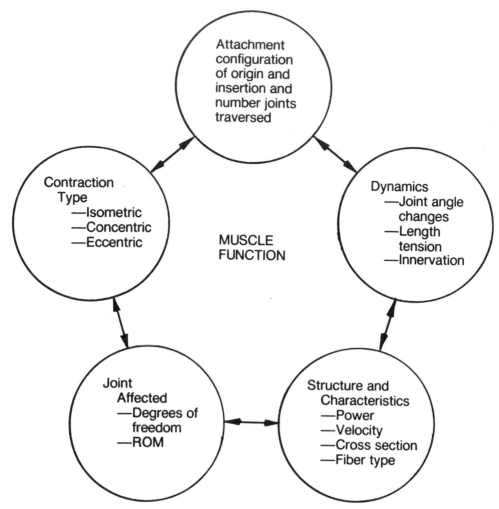

Figure 2.5.   Diagram of the factors influencing and/or determining the function of in vivo human muscle.

elastic component is the *SE* portion of the model and can be considered to be the tendinous portion of the neuromuscular unit. These components exist in every muscle, but exactly how these various elements relate to each other determines the length-tension relationship for a given muscle.

To explain the length-tension relationship the contribution of each of the elements must be evaluated. Referring to Figure 2.7*B*, consider an attempt to lengthen muscle. To do so move to the right on the abscissa. When this is done, passive tension, indicated by the r curve, arises within the muscle. The total tension, shown as a, is available under conditions of contraction of muscle. This represents the combined effect of the passive (r) and the contractile (d) elements. Note that the curve generated by the contractile element (d) is the tension achieved under different lengths by the contractile component, i.e., the actin and myosin filaments. However, this contractile element curve is not totally discernible because as contractions are performed at different lengths the passive elements (r) intervene. Thus, the tension shown by curve a is the result of the passive plus the contractile components, or a = d + r.

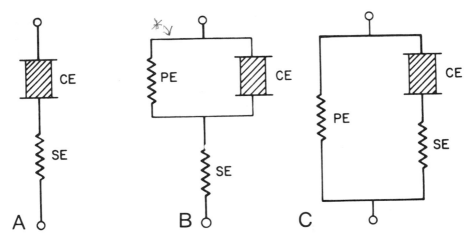

Figure 2.6. Several examples of models of human muscles. (A) According to the Hill model the series elastic (SE) and the contractile element (CE) are in series. (B) In the Voight model a parallel element (PE) has been added in parallel to CE. (C) In the Maxwell model note that the PE is in parallel with both CE and SE. (Reprinted with permission from Phillips CA, Petrofsky JS. The passive elastic force-velocity relationship of cat skeletal muscle: influence upon the maximal contractile element velocity. *J Biomech* 14:400, copyright 1981, Pergamon Press, Ltd.)

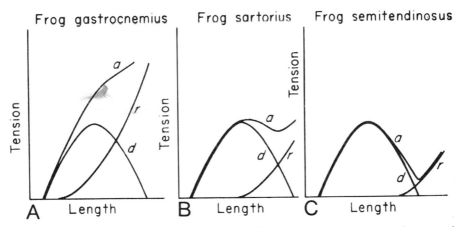

Figure 2.7. Length-tension curves for three different muscles. See text for complete description. (From Wilkie DR: *Muscle.* New York, St. Martins Press, 1968, p 30.)

On review of the length-tension relationships for the three different muscles in Figure 2.7, one readily notes the difference in configuration. Differences in the shape of the curve are accounted for by the shifting of the passive element to the left, or in other words, as muscle length is increased, passive tension is a factor earlier in the lengthening process. Since the total tension a is a result of r + d there are concurrent changes in a that are reflective of the shifting of the passive element to the left. Thus, the gastrocnemius muscle would have a much greater total tension-generating capability than semitendinosus at equivalent lengths of the respective muscles (38).

Configuration of the length-tension curve also varies between animals. Goldspink and White have respectively presented length-tension and resting tension diagrams for the bumblebee, locust, frog, and snail (11, 37). Two things are apparent from these figures. First, in Figure 2.8, the net voluntary tension curve is contained along a very short length axis. Second, in Figure 2.9, the passive ·elements have varying degrees of slope. Considering these two factors in relationship to the functions performed by each animal it is not remarkable that the snail moves at a slow pace, while the bumblebee is capable of sustaining wing motions upwards of 600 Hz (11).

These characteristics vary across muscles, not only in lower animal forms but also in humans. For example, cardiac muscle will more closely simulate the frog gastrocnemius than the semitendinosus because of functional requirements related to cardiac output. Intact human muscle has been difficult to evaluate in vivo for obvious reasons, but work published by Ralston indicates that characteristics identified in animals have similar features in humans. Subjects in their experiments were amputees who had undergone a cineplastic procedure. In this instance surgery places a tunnel through the muscle tendon so that a cable or other mechanical mechanism can be permanently attached. Thus, a direct attachment to muscle was possible. Subsequently, Ralston et al were able to evaluate the passive component and other features associated with tension

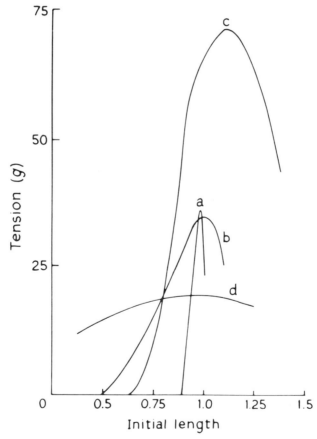

Figure 2.8. The length/active tension curves are shown for a variety of muscles. The tensions cannot be directly compared because they are not in grams per unit cross section. Bumblebee flight muscle is *a*, *b* is locust flight muscle, *c* is frog sartorius muscle, and *d* is snail pharynx retractor muscle. (From Alexander R McN, Goldspink G: *Mechanics and Energetics of Animal Locomotion.* New York, Wiley, 1977, p 7.)

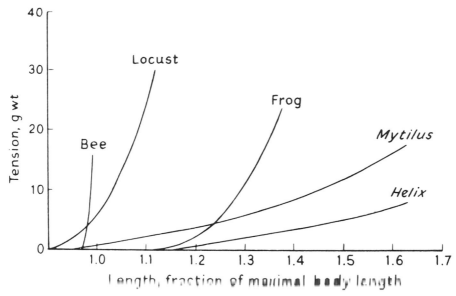

Figure 2.9. Resting length/passive tension curves for the muscles shown in Figure 2.8 and the mytilus. The combined curves of Figures 2.8 and 2.9 would form similar active and resting tension curves as for those shown in Figure 2.7 accounting for the mechanics of each of the muscles. (From Alexander R McN, Goldspink G: *Mechanics and Energetics of Animal Locomotion.* New York, Wiley, 1977, p 40.)

development at various biceps brachii muscle lengths (26). That the passive components for human muscles vary has been demonstrated and graphically displayed by Yamada (Fig. 2.10) (41).

Length-tension factors must also be considered in surgical procedures and in therapeutic programs. Outright releases, tenodeses, and transfers of muscles offer primary examples. The pes anserinus transfer serves as a good example of the importance of appropriate length. In this case the common tendon is adjusted for the expressed purpose of limiting external tibial rotation and providing stability to the medial aspect of the knee. Thus, the success of transfers is very dependent on correct length; otherwise, the patient may not have sufficient active or passive tension because the muscle is too short. In all cases therapists need to be cognizant of lengthening muscle for the purpose of eliminating contracture, yet conversely avoiding excessive lengthening that may remove the musculotendinous unit from the tension-generating range. Specific examples as applied to joints will be presented in later chapters.

Also of interest is that in 1966 Gordon et al were able to study the length-tension curve at the sarcomere level (12). A schematic summary of results is shown in Figure 2.11. The arrows along part A show the various stages of overlap portrayed in section B of the figure. Assuming similar findings hold true for all other sarcomeres a large population of such curves would produce the dome-shaped configuration of the contractile component of the length-tension relationship for a total muscle (Fig. 2.7).

There are several specific applications and implications arising from the length-tension relationship. The first is the influence of precontraction stretch. Figure 2.12 shows the effect of the passive or elastic element on muscle action and ultimate tension output. Note, however, that the figure ignores the concept of

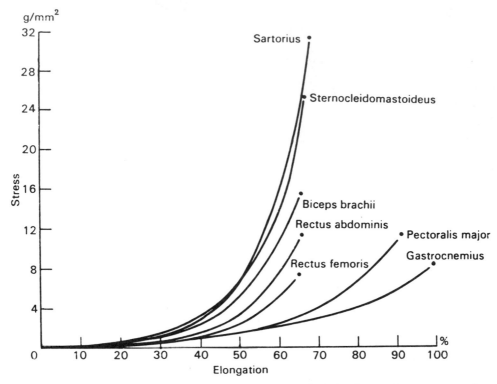

Figure 2.10. Stress-elongation curves for tension of skeletal muscle in 29 yr olds. Practically, stress is equivalent to tension and elongation equal to length. Note the variation between muscles. (From Yamada H: In Evans FG (ed): *Strength of Biological Materials*, p 95. © 1970, Williams & Wilkins, Baltimore.)

viscosity that really exists because of the fluid elements within the muscle. This viscosity, influenced by factors such as temperature and amount of body fluids, is difficult to determine. However, for the sake of a more complete model of muscle, inclusion is well warranted. Note that in *B* the figure shows that the contractile component has shortened and stretched the series elastic component, producing the tension shown on the dial. In Figure 2.12C a quick stretch has been applied to the muscular unit, while at the same time the contractile component is shortening the same degree as shown in *B*. The ultimate result is an increase in total tension output. Thus, by applying stretch or by lengthening the muscle during the course of the contraction a greater amount of tension can be generated. This concept of precontraction stretch is applied in many therapeutic situations and will be elucidated in later chapters.

It is well-known that elastic energy can, in fact, be stored and transformed into kinetic energy. Such was the case in Figure 2.12 when stretch was applied as the contraction occurred. Other examples can be located. Alexander and Goldspink state that fleas have a substance known as resilin. This near perfect rubber material, when stretched or deformed, can rapidly return to its original state. Thus, muscle is used to develop tension over a long period of time. Then, with a quick tension release the flea performs a tremendous leap (11).

Asmussen and Bonde-Petersen have evaluated similar characteristics in humans. They compared the squat jump, a jump preceded by a rapid counter movement to stretch the muscle, and a jump from a height. Their findings

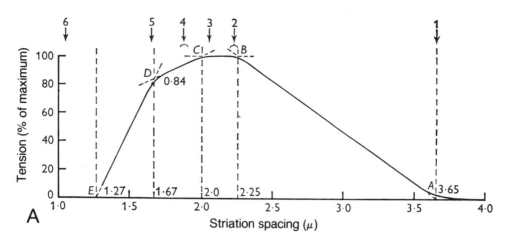

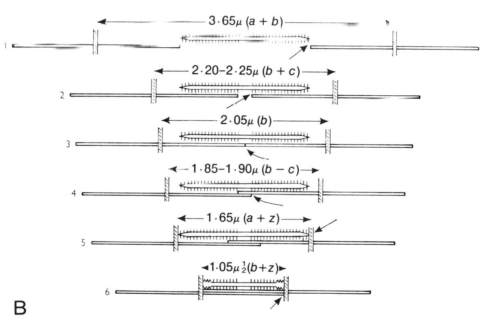

Figure 2.11. Composite showing the relationship of sarcomere length to the length-tension curve. Length of the various elements equals 1.60 μm for a, 2.05 for b, 0.015-2 for c, and 0.05 for z. See text for complete explanation. (From Gordon AM, Huxley AF, Julian FT: The variation in isometric tension with sarcomere length in vertebrate muscle fibers. *J Physiol* 184:185–186, 1966.)

showed that the countermovement jump was 22% higher than the jump from a static position. Likewise, the jump from a height was 3 to 13% higher (4). In other work these same investigators have calculated that in humans 35 to 53% of the energy absorbed during the negative phase is reused during positive work (3). Most recently Bosco et al have shown that concentric contraction performance can be attributed to a combination of elastic energy and myoelectric potentiation of muscle activation (8). Thus, these factors become important any time that motion causes the muscle to undergo lengthening prior to contraction.

Another significant feature related to the length-tension relationship is the

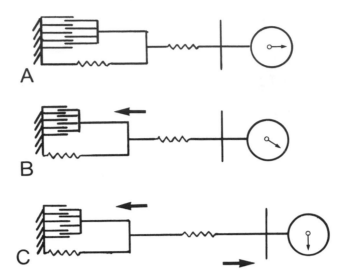

Figure 2.12.   Influence of elongation upon the ultimate tension generated in muscle. (A) Model of resting muscle. (B) Generation of isometric tension. Note that the two attachments of the muscle have not been separated. (C) Contraction of the contractile component with simultaneous lengthening of the muscle increasing the tension available.

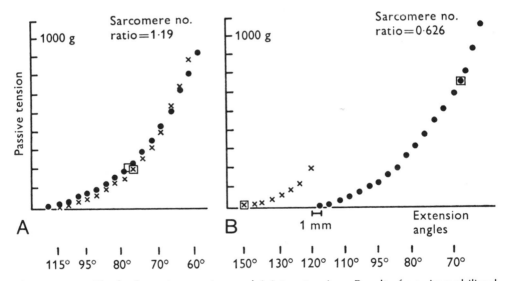

Figure 2.13.   Plots of passive tension and joint extension. Results from immobilized muscle are shown with an x and contralateral controls with an ●. Larger angles produced shorter muscles; thus, the results for muscles immobilized in the lengthened position are in the left-hand portion of the figure, and those for shortened muscle are in the right-hand segment. Further description is contained in the text. (From Tabary JC, Tabary C, Tardieu C, et al: Physiological and structural changes in the cat's soleus muscle due to immobilization at different lengths by plaster casts. *J Physiol (Lond)* 224:234, 1972.)

influence of immobilization. Shown in Figure 2.13 is the effect, on passive elements, of immobilization in a lengthened position (A) versus the shortened position (B) (32). This experiment, performed on cat soleus muscle, indicated that the passive element of the muscle immobilized in a shortened position (curve x in Fig. 2.13B) shifted to the left. Recalling the influence of shift of the passive element (Fig. 2.7) the result would be a tendency to increase total tension available as length was increased. Given the interrelationship between muscle tension and length changes, tissue immobilized in a shortened position, such as during casting, may in fact produce similar clinical results. In fact, changes in musculotendinous lengths are known to be the cause of limitations in range of motion when joints are released from immobilization. Crawford, also using immobilization, has produced similar effects in the overall muscle lengths of rabbits, subsequently producing marked changes in length-tension curves (10).

Further, investigations have determined that the number of sarcomeres significantly decrease, while mature muscles (32) or young developing muscles are immobilized in a shortened position (10). Conversely, sarcomeres are added during immobilization in the lengthened position in animal adult muscle but not in very young muscles or during recovery following immobilization in a shortened position (39). Also of interest is the recent study of Tabary et al, which has shown a 25% decrease in the number of sarcomeres after only 12 hr of electrical stimulation, but only if the muscle was concurrently allowed to assume a shortened position (33). On the other hand, if the muscle was prevented from shortening, no decrease in sarcomere numbers or hypoextensibility occurred (10). These results are of significance to the therapist, since the implication is that an elongation tension is needed to facilitate the return of sarcomeres and the subsequent length-tension relationship inherent to normal function.

Further evidence is available from studies of myofibrillar content. In a very recent study, Jokl and Konstadt showed that immobilization in the shortened position caused the greatest degree of atrophy (16). In general, the least changes occurred in the lengthened position. Assuming that Sargent's data can be related to patient care situations would mean that by 6 weeks after removal from immobilization, the mean muscle fiber area of the leg recovering postinjury would be at approximately 75% of the area of the injured leg (27). And, since Booth has shown differences in mechanical and physiological characteristics and fiber numbers between slow and fast-twitch muscle fibers as a result of immobilization, the implication may well be that therapists need to rehabilitate muscles using training programs that offer higher degrees of specificity and/or variations in restrictive load, duration of contraction, and velocity of contraction (7). Virtually no studies have been completed as to the effects of these training programs on patients.

Force-Velocity

The basic force-velocity relationship uncovered by Hill is shown in Figure 2.14. V_0 stands for the maximum velocity of shortening while P_0 signifies the maximum load or force. Subsequently, the figure demonstrates that at maximum velocity muscle is capable of lifting the lightest load, while as the velocity approaches zero the maximum load can be lifted. At P_0 there is zero velocity, and thus the condition of isometric contraction. The dotted line superimposed on the curve is the mechanical power produced. Such a relationship is derived by substituting the formula: velocity = d/t into the power = fd/t relationship so that P = FV. Note that the maximum mechanical power is available at approximately 1/3 maximum velocity and 1/3 maximum load or force (40).

Because the cross section of the gastrocnemius is greater than that of the semitendinosus muscle, the gastrocnemius would produce greater force than the semitendinosus. If velocity of contraction (d/t) was held constant clearly the

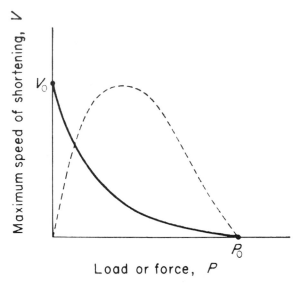

Figure 2.14. Force-velocity and power curves for muscle. See text for further details. (From Wilkie DR: *Muscle*. New York, St. Martins Press, 1968, p 33.)

greater power would be generated by the gastrocnemius muscle because the f would be greater. Recall also, from Chapter 1, that the degree of shortening is influenced by angle of fiber insertion and that the pennate muscle shortens less per unit time than does the fusiform muscle. The result is a tendency for velocity for pennate muscles to be somewhat less than that for the fusiform type of muscle. The specific power capabilities of any muscle are, therefore, determined by the contractile properties and mechanisms that are responsible for the force and the velocity. The product of the force multipled by the respective velocity produces the power or *dashed curve* shown in Figure 2.14.

A practical example of how this force-velocity relationship is manifested in performance is during bicycle riding. If an individual attempts to initiate pedaling on a steep upgrade it is usually impossible to turn the crank, because sufficient tension cannot be generated at the low velocity required. Conversely, when descending a steep grade the bicycle is shifted into a higher gear so that the velocity of the extremities can exert an effective force on the crank. Other examples of this fundamental relationship can be established for isokinetic testing, whereby the clinician has an opportunity to control or adjust the velocity of the angular movement. In most instances, however, velocities for patient care circumstances are slow, thus tending to produce far less than optimal power.

Figure 2.15 from the work of Komi shows the force-velocity relationship for elbow flexor musculature for concentric and eccentric contractions. Although the tension and velocity scales have been inverted on the graph, as compared to the previous figure, the relationship is unaltered. Note that the vertical line in the center of the graph indicates an isometric condition. Concentric work, when the muscle shortens, is to the right of the graph. Conversely, eccentric contraction is to the left. Observe that at the highest velocity of concentric work the lowest possible tension is achieved. During the eccentric contraction the highest tension available is at the highest velocity, while the isometric value is recorded at approximately 31 kgf. In retrospect, these data are as we would expect, since eccentric work is, in fact, stretching the muscle concurrently while a contractile

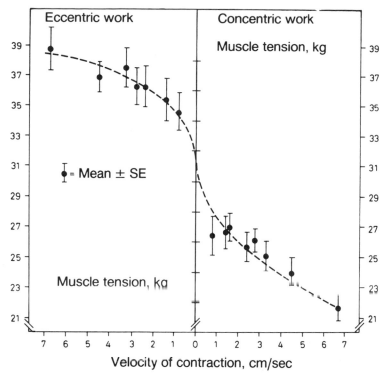

Figure 2.15.   Force-velocity curve for elbow flexor muscles. Further explanation is contained in the text. (From Komi PV: Measurement of the force-velocity relationship in human muscle under concentric and eccentric contractions. In Cerquigliani S (ed): *Biomechanics III*. Basel, Switzerland, Karger, 1973, p 227.)

component is attempting to shorten the entire neuromuscular unit. Since it has been established that humans can move at over 1000°/sec, the 7 cm/sec velocity (corresponding to approximately 120°/sec) represents only a limited range of the velocity available to human muscle (17).

Other exercise physiology studies have shown that the energy required by eccentric contractions is far less than those created by concentric exercise (1). For example, it is well-known to be easier to descend stairs than to ascend a similar flight of stairs or to control a specific therapeutic load while lengthening muscle as opposed to shortening the muscle. These specific examples demonstrate the ability of muscle to utilize the elastic components during lengthening contractions.

Force-Time

The fundamental relationship of force and time is demonstrated in Figure 2.16 (30). Included are several measures used in evaluating force-time curves. This curve applies to isometric contractions and can be explained on the basis of muscle structure. As the contraction is initiated the contractile component proceeds to stretch the elastic components within the muscle. During that phase there is a nonlinear increase in the force production created. Once the elastic components have been "pulled out," the development of force will reach an essentially linear stage around the point of inflection through which the slope or tangent line has been drawn. The maximum is reached as the contractile

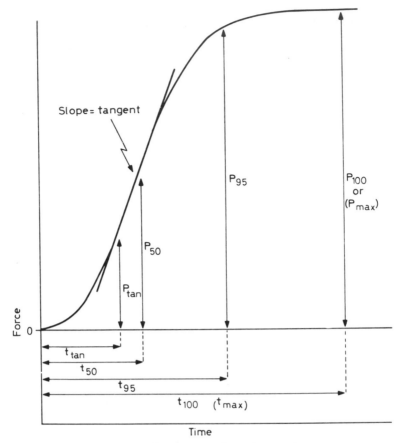

Figure 2.16.   Force-time curve for human muscle and several common measures used to evaluate tension generation and maintenance. (From Stothart JP: Relationship between selected biomechanical parameters of static and dynamic muscle performance. In Cerquigliani S (ed): *Biomechanics III*. Basel, Switzerland, Karger, 1973, p 212.)

component can generate no greater tension by exerting force through the series elastic component. Studies involving training have indicated that maximum tension can be generated in approximately 300 msec (31).

The rapid development of force is important in at least selected circumstances of pathological movement or in recovery of normal movement capabilities. And, although not a primary factor in low velocity activities such as gait, the development of adequate amounts of tension becomes an important consideration when relating temporal events to injury or reinjury prevention. Specific rapid tension development associated with athletic requirements may also be pertinent when patients attempt to complete an effective rehabilitation program that will allow return to competition.

Finally, realize that as the joint angle is varied the force-time curve will vary in P_0 (maximum tension) reached. Recall that at angles of muscle insertion less than 90° a component of the force will be transmitted to compress the joint. Consequently, less tension can go towards creating the turning moment, thus resulting in a lower P_0 value measured. It is for this reason that moments should be used as the standard and comparative measure within and between patients. Also recall that at greater than 90° a component of the muscular tension is distracting the joint and, therefore, changes the features of the force-time curve.

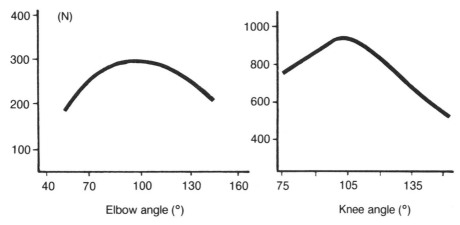

Figure 2.17. Average maximal isometric force curve for male subjects plotted versus elbow and knee angle, respectively. (From Komi PV: Neuromuscular performance: factors influencing force and speed production. *Scand J Sports Sci* 1:4, 1979.)

Summary

Production of effective and appropriate muscularly generated moments depends, then, on a number of factors. Tension available is highly dependent upon the length at which muscle is required to contract as well as in the direction (i.e., concentric, isometric, or eccentric) of contraction. Velocity is a third prime variable that clinicians must take into account in applying knowledge to patient care situations. How these factors interact will determine the ultimate or final torque produced in the temporal sequence allowed. An example is shown in Figure 2.17 for the elbow and knee (18). Note that the force output varies significantly throughout the range of motion, recognizing that this mechanical curve is dependent on the angle of insertion and the joint angle at every given point in the range of motion. While only the effective or resultant force is what ultimately matters, an understanding of how these factors interact is essential to understand normal human motion and how this motion may be ultimately disturbed in the pathological circumstance.

NEURAL CONTROL

Movement is intimately controlled by neural mechanisms. There are known central and peripheral influences that modify or have some responsibility in the production of movement and its control. Central influences would include visual and vestibular systems, while peripheral influences would include free nerve endings, ligaments, and capsules as well as Pacinian corpuscles. Golgi tendon organs, located primarily at musculotendinous junctions, in the aponeurosis and in tendons, appear to be primarily tension-sensitive. They are less affected by passive stretch because they are located in inelastic tendons that lengthen little in comparison to muscle. Also central to the control of movement are the flexion, withdrawal, and cutaneous reflexes.

Of considerable importance is the stretch reflex, also known as the myotatic reflex. Apparently the reflex continuously activates extensor and axial muscles and results in counteraction of the force of gravity. The reflex may also contribute to maintenance of upright posture. The primary organ responsible for effecting this reflex appears to be the muscle spindle.

The spindle has the role of perceiving length or change in length of muscle.

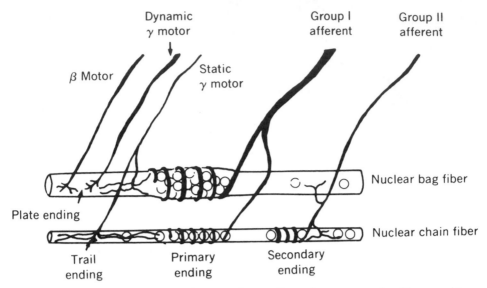

Figure 2.18. Schematic view of the muscle spindle and accompanying fibers and innervation. Full detail is provided in the text. (From Harris DA, Henneman E: Feedback: their efferent signals from muscle and control. In Mountcastle VB (ed): *Medical Physiology*. St. Louis, CV Mosby, 1980, p 705.)

Distribution of spindles has been studied fairly extensively, revealing that high populations appear in the hand and back extensors as compared to few in the diaphragm and shoulder area.

The muscle spindle (Fig. 2.18) is located within the muscle in parallel to the gross muscle fibers (13). Within the capsule of the spindle are 10 to 12 striated "intrafusal" muscle fibers composed of two fiber types—nuclear chain and nuclear bag fibers. Both are contractile at either pole and noncontractile in the nucleated central region. Two types of sensory fibers originate from the intrafusal muscles. The Ia afferents, also called primary, annulospiral, or nuclear bag, originate from the central nucleated region of the intrafusal fiber and project to the spinal cord through very large diameter fibers. The II or secondary afferents, also called flower spray or myotube, originate more diffusely from the polar regions of the intrafusal fibers and project to the cord through medium sized fibers. Sensory discharge from the spindle is produced by stretch of the gross muscle (increased muscle length) which also stretches the spindle intrafusal fibers, depolarizes the terminal endings of the spindle afferents, and causes action potentials to be transmitted centrally along the afferent fibers. The primary afferents discharge to stretch at a lower threshold than do the secondary afferents and show both an initial burst of rapid discharge (dynamic component) and a somewhat less rapid sustained increase in discharge (static component).

The intrafusal fibers receive motor innervation from small γ-motoneurons (also called fusimotor, γ-efferent), interspersed among the large α-motoneurons of the spinal cord ventral horn. The γ-fibers terminate on the striated polar regions of the intrafusal muscle fibers, and γ-motorneurons discharge produces intrafusal muscle contraction; the gammas cause no direct change in the gross muscle tension.

Discharge of the γ-motoneurons produces contraction of the striated polar regions of the intrafusal muscle fibers which, in turn, stretches the central noncontractile region and depolarizes the afferent terminals. The resultant spindle discharge is thus a direct effect of γ-motoneuron excitation of the intrafusal fibers. If the γ-motoneurons are very active, the resultant intrafusal fiber contractions may be sufficient to overcome the slack resulting from gross muscle contraction and thus prevent spindle discharge cessation. The amount of spindle discharge which is due to γ-motoneuron activation of the intrafusal fibers is called the gamma bias of the spindle (5, 22, 23).

Reflex Anatomy

The stretch reflex is elicited by muscle stretch sufficient to discharge the primary spindle afferents. The large myelinated primary afferent fibers enter the dorsomedial portion of the spinal cord dorsal horn and project directly, or monosynaptically, onto homonymous α-motoneurons (neurons innervating the muscle from which the spindle discharge originated) to produce contraction of the homonymous muscle; concurrent monosynaptic reflex activation of the synergist muscle also occurs, which results in stabilization of the joint across which the synergists attach. Contralateral influences have also more recently been recognized. Many extensor and axial muscles are continuously activated by this stretch reflex circuit (Fig. 2.19). The group IIs have been shown to contribute a monosynaptic excitation to homonymous muscle (29). Functional implications are currently being debated. Another form of innervation has been demonstrated in a wide variety of mammalian muscles. β-fibers distribute branches of given fibers to both intrafusal and extrafusal muscle fibers. For more complete descriptions current neurophysiology texts should be consulted.

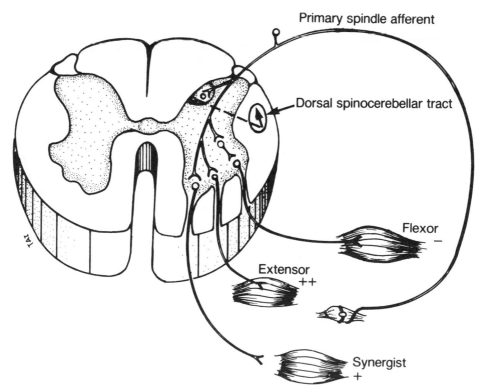

Figure 2.19.   Diagram of the neuronal connections associated with the stretch reflex.

Contraction Effects

During contraction of the gross muscle, the muscle shortens and the muscle spindles go "slack." As a result, the intrafusal fibers are no longer stretched, and the spindle afferent discharge ceases. Following contraction the muscle returns to precontraction length, as do the intrafusal fibers. When the intrafusal fiber stretch is sufficient to depolarize the afferent terminals, the spindle sensory discharge resumes.

Gamma Regulation of Spindle Discharge

The small γ-motoneurons, interspersed with the α-motoneurons throughout the motor pools of the spinal cord, have control connections similar to the α-motoneurons with the exception of the primary spindle afferents which do not project to the γ-motoneurons, i.e., there is no monosynaptic reflex from the muscle spindles to the γ-motoneurons. Cutaneous stimuli, for example, produce reflex discharges of the γ-motoneurons, and descending projections from higher centers produce excitation of inhibition of gamma discharge. In general, γ- and α-motoneurons innervating the same muscle are activated in the same direction of excitation or inhibition by an incoming stimulus (alpha-gamma linkage), but the γ-motoneurons respond at lower thresholds than do the α-motoneurons.

Practical examples of spindle-modulated effects are seen in the assumption of postures. In the lower leg during standing, spindles in the anterior compartment perceive stretch as the body sways posteriorly. Muscle contraction of the dorsiflexors ensues, bringing the body more anteriorly over the supporting foot. Because the same mechanism operates in the triceps surae the constant sagittal plane sway is closely monitored and controlled. Spindle control in head posture is obvious in those attending events that lead to sleep while in the seated position. As sleep (and relaxation) ensues, posterior cervical muscles lengthen, allowing the head to drop forward. As the spindles are sufficiently stretched the posterior neck muscles contract, and the head can be observed to abruptly return to the upright position.

Modulation by the spindle is also responsible for other features of interest to the clinician. For example, muscle stiffness, defined as a change in force divided by the corresponding change in length, will determine the effect of both external and internal disturbances on motion production. Because muscle contains elastic elements, viscous elements, and spindle control, the behavior of muscle is fundamentally nonlinear except under restricted experimental conditions. So, to predict the movement resulting from a given contraction, conditions such as level of motor unit activation and firing rate, as well as initial length and contraction velocity, must be taken into account. Further, the action of antagonistic muscle must also be considered. Thus, a combination of length and force feedback would tend to regulate stiffness (since these are the two factors involved). One example of a model used to describe the interactions is presented in Figure 2.20 (6).

Clinical Correlations

A phasically induced stretch reflex is a common neurological test of motor function and is termed a tendon jerk or knee jerk. A tap on the tendon of the tested muscle stretches the muscle and produces a phasic, synchronous discharge of primary spindle afferents which in turn triggers the monosynaptic stretch reflex. A hyperactive tendon jerk (hyperactive stretch reflexes) on one

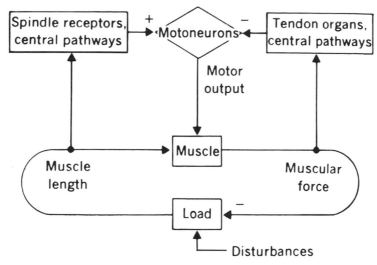

Figure 2.20. Schematic view of the role of muscle length and force in regulating muscle stiffness. (From Binder MD, Houk JC, Nichols TR, et al: Properties and segmental actions of mammalian muscle receptors: an update. Fed Proc 41:2915, 1981.)

side of the body is generally indicative of damage in the motor pathways descending from the cortex. The increased resistance to passive movement due to hyperactive stretch reflexes is termed spasticity. In the hyperreflexic patient, if a constant stretch is applied to the muscle and a tendon tap is superimposed, not one but a series of tendon jerk reflexes results. This repetitive jerking is called clonus and reflects the highly sensitive state of the α-motoneurons to synchronous afferent volleys.

Summary

The neural input from the muscle is constantly a factor in determining the state of responsiveness or what some may call muscle tone. That these neural influences play a primary role in normal and pathological motion cannot be overemphasized. This chapter has also discussed the importance of muscle length, contraction type, velocity of contraction, and other factors as they influence muscle tension. Throughout the remainder of this volume these fundamentals of muscle mechanics will be reinforced with examples applied to kinesiology and pathokinesiology.

References

1. Abbott BC, Bigland B, Ritchie JM: The physiological cost of negative work. J Physiol 117:380–390, 1952.
2. Alexander RM: Mechanics of skeleton and tendons. In Brooks VB (ed): Handbook of Physiology. Bethesda, MD, American Physiological Society, 1981, vol 4, p 17.
3. Asmussen E, Bonde Petersen F: Apparent efficiency and storage of elastic energy in human muscles during exercise. Acta Physiol Scand 92:537–545, 1974.
4. Asmussen E, Bonde-Petersen F: Storage of elastic energy in skeletal muscles in man. Acta Physiol Scand 91:385–392, 1972.
5. Basic Neurology Syllabus. Winter-Spring, University of California, Los Angeles, 1977.
6. Binder MD, Houk JC, Nichols TR, et al: Properties and segmental actions of mammalian muscle receptors: an update. Fed Proc 41:2907–2918, 1982.
7. Booth FW, Seider MJ: Effects of disuse by limb immobilization on different muscle fiber types. In Pette D (ed): Plasticity of Muscle. New York, de Gruyter, 1980, pp 373–383.

8. Bosco C, Tarkka I, Komi PV: Effect of elastic energy and myoelectrical potentiation of triceps surae during stretch-shortening cycle exercise. *Int J Sports Med* 3:137–140, 1982.
9. Bouisset S: EMG and muscle force in normal motor activities. In Desmedt JE (ed): *New Developments in Electromyography and Clinical Neurophysiology*. Basel, Switzerland, Karger, 1973, vol 1.
10. Crawford GNC: The growth of striated muscle immobilized in extension, *J Anat* 114:165–183, 1973.
11. Goldspink G: Design of muscles in relation to location. In Alexander RMcN, Goldspink G: *Mechanics and Energetics of Animal Locomotion*. London, Chapman and Hall, 1977.
12. Gordon AM, Huxley AF, Julian FT: The variation in isometric tension with sarcomere length in vertebrate muscle fibers. *J Physiol (Lond)* 184:170–192, 1966.
13. Harris DA, Henneman E: Feedback: their efferent signals from muscle and control. In Mountcastle VB: *Medical Physiology*. St. Louis, CV Mosby, 1980, pp 703–717.
14. Hill AV: Heat and shortening and the dynamic constants of muscle. *Proc R Soc Lond* [Biol] 126:136–195, 1938.
15. Jackson KM, Joseph J, Wyard SJ: Sequential muscular contraction. *J Biomech* 10:97–106, 1977.
16. Jokl P, Konstadt S: The effect of limb immobilization on muscle function and protein composition. *Transactions of the 28th Annual Orthopedic Research Society*. New Orleans, January 19–21, 1982. Chicago, Dependable Printing, 1982, p 266.
17. Komi PV: Measurement of the force-velocity relationship in human muscle under concentric and eccentric contractions. In Cerquiglini S (ed): *Biomechanics III*. Basel, Switzerland, Karger, 1973, pp 224–229.
18. Komi PV: Neuromuscular performance: factors influencing force and speed production. *Scand J Sports Sci* 1:2–15, 1979.
19. Lehmkuhl LD, Smith LK: *Brunnstrom's Clinical Kinesiology*. Philadelphia, FA Davis, 1983.
20. MacConaill MA: The movements of bones and joints. 2. Function of the musculature. *J Bone Joint Surg* [Br] 31:100–104, 1949.
21. MacConaill MA, Basmajian JV: *Muscles and Movements: A Basis for Human Kinesiology*. New York, Krieger, 1977.
22. Matthews PBC: *Mammalian Muscle Receptors and Their Central Actions*. London, Arnold, 1972.
23. Matthews PBC: Muscle spindles: their messages and their fusimotor supply. In Brooks VB (ed): *Handbook of Physiology*. Bethesda, MD, American Physiological Society 1981, vol 4.
24. O'Connel AL, Gowitzke B: *Understanding the Scientific Bases of Human Movement*. Baltimore, Williams & Wilkins, 1972.
25. Phillips CA, Petrofsky JS: The passive elastic force-velocity relationship of cat skeletal muscle: influence upon the maximal contractile element velocity. *J Biomech* 14:399–404, 1981.
26. Ralston HJ, Inman VT, Strait LA, et al: Mechanics of human isolated voluntary muscle. *Am J Physiol* 151:612–620, 1947.
27. Sargent AJ, Davies CTM, Edwards RHT, et al: Functional and structural changes after disuse of human muscle. *Clin Sci Mol Med* 52:337–342, 1977.
28. Spector SA, Simard CP, Fournier M, et al: Architectural alterations of rat hind-limb skeletal muscles immobilized at different lengths. *Exp Neurol* 76:94–110, 1982.
29. Stauffer EK, Watt DGD, Taylor A, et al: Analysis of muscle receptor connections by spike-triggered averaging. 2. Spindle group II afferents. *J Neurophysiol* 39:1393–1402, 1976.
30. Stothart JP: Relationship between selected biomechanical parameters of static and dynamic muscle performance. In Cerquigliani S (ed): *Biomechanics III*. Basel, Switzerland, Karger, 1973, pp 210–217.
31. Sukop J, Nelson RC: Effects of isometrical training in the force-time characteristics of muscle contractions. In Nelson RC, Morehouse CA (eds): *Biomechanics IV*. Baltimore, University Park Press, 1974, pp 440–447.
32. Tabary JC, Tabary C, Tardieu C, et al: Physiological and structural changes in the cat's soleus muscle due to immobilization at different lengths by plaster casts. *J Physiol (Lond)* 224:231–244, 1972.

33. Tabary JC, Tardieu C, Tardieu G, et al: Experimental rapid sarcomere loss with concomitant hypoextensibility. *Muscle Nerve* 4:198–203, 1981.
34. Thorsten IH, Halkjaer-Kristensen J: Force-velocity relationships in the human quadriceps muscle. *Scand J Rehabil Med* 11:85–89, 1979.
35. Tricker RAR, Tricker BJK: *The Science of Human Movement*. New York, Elsevier, 1967.
36. Warwick R, Williams PL (eds): *Gray's Anatomy*, 36th British Ed. Philadelphia, WB Saunders, 1980.
37. White DCS: Muscle mechanics. In Alexander RMcN, Goldspink G (eds): *Mechanics and Energetics of Animal Locomotion*. London, Chapman and Hall, 1977.
38. Wilkie DR: *Muscle*. New York, St. Martins Press, 1968.
39. Williams PE, Goldspink G: The effect of immobilization on the longitudinal growth of striated muscle fibres. *J Anat* 116:45–55, 1973.
40. Winter DA: *Biomechanics of Human Movement*. New York, Wiley, 1979.
41. Yamada H: Mechanical properties of locomotor organs and tissues. In Evans FG (ed): *Strength of Biological Materials*. Baltimore, Williams & Wilkins, 1970.

3

Articular Mechanics and Function

The function of individual joints and the collective actions of many joints are ʷ ᵃⁿⁱᵐⁱᵗᵉᵈ ᶠᵒʳ the ʰᵃⁿᵍᵉ ᵒᶠ ʰᵘᵐᵃⁿ ᵐᵒᵗⁱᵒⁿˢ ᵖᵒˢˢⁱᵇˡᵉ ᴬˡᵗʰᵒᵘᵍʰ ʳᵉᶠᵉʳ ᵃᵖᵖᵉᵃʳⁱⁿᵍ as remarkably simple in both form and function, any joint is a complex anatomical structure with a specific set of surfaces, all of which contribute to gross or finite movements. This chapter will focus on the structure of the typical diarthrosis and thoroughly discuss the mechanics associated with the movements of the articular surfaces of the joint. The concept of the instant center of rotation will be elucidated, and theories of lubrication will be presented in terms of their impact on function. Representative pathologies and their influence upon joint function and dysfunction will also be included.

CLASSIFICATION SYSTEMS
General Terminology

Various classification systems have been used for many years, all for purposes of clarifying joint function. The most frequently considered factors taken into account in adoption of any of the current systems in use have included: (a) the complexity and number of structures, (b) number and distribution of the axes, (c) geometric form, and (d) movements permitted. Using these factors Steindler classified joints as simple and composite, discussing simple cylindrical joints such as the ankle or screw surfaces whereby one bone moves in a progressive direction while also moving circularly. Steindler also discusses the oval surface, semicircles rotating about an axis as in the shoulder, and the saddle-like surfaces as found in the carpal-metacarpal joint of the thumb (28). In presenting another view MacConaill has stated that all joints should be classified as simple, compound, and complex. Simple is a result of two articulating surfaces, compound includes three articulating surfaces, and complex joints include surfaces as well as an intercapsular disc, meniscus, or fibrocartilage (20).

The most frequent designation of joint type is based on the form and function as they occur in the human body. Seven basic types have been identified.

plane variety—consists of flat or fairly flat surfaces such as the intermetatarsal or in some of the intercarpal joints.
hinge joint or ginglymus—a uniaxial joint with strong collateral ligaments. Examples appear in the interphalangeal and ulnohumeral joints.

pivot joint—these are limited to rotation, but also have an osteoligamentous ring. These joints are usually uniaxial, such as the radioulnar joint.

condylar joint—the principal movement is in one plane, but the motion also includes a small amount of rotation. The knee and temporomandibular joint are frequently used as examples.

ellipsoid or biaxial joint—joint between one convex articular surface and one concave articular surface with motion possible in two planes. Typically the rotation is limited. Examples are the radiocarpal and the metacarpal-phalangeal joints.

saddle or sellar joints—biaxial joints with surfaces that are concavoconvex. Either surface has a convexity, but 90° to either a concave surface exists. Motions are primarily in two directions, but with some rotation existing as a byproduct motion.

ball and socket, or spheroidal joint—this type is a multiaxial, egg-shaped joint, such as the hip or shoulder (30).

Other terms occasionally used include synchrondosis, meaning that cartilaginous structures are included within the joint. A schindylesis means that there is one bone with a long process that fits into a groove, for example the vomer bone in the nose. A gomphosis means that there is a peg inserted into a socket such as for the teeth. Of some interest to therapists are the types of amphiarthroses. In general, the amphiarthrosis is a limited motion articulation connected by fibrocartilage, or in the case of the synarthrosis, by ligaments. This amphiarthrosis has two varieties, symphysis and syndesmosis, the former being a joint with an all cartilaginous junction and no capsular or synovial membrane. They all lie in the midline of the body. Examples are the sternomanubrium joint and the pubic symphysis. The syndesmosis is defined as a closely interposed joint attached by ligaments (30).

Geometry and Mechanics

MacConaill would maintain that virtually all joints have a convex and a concave surface. The ovoid, or egg shape, adequately describes the contours. In addition, he would state that there are sellar, or saddle-shaped, surfaces which are concavoconvex (Fig. 3.1). Although the surfaces may vary in degree of curvature, there are no true flat or other kinds of joints existing in the human body. These considerations will be discussed later under the heading of osteokinematics.

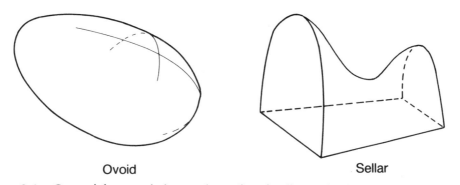

Ovoid   Sellar

Figure 3.1.   General form and shape of ovoid and sellar surfaces. (From Kessler RM, Hertling D: *Management of Musculoskeletal Disorders.* New York, Harper & Row, 1983, p 13.)

Examples of joints composed of a convex and a concave surface are the carpo-metacarpal joint of the thumb, the ankle, and the calcaneocuboid joints.

Kaltenborn, in a treatise on Manual Therapy for the Extremity Joints, provides a somewhat different classification scheme. In classifying bony connections into synarthroses and diarthroses he further subdivides the diarthrosis into full joints or synovial joints and half joints or symphyses with a partial joint space. Articulations are further divided according to whether the range of motion exceeds 10°. The full joints, i.e., with a range greater than 10°, are subclassified into anatomically and mechanically simple or compound joints. Table 3.1 shows a schematic view of the system (14). Another system, shown in Table 3.2, has been proposed by Wadsworth (29).

A purely mechanical approach may also be taken when considering joint function. Such is shown in Figure 3.2. In these cases the motions allowed are perfectly described based on the motion allowed in the mechanical system. A through C show single degree of freedom systems. Although C may be interpreted to have more than a single degree, in effect the motion of the nut can be described by either the distance moved (z) or the number of revolutions needed to perform the excursion. D shows a double hinge mechanism, such as in automobile transmission systems. E also has two degrees of freedom, since the block can both rotate or slide along it. Therefore, two quantities are needed to specify the position. F, as the ball-and-socket joint requires three quantities to specify the position of the joint (1).

However, by far, the diarthrosis is the joint of most interest to investigators and clinicians. Because the features of these synovial joints are critical to the understanding of joint function, key characteristics will be described in the next section.

STRUCTURE OF SYNOVIAL JOINTS

The diarthrosis, or typical synovial joint has several components fundamental to structure. In turn, the structure may also influence mechanics, leading to the production of pathology as manifested in abnormal kinematics and/or kinetics. A primary structure, the articular cartilage, will be dealt with extensively in this chapter. Other components, including the disc, capsule, and the synovial membrane and fluid, will be dealt with less extensively but discussed in terms of importance to the understanding of pathological motion.

Articular Cartilage

Many functions have been ascribed to this aneural, alymphatic, and avascular mass nourished by synovial fluid. According to Mow et al (25), the main functions are to distribute loads over the joint surfaces so that the contact stresses are decreased and to allow movement with minimum friction and wear. At least indirectly the articular cartilage thus prevents damage to bone that might occur because of excessively large stress or energy inputs or from abrasive wear (15). In effect, cartilage, because of its constituents, can distribute stress more uniformly and increase the contact area across a joint. In fact, Evans and King, as reported by Kempson, have shown that the elastic modulus (i.e., stiffness) is less for cartilage than for bone, ranging from 2 to 15 meganewtons/m^2 as compared to 300 meganewtons/m^2 (16). Weightman and Kempson demonstrated in 1979 that cartilage can effectively reduce the maximum contact stress in a joint by 50% or more (32).

Table 3.1. Classification of Joints According to Kaltenborn

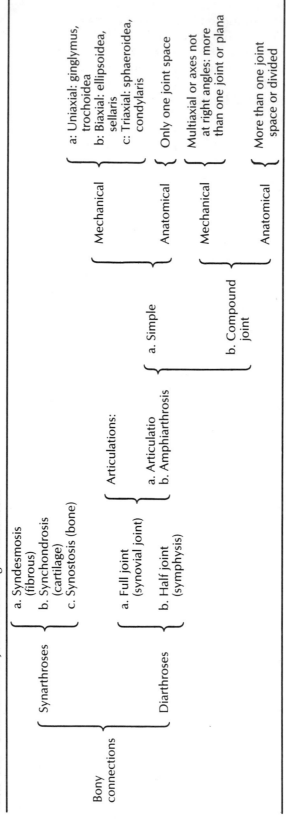

Bony connections

Synarthroses
  a. Syndesmosis (fibrous)
  b. Synchondrosis (cartilage)
  c. Synostosis (bone)

Diarthroses
  a. Full joint (synovial joint)
  b. Half joint (symphysis)

Articulations:
  a. Articulatio
  b. Amphiarthrosis

a. Simple

b. Compound joint

Mechanical
  a: Uniaxial: ginglymus, trochoidea
  b: Biaxial: ellipsoidea, sellaris
  c: Triaxial: sphaeroidea, condylaris

Anatomical
  Only one joint space

Mechanical
  Multiaxial or axes not at right angles: more than one joint or plana

Anatomical
  More than one joint space or divided

50

Table 3.2. Classification of Joints According to Wadsworth

Synarthroses —
  Fibrous
    Suture—allows no movement
    Syndesmosis—permits minimal movement
  Cartilaginous
    Synchrondrosis—temporary (epiphyseal plate)
    Symphysis—fibrocartilage

Diarthroses —
  Uniaxial
    Ginglymus (hinge)
    Trochoid (pivot)
    Condylar
  Biaxial
    Ellipsoid
    Sellar (saddle)
  Multiaxial
    Spheroid (ball and socket)
  Plane

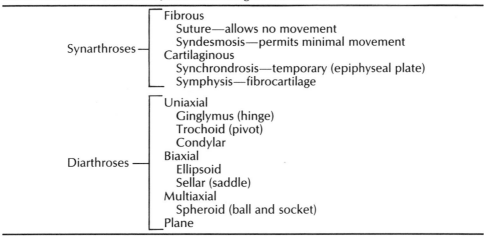

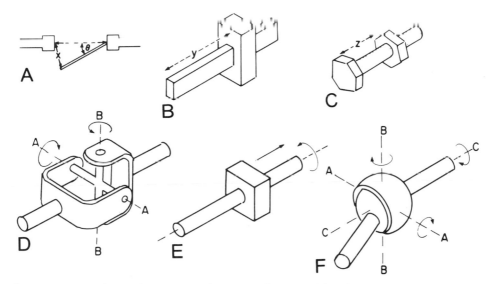

Figure 3.2. Mechanical systems with varying degrees of freedom. Distances are labeled with x, y, and z. Further description is contained in the text. (From Alexander RM: Mechanics of skeleton and tendons. In Brooks VB (ed): *Handbook of Physiology*, Section 1: The Nervous System. Bethesda, MD, American Physiological Society, 1981, vol 2, p 19.)

The components of articular cartilage are responsible for adequately serving the designated functions. Included among the key features is that 60 to 80% of the tissue is water. Of the 20 to 40% of the wet weight made up by solid matrix, collagen fibers compose 60% and proteoglycan gel 40% of the volume (25). The collagen fibers, having important tensile, stiffness, and strength properties provide a fibrous ultrastructure for the articular cartilage. Thickness may vary from 1 to 7 mm (30). Edwards and Chrisman thoroughly described four zones based upon cellular arrangement (5). Outermost on the articular surface, the gliding zone is made up of two layers, the superficial and the tangential (Fig. 3.3) (33). The superficial contains only collagen and is only 200 μm thick. Principally, the collagen is randomly oriented in flat bundles of very fine fibrils. The tangential

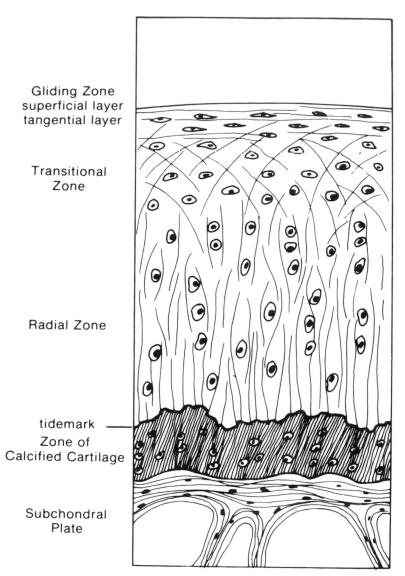

Gliding Zone
superficial layer
tangential layer

Transitional
Zone

Radial Zone

tidemark
Zone of
Calcified Cartilage

Subchondral
Plate

Figure 3.3. Depiction of the zones of adult articular cartilage. (From Edwards CC, Chrisman OD: Articular cartilage. In Albright JA, Brand RA (eds): *The Scientific Basis of Orthopedics*. New York, Appleton-Century-Crofts, 1979, p 316.)

layer, comprising between 10 and 20% of the total cartilaginous thickness, is densely packed fibrils running parallel to the joint surface (25). One of the primary purposes of this arrangement appears to be for protection of the cartilage surface. The next deepest layer, the transitional zone, demonstrates an oblique orientation of the collagen bundles. This section makes up approximately 40 to 60% of the total depth of the cartilage. The radial zone contains more vertical orientation of the collagen bundles and a columnar arrangement of the cartilage cells. Next deepest is the tidemark, a 2- to 5-μm thickness of dense collagen bands of collagen fibers running parallel with the articular surface. Redler et al feel that the undulating pattern demonstrated may afford resistance to the shear stress in the joint (27). The zone of calcified cartilage, between the tidemark and the subchondral bone, is the precursor to the subchondral endplate composed of dense cortical bone.

The other major constituent, the proteoglycan gel, has a high affinity for water. Because of the negative charge associated with these long flexible chains of disaccharides there is an apparent affinity for an osmotic swelling pressure that in effect produces a preload in the cartilage. Mow et al state that just how the proteoglycans and collagen fibers interact has really not been absolutely determined (25). It is known, however, that even when no stress is applied to the cartilage the collagen fibers are in tension. The relatively complex interaction between these two constituents is beyond the scope of this volume, and the reader is referred to the work of Maroudas (23). The swelling pressures, gradients, and permeability factors allow viewing of the cartilage as a fluid-filled porous medium. The mechanical features of this medium, which can be likened to a water-saturated sponge, become difficult to analyze on a mechanical basis.

The primary features determining the biomechanical properties are the structure of the collagen and the permeability of the tissues. Edwards and Chrisman, citing the Simon et al work from 1973, have stated that the thickness of the cartilage is related to the degree of congruence in the joint surfaces. Subsequently, the ankle and ulnohumeral articular cartilage is thin as compared to the hip and knee (5). Cell configuration also appears to play a role, since Kempson et al have shown that the tensile stiffness in the superficial layers of cartilage was 20 times greater than in the deepest zones (17). The 1898 study by Hultkrantz, as cited by Kempson, showed a split line pattern of collagen fiber alignment in the superficial layers. In verifying this work, Kempson et al evaluated the tensile stress-strain features in directions parallel and perpendicular to the split line pattern. Those specimens tested with parallel orientation had increased stiffness, while the perpendicularly oriented specimens were less stiff (18). Thus, fiber orientation represents the ability of the cartilage to resist the maximum tensile strain produced by the compression and friction produced at the joint (31). Perhaps this most superficial layer of dense collagen serves as a tough, protective surface for the remainder of the tissue. While the more random orientation of the deeper fibers resists compressive loading there is still some allowance for resiliency (5).

Cartilagenous resistance to deformation is also known to vary over the articular surface (7). Kempson demonstrated that the stiffest cartilage occurred in regions where the highest loads would be expected (18). In fact, there is a decrease in tensile stiffness and strength with increased distance from the surface of normal adult articular cartilage (17). Mow et al have produced a stress-strain curve for articular cartilage strips. The relationship, which may be described by an exponential function, is shown in Figure 3.4 (25). During the lower levels of strain the collagen fibers are brought into alignment. As strain increases the slope increases, showing the true tensile stiffness of cartilage.

As indicated previously, articular cartilage has a large amount of water retained within the tissue. The proteoglycans are largely responsible for holding water but are also a key factor in holding the water osmotically and through controlling matrix permeability. This control of "swelling pressure" amounts to restrictions associated with fluid flow (26). Therefore, by controlling this flow the mechanical characteristics are influenced. For example, during a prolonged mechanical load, fluid will move within the tissue as well as be exuded by the tissue (22). So, as the rate of exudation varies over time the creep characteristics of the articular

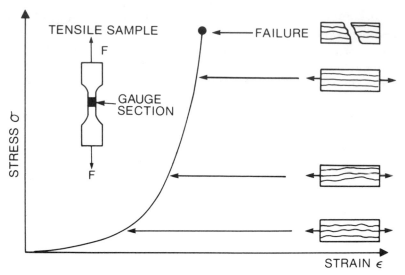

Figure 3.4.   Stress-strain curve for strips of articular cartilage. (From Mow WC, Roth V, Armstrong CG: Biomechanics of joint cartilage. In Frankel VH, Nordin M: *Basic Biomechanics of the Skeletal System.* Philadelphia, Lea & Febiger, 1980, p 71.)

cartilage present different features than those of other viscoelastic materials (25). Further, because of the low permeability the behavior is also dependent upon the rate at which loads are applied and removed. In rapid loading little time is available for exchange of fluid, so the cartilage acts as an elastic material. Conversely, during prolonged loading, such as standing, deformation will occur with time, squeezing fluid out. In either case, as the load is removed the cartilage will return to the original configuration. Further details on this topic can be found in a 1978 volume containing a chapter by Kempson on the mechanical properties of articular cartilage (15).

Discs, Synovial Membrane, and Fluid

Contained within many synovial joints are fibrocartilaginous structures known as discs or menisci. According to *Gray's Anatomy* the latter term should be applied only to incomplete discs, such as those found in the knee joint (30). At any rate these largely avascular, aneural structures are composed largely of fibrous tissue with interconnections to the fibrous capsule. Based on a comprehensive review of available literature Ghadially states that few studies on the fine structure of discs and menisci have been reported (9). The precise functional role is as yet unclear, in spite of numerous suggestions. Among the possible functions are load absorption and distribution, improvement of fit of surfaces, limitations of joint translatory motions, protection of the edges of articular surfaces, and lubrication (30). Regardless of their exact role these structures play an intimate part in both joint kinetics and joint kinematics. Further discussion of their influence on pathology will be provided later in this chapter.

Capsule

Generalized white connective fibrous tissue makes up the continuous series of attachments connecting the bony segments contributing to the joint. Hettinga states that the capsule consists of two parts (11, 12). The outer layer, blending into the periosteum and perichondrium, does not extend over the articular cartilage. Serving a protective function while enclosing the synovial membrane, this portion is often reinforced by tendons or slips from tendons (12). Thickenings of the capsule are frequently encountered and located for purposes of providing increased support and/or stability to the joint. Because these thickenings, known as ligaments, are important to joint kinematics and kinetics by virtue of inherent tensile properties, their function will be discussed in subsequent chapters describing the joints (30).

The other portion of the capsule, the synovial membrane, consists of loose, highly vascularized connective tissue. The membrane encloses any bony surfaces, ligaments, or tendons that are intercapsular. The membrane is nonexistent, however, over the surfaces of discs or menisci and stops at the margins of the articular cartilage. In addition, the cellular substructure allows for location of fat pads and vascular connective tissues that are important for joint function and nutrition. Of rather specific interest is the synovial intima, because the cells that produce and absorb the synovial fluid are located here. The fluid, essential to joint function, is clear or pale yellow, slightly alkaline and viscous in nature. These features are a result of the fluid being a dialysate of blood plasma with mucin added (30). The physical proportions, as evaluated by a number of studies, have shown the fluid to be nonnewtonian. That is, fluids may demonstrate increasing viscosity with increasing shear rate or decreasing viscosity with increasing shear rate. The former, known as a dilatant fluid, is best represented by putty. At low shear rates, completed by hand molding the putty, the material is pliable, while thrown at high speeds the material has high viscosity, i.e., it is hard. Conversely, a fluid such as catsup is thixotropic, demonstrating decreasing viscosity with increasing shear rates. Features of this fluid are best remembered by recalling that the initial flow of catsup from the bottle is far more difficult than the continuation of the flow. Because synovial fluid behaves like a thixotropic fluid the behavior is described as nonnewtonian. Figure 3.5 shows the effects of shear rate on shear stress and viscosity (2). Functions of the synovial fluid are believed to be provision of a liquid environment, maintenance of nutrition for the articular cartilage, discs or menisci, and provision of a lubricant (30).

LUBRICATION

In an excellent chapter on joint lubrication Brand points out the efficiency of animal joints. In the best, well oiled metal surfaces the coefficient of friction is of the order of 0.05, and for a skate on ice about 0.03. Joints, however, are capable of coefficients in the range of 0.005 to 0.01. Maintenance of these low coefficients is contingent upon synovial fluid, smooth articular surfaces, and appropriate mechanisms for effective lubrication (2). These considerations require the study of deformation of surfaces and flow of matter (rheology) and the study of friction, lubrication, and wear (tribology).

Many types of lubrication mechanisms exist, although Mow et al maintain that two fundamental types exist (25). One type, boundary lubrication, occurs when a layer of lubricant molecules exists between the two surfaces. During motion the molecules slide over each other, preventing adhesion and abrasion. Evidence exists that synovial fluid can, at least under some conditions, act as a boundary lubricant. Under conditions of lower load and higher speed there appears to be greater likelihood that fluid film lubrication exists. In this case a much greater film of lubricant forces a greater separation of the joint surfaces. The pressure in

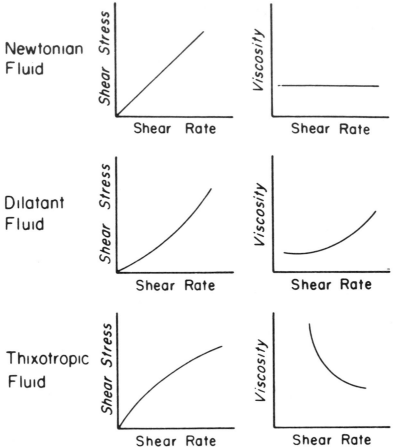

Figure 3.5. Effects of shear rate on shear stress and viscosity for various fluids. See text for complete details. (From Brand RA: Joint lubrication. In Albright JA, Brand RA (eds): *The Scientific Basis of Orthopedics.* New York, Appleton-Century-Crofts, 1979, p 350.)

the fluid thus supports the load bearing and under stationary conditions is known as hydrostatic lubrication. In dynamic circumstances fluid creates a lifting effect as it is pulled between the two surfaces (hydrodynamic lubrication). However, if the surfaces are being compressed together, such as in the knee during standing posture, fluid is squeezed out from the area between the two surfaces. In these latter two cases, the thickness, extent, and load-bearing abilities of the fluid film are determined by viscosity, the shape of the joint surfaces, and the velocity of the relative motion of the joint surfaces. But, because the articular cartilage is relatively soft, deformation may occur, therefore changing the contact area and geometry and subsequently altering the fluid conditions. These circumstances produce hydrodynamic lubrication (25). Brand points out that boundary lubrication may be augmented by boosted lubrication due to cartilage porosity. This may also be governed by molecular size. The effect is to increase the viscosity of the fluid. Brand also points out that during high shear the boundary level may be destroyed, and, therefore, convert the lubrication mechanism back to the hydrostatic version that is characteristic of low speed and heavy load bearings (2).

In summary, mechanical transport of fluids, from a time perspective, is reasonable. However, the molecular restrictions are questionable. It seems unlikely that a single mode of lubrication can effectively respond to the large number of variables, such as load, velocity, viscosity, and geometry of bony surfaces, for which we must account. These mechanisms do, however, play a role in normal and abnormal joint kinetics and kinematics (25). Demonstration of these concepts will follow in subsequent chapters.

STRUCTURE AND FUNCTIONAL MECHANICS
General Considerations

Accurate description of joint motion, arthrokinematics, has been difficult to achieve. Because of variance in surface geometry among joints different degrees of motions are known to occur. Steindler addressed several types of motion, including subfactoring of gliding motion into surface and linear types. To fit his criterion for rocking or rolling motion, equidistant points were required to touch each other in the course of the motion. Further, Steindler classified rocking combined with gliding. Axial rotation was also listed under types of joint movement (28).

Angular movement or rotations are also frequently used both clinically and in the literature to describe range of motion in degrees. Circumduction is also used, conceded to be motion accomplished by a combination of motions in the three cardinal planes. Now, based on strong clinical and experimental evidence, there is consensus that both translatory and angular motions occur during virtually all joint motions. The evidence for this statement will be presented in each respective joint chapter, but for the present consider the geometry of the articular surfaces and their impact upon joint motion.

Surface Geometry and Motion

The most extensive student and author of joint geometry and resultant mechanics has been MacConaill. He maintains, with sound anatomic and geometric data, that articular surfaces are never flat. Rather, surfaces are ovoids or compounded by more than one ovoid surface. If convex in all one direction they are referred to as a male surface. Likewise, concave shapes are referred to as female surfaces. The other type of surface is the sellar or saddle-shaped surface, described as being concave in one direction and convex in another plane (Fig. 3.1). Although the surfaces may vary in degree of curvature, there are not true flat or other kinds of joints existing in the human body.

Movements of the bones upon each other are then described by ovoids of motion, and MacConaill uses a specific set of terminology to describe the motion. In essence, specific paths are described upon the articular surface, and, because the surface is not flat, the displacements follow a curved path, labeled as a chord or an arc. Further, all motions are classified around a "true" mechanical axis. Motions around this axis are labeled as spins, while all other motions are swings. Without going into great detail, the spins that accompany certain varieties of swings are called conjunct rotations. These rotations are inherent to the joint surfaces and a result of the concave and convex surfaces interacting as the motion is completed. Reference to a number of sources is possible for complete descriptions of the geometry and mechanics (20, 21).

There are several key points that should be made when considering joint geometry. The first is that joint geometry is responsible for the available motions.

Positioning the joint, or surfaces, in different configurations has a definite effect. Considering two ovoid surfaces one readily discovers that there is only one single position of best fit of the two surfaces. In this configuration, known as the close packed position, the bones are in maximum congruence, implying that the area of contact is at a maximum. The joint is compressed by virtue of the fact that the capsule and ligaments are spiralized and tense. In this situation the surface cannot be separated by distractive force, but the position does subject the joint to possible damage. Typically, the close packed position occurs at one extreme of most habitual movements of the joint. As examples, close packed position is achieved at full extension of the knee, wrist, and interphalangeal joints, and at full dorsiflexion of the ankle.

All other positions of the joint are known as the loose packed position, allowing for motions referred to as spin, roll, and glide. Compared to the close packed position this loose packed configuration has decreased the contact area of the articular surfaces. Frequent changes in contact areas serve to decrease friction and minimize the possibility of cartilaginous erosion. The loose packed position also provides for efficient joint lubrication and increases the available range of motion.

Because joints are maintained in the loose packed position during most of the range of motion as conventionally known there are motions known as joint play or intrinsic motions (30). A simple demonstration of these motions can be provided by considering two ovoid surfaces. Figure 3.6A shows a force applied in the direction of the shaft of the bone, thus creating a shear force or glide at the articular surface. Segment B of Figure 3.6 shows the humerus being driven posteriorly on the glenoid, thus creating a shear force or glide in a direction perpendicular to that in part A of the figure. Finally, in part C, the humeral head is being distracted from the glenoid through the application of a force applied to the inner, proximal surface of the humerus. These motions, although shown to exist through application of external forces, are part of the natural arthrokinematics of the articular surfaces. These intrinsic, or joint play, movements give yet three more degrees of freedom to the joints. Added to the three primary motions available in the cardinal planes shown to exist in virtually every joint

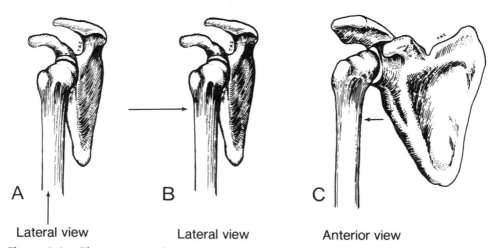

A   B   C

Lateral view   Lateral view   Anterior view

Figure 3.6. Three views of a joint consisting of one ovoid and one sellar surface. A description of the motions resulting from the forces, represented as vectors, is contained in the text.

(Chapter 2 and subsequent chapters), a total of 6° of freedom is available. That each of these degrees of freedom is therapeutically important has been shown by Mennell and other clinicians (19, 24).

A second consideration relates directly to movement. Strong clinical implications also result from findings as to how one surface moves on the other. To consider the events, move the female, or concave, surface over the stationary male surface. When this motion is performed the female surface will roll and slide in the same direction as the distal end of the extremity. When the male surface is moved upon the female surface slide and roll will occur in opposite directions. The direct result is that there is an increase in the amount of angular motion possible without increasing the size of the articular surfaces. A specific example of how these mechanisms work is shown in Figure 3.7 (30).

Therapeutic Implications

For therapeutic purposes, therapists must be aware of the mechanics because the technique of application will determine the resultant motions between two articular surfaces. Use, as an example, a joint limited to 60° of flexion as shown in Figure 3.8. Note the shape of the surfaces. Now assume that passive motion is to be manually applied to the bone containing the concave (female) surface. If the force is applied on the distal aspect of this segment and the joint motion is firmly restricted, say by collagenous structures, the effect can be a levering of the female surface in a direction opposite to that desired in normal arthrokinematics (Fig. 3.8B). Now consider the case shown in Figure 3.8C, where the force application is close to the joint under consideration. In this circumstance the segment can only move in the same direction as the required rolling. Therefore, the latter situation is to be much preferred because the normal arthrokinematics are produced by the therapeutic effort.

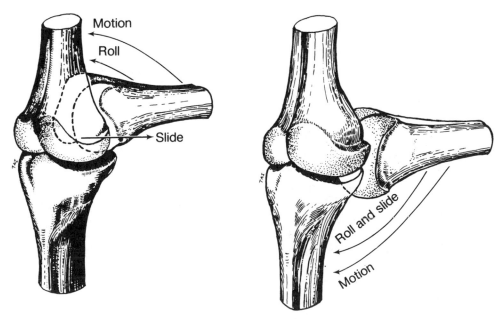

Figure 3.7.   Representation of the dependency of the nature of the joint surfaces upon the motions that occur between bony surfaces. See text for a complete description.

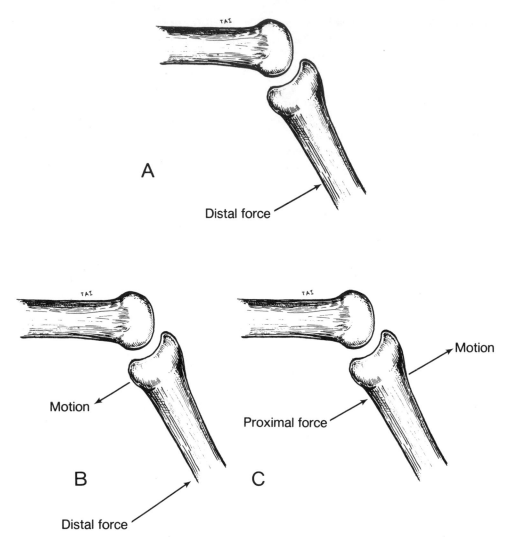

Figure 3.8. Schematic representation of the effects of incorrect and correct applications of forces when considering the arthrokinematics. Complete discussion of the figure is contained in the text.

LINKS AND CHAINS

Use of the terms link and chain has arisen from descriptions of collective joint actions. In most practical situations multiple segments move, and the joints are considered to be the centers for the connections of the various links. Therefore, this concept serves a useful purpose in describing the kinematics of a multiseg- ment model. Certain assumptions, however, are necessary for effective use of the link segment model (10). The technique, detailed by Dempster and discussed in Chapter 1, is considered useful (4). Gowitzke and Milner and Steindler all discuss chains, differentiating between the closed and open systems. The closed system is operational when the situation is such that when one link moves all the other links will move in a predictable pattern (Fig. 3.9). Conversely open systems result when the segment is not fixed, i.e., as the leg moves during the swing phase of gait (10, 28). Thus, open systems are the rule for the upper

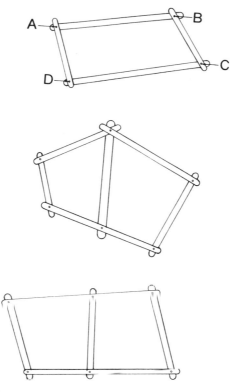

Figure 3.9. Examples of types of closed kinematic chains in which the joints shown are pinned and freely movable. The joints fixed, i.e., A, A and D, or other combinations, determine the resultant ranges of motion. (From Gowitzke BA, Milner M: *Understanding the Scientific Bases of Human Movement,* p 2. © 1980, Williams & Wilkins, Baltimore.)

extremity. And, in gait the lower extremities operate with closed kinetic and kinematic chains only to produce open chains during the swing phase of the extremity. In effect, then, rotatory motion at the joints turns into translatory motion of the whole body.

INSTANT CENTER OF ROTATION

The instant center of rotation is defined as the location of a point, resulting from the construction of an intersection of two axes perpendicular to the plane of motion. The concept is frequently used in defining motion of two segments and has been adequately determined for many joints. Use of the instant center of rotation (ICR) is valuable in the correct determination of the axis around which to consider motion at any point in time. Specifically, there are a number of techniques available for determining the ICR. Figure 3.10 shows a graphic technique when a segment has been moved from one location to another. Note that the landmarks selected must be readily identifiable in both positions, thus placing constraints on the ICR determinations. ICRs relative to other bony segments may also be determined. As White and Panjabi point out the ICR of any kind of plane motion, translation, rotation, or combinations of the two can be described. For other planes, similar procedures are followed (34). Frankel and Burstein present an excellent discussion of the procedures involved in determining the joint ICRs (6). One illustration for the knee is shown in Figure 3.11.

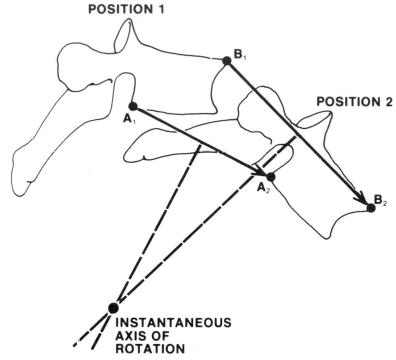

Figure 3.10.   The method for construction of the instantaneous axis of rotation. The same vertebrae has been moved from one position to the other. Note that the location, in this case, is not contained within the motion segment being considered. (From White AA, Panjabi MM: *Clinical Biomechanics of the Spine.* Philadelphia, JB Lippincott, 1978, p 479.)

PATHOLOGY AS AFFECTING JOINTS

There are several reasons why pathology frequently affects joints or the materials responsible for maintaining the integrity of the joint. Articular cartilage, by virtue of location on the ends of the bones, is subject to wear because of the cyclic loading that must be tolerated to accomplish the normal activities of daily living. Affections of the synovium will also profoundly affect the frictional factors, while trauma effectively stresses the collagenous tissues in and around the synovial joint. Each of these pathological effects will be discussed in this chapter, and many will be elaborated on in subsequent chapters on the individual joints.

According to Mow et al wear is the removal of material from solid surfaces by means of mechanical action. Interfascial wear can take place either by adhesion or by abrasion. The former takes place when fragments are torn from one surface and adhere to another. Abrasion can occur if a soft surface is scraped by a harder surface, be it from loose particles or from an opposing surface. There is evidence that once there is destruction of the surface further softening of deeper layers of the cartilage will occur. Thus, fluid movement may be altered, destroying the normal relationships and further exacerbating the abrasion process. The other type of wear, fatigue, is due to repetitive loading of the cartilage. Most injuries of this type are thought to be due to the solid matrix and/or to the fluid flow mechanisms (25). Two investigators have hypothesized that the cartilaginous failure is due to tensile failure of the collagen framework (8, 30). Defects frequently seen are splitting, or fibrillation, and erosion. There is little evidence

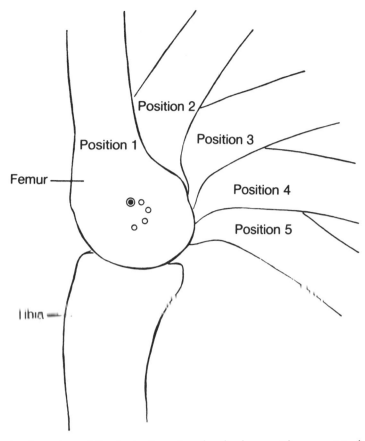

Figure 3.11.   Location of the instant centers for the knee with respect to both the tibia and the femur. The *solid circle* is the instant center for position 1. (From Frankel VH, Burstein AH: *Orthopedic Biomechanics,* Philadelphia, Lea & Febiger, 1970, p 138.)

that one type of wear is the cause of cartilaginous injury. Perhaps all mechanisms exist, but they are specific to the features of any given joint (25).

There have been numerous factors identified as playing a role in joint wear. Among these factors are stress magnitude, number of applied stresses, and the molecular and microscopic structure of the solid matrix. For example, diminished joint contact areas often produce increased stresses at particular locations in the joint, such as produced following simple menisectomies of the knee. These increased stresses also make maintenance of the fluid film barrier more difficult, therefore increasing the chances for wear. Occupations requiring repetitive loadings may also contribute to wear mechanisms, there being some evidence among certain types of workers and athletic performers. Finally, rheumatoid arthritis may predispose patients to alterations in the matrix, leading to ultimate degeneration of the cartilage (25).

Some evidence exists that cartilage is capable, under certain circumstances, of healing by formation of fibrocartilage. Even in cases of complete fracture, fibrous tissue with an overlay of polysaccharides may closely resemble the original hyaline cartilage. Hettinga details many of the gross and cellular changes that occur due to injury of the cartilage. Caution must be exercised in dealing with these injuries so that the regeneration process may proceed without sacrificing joint mobility (13).

Interarticular discs are frequently injured, primarily in the knee. As to be expected most injuries result from the application of greater stresses than the tissue can tolerate. Rotation and/or medial-lateral stress applied to this joint while bearing body weight is the classic position for the production of the torn meniscus. And, because of the avascular nature of the fibrocartilage, primarily in the central portions, healing does not occur. Peripheral displacements are complicated by concurrent injury of the synovium, leading to effusion. Healing of the peripheral portion of the meniscus is accomplished by infiltration of fibrous tissue (3).

Injuries to the capsule are of importance because involvement of the synovial membrane can potentially produce chronic effusions and long-term disabilities of considerable magnitude. Hettinga summarizes the inflammatory responses to be a proliferation of surface cells, an increase in the vascularity, and a gradual fibrosis of the subsynovial tissue. Posttraumatic synovitis may also be differentiated from other inflammatory and degenerative changes. In this case the synovial membrane has become thicker. Synovial fluid changes also appear, as do changes in the blood vessels. Fibrosis of the synovial membrane was concurrently noted as mature, densely packed collagen fibers formed up to the synovial surface. Continuation of the symptoms also has been blamed for other cellular and functional changes (12).

Lubrication of artificial joint surfaces has also been of some interest. Brand discusses the work relative to the findings and their influence on joint mechanics. Although indicating that lubrication problems are of less magnitude than other changes that occur, considerable work has been done on polyvinylpyrrolidone and silicone oil. Each has been demonstrated to be less effective than synovial fluid, however, indicating that further work needs to be done before fruitful results are available (2).

SUMMARY

Diarthrodial joints are of importance because of the dependency of the human body upon their delivering normal motion. Normal mechanics are frequently negated by traumatic or degenerative processes, thereby creating pathological motion that must be treated with anticipation of correction. While many pathologies are specific to individual joints this chapter has discussed the basic structure and function of joints so that each can be more thoroughly discussed in subsequent chapters.

References

1. Alexander RM: Mechanics of skeleton and tendons. In Brooks VB (ed): *Handbook of Physiology*, Section 1: The Nervous System. Bethesda, MD, American Physiological Society, 1981, vol 2, p 17.
2. Brand RA: Joint lubrication. In Albright JA, Brand RA (eds): *The Scientific Basis of Orthopedics*. New York, Appleton-Century-Crofts, 1979.
3. Calliet R: *Soft Tissue Pain and Disability*. Philadelphia, FA Davis, 1977.
4. Dempster W: Space Requirements of the Seated Operator, WADC Technical Report 55-159. Washington, DC, Office of Technical Services, US Department of Commerce, July 1955.
5. Edwards CC, Chrisman OD: Articular cartilage. In Albright JA, Brand RA (eds): *The Scientific Basis of Orthopedics*. New York, Appleton-Century-Crofts, 1979.
6. Frankel VH, Burstein AH: *Orthopedic Biomechanics*. Philadelphia, Lea & Febiger, 1970.
7. Frankel VH, Nordin M: *Basic Biomechanics of the Skeletal System*, Philadelphia, Lea & Febiger, 1980.

8. Freeman MAR: The fatigue of cartilage in the pathogenesis of osteoarthritis. *Acta Orthop Scand* 46:323–328, 1975.

9. Ghadially FN: Fine structure of joints. In Sokoloff L (ed): *The Joints and Synovial Fluid*, New York, Academic Press, 1979, vol 1.

10. Gowitzke BA, Milner M: *Understanding the Scientific Bases of Human Movement*. Baltimore, Williams & Wilkins, 1980.

11. Hettinga DL: I. Normal joint structures and their reaction to injury. *J. Orthop Sports Phys Ther* 1:16–22, 1979.

12. Hettinga DL: II. Normal joint structure and their reaction to injury. *J Orthop Sports Phys Ther* 1:83–88, 1979.

13. Hettinga DL: III. Normal joint structure and their reaction to injury. *J Orthop Sports Phys Ther* 2:178–185, 1980.

14. Kaltenborn FM: *Manual Therapy for the Extremity Joints*. Oslo, Norway, Olaf Norlis Bokhandel, 1976.

15. Kempson GE: Mechanical properties of articular cartilage. In Freeman MAR (ed): *Adult Articular Cartilage*. London, Pitman, 1973.

16. Kempson GE: The mechanical properties of articular cartilage. In: Sokoloff L (ed): *The Joints and Synovial Fluid*. New York, Academic Press, 1978, vol 2.

17. Kempson GE, Freeman MAR, Swanson SAV: Tensile properties of articular cartilage. *Nature* 220:1127–1128, 1968.

18. Kempson GE, Spivery CJ, Swanson SAV, et al: Patterns of cartilage stiffness in normal and degenerate human femoral heads. *J Biomech* 4:597–609, 1971.

19. Kessler RM, Hertling D: *Management of Musculoskeletal Disorders*. Philadelphia, Harper & Row, 1983.

20. MacConaill MA: The movements of bones and joints: 5. The significance of shape. *J Bone Joint Surg [Br]*: 35:290–297, 1953.

21. MacConaill MA, Basmajian JV: *Muscles and Movements: A Basis for Human Kinesiology*. Baltimore, Williams & Wilkins, 1969.

22. Maroudas A: Physico-chemical properties of articular cartilage. In: Freeman MAR (ed): *Adult Articular Cartilage*. London, Pitman, 1973.

23. Maroudas A: Balance between swelling pressure and collagen tension in normal and degenerate cartilage. *Nature* 260:808–809, 1976.

24. Mennell JMc: *Joint Pain*. London, Churchill, 1964.

25. Mow VC, Roth V, Armstrong CG: Biomechanics of joint cartilage. In Frankel VH, Nordin M: *Basic Biomechanics of the Skeletal System*. Philadelphia, Lea & Febiger, 1980.

26. Mulholland R: Lateral hydraulic permeability and morphology of articular cartilage in normal and osteoarthrosic cartilage. *Proceedings of the Symposium of the Institute of Orthopaedics*, London, 1974

27. Redler I, Mow VC, Mansell J: Ultrastructural changes in aging human articular cartilage. *J Bone Joint Surg [Am]* 57A:575, 1975.

28. Steindler A: *Kinesiology of the Human Body under Normal and Pathological Conditions*. Springfield, IL, Charles C Thomas, 1955.

29. Wadsworth C: Fundamentals of Orthopedics, University of Iowa, Iowa City, IA, 1984.

30. Warwick R, Williams PL: *Gray's Anatomy*, ed 36. Philadelphia, WB Saunders, 1980.

31. Weightman B: Tensile fatigue of human articular cartilage. *J Biomech* 9:193–200, 1976.

32. Weightman BO, Kempson GE: Load carriage. In Freeman MAR (ed): *Adult Articular Cartilage*. London, Pitman, 1979.

33. Weiss C, Rosenberg L, Helfet AJ: An ultrastructural study of normal young adult human articular cartilage. *J Bone Joint Surg [Am]* 50:663–674, 1968.

34. White AA, Panjabi MM: *Clinical Biomechanics of the Spine*. Philadelphia, JB Lippincott, 1978.

4

Material Properties of Biological Tissues

An understanding of materials and their properties is important because most therapists will deal with many pathologies produced by acute loading. Other tissue failures will result from long-term or acute loads and stresses. Material properties are specifically a factor in joint prostheses and their retention in the human body. The properties of tissue are also very significant in cases of burns and in such common afflictions as capsulitis. Lumbar discs, in particular, are known to rupture and be subject to degenerative processes. Further, fracture repair and the management of scoliosis are affected by applied forces. This chapter will present basic definitions necessary to understand the reactions of biological tissues to applied forces. Properties of tissues, including bone, muscle, ligament, and cartilage, will be discussed. Finally, how the properties affect normal and pathological motion will be presented.

FORCES, LOADS, AND STRESS
Definitions

Biological materials are constantly subjected to contact or remote forces. By definition, a force is the action or effect of one body on another (3). Because, as noted in Chapter 1, these forces are vector quantities, they have magnitude, a point and line of application, and direction. Recall also from Chapter 1 that where the force is applied will determine whether rotational or linear movement will potentially or actually occur.

Included as forces can be a push or pull, a tendency to compress, or an application of tension to a structure. Five types of forces have been identified, including:

Compression—the act of pressing together.
Tension—defined as the normal force tending to stretch or pull a body apart.
Bending—known as deformation due to loading of a structure when load is applied at an area where there is not direct support.
Torsion—the force tending to twist a body.
Shear—considered to be forces that act like the cutting action of a scissors. That is, the force is applied parallel to the surface or plane within an object. Representations of these forces are shown in Figure 4.1 (11).

Two other terms are commonly encountered when forces are described. The first, normal, means that force is applied perpendicular to a surface or a plane

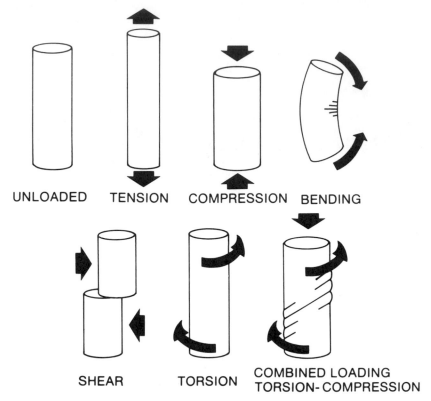

Figure 4.1.   Representation of various loading modes. (From Frankel VH, Nordin M: *Basic Biomechanics of the Skeletal System*. Philadelphia, Lea & Febiger, 1980, p 23.)

within an object. An example of normal loads are shown in the tension and compression modes in Figure 4.1. The other term is axial, meaning applied along the long axis of the body or object being considered. In the case of Figure 4.1 both the tension and compression modes are also axial since they are applied along the long axis.

Applications

Examples of ways that these forces are applied to biological tissues may be helpful in understanding and recalling the effect of the force. Prior to doing so, however, some understanding of stress and strain is necessary.

Stress is defined as the intermolecular resistance within a body to the deforming actions of an outside force. The symbol used for identification is the greek letter sigma (σ). Strain is a measure of deformation, describing the change in the dimensions of a body as a result of load application. Designation is by means of epsilon (ϵ). For both stress and strain two types are possible. By definition, recall that normal stress or strain occurs perpendicular to the plane of the cross section of the loaded object. Shear stress or strain occurs parallel to the plane of the applied load (Fig. 4.2).

When loading (defined as the application of a force and/or moment to a structure) is applied to produce compression the structure shortens and widens. Both compressive stress and strain occur within the structure, and according to Frankel and Nordin, maximal compressive stress occurs on a plane perpendicular to the applied load (11). The skeletal system is commonly loaded in compression

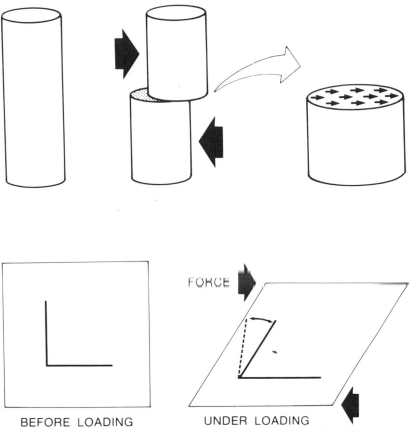

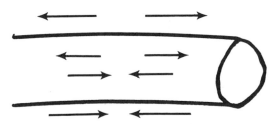

Figure 4.2. Shear loading and the stress and strain occurring within the structure. The bottom two structures show that when loading occurs in shear, lines change their orientation, the angle formed becoming obtuse or acute. This change indicates shear. (From Frankel VH, Nordin M: *Basic Biomechanics of the Skeletal System.* Philadelphia, Lea & Febiger, 1980, p 28.)

Figure 4.3. Bone undergoing bending.

during weight bearing by the lower extremities, but note that any time a structure is undergoing bending, compression must always occur on the concave surface (Fig. 4.3). Muscle contractions across joints that are fully extended also are responsible for increasing compressive load across joints. Specific examples of the effect of this mechanism will be discussed in the chapters on each of the joints.

In tension, stress and strain also occur in materials. Maximal tensile stress occurs, as for compression, in a plane perpendicular to the applied load as the structure now narrows and elongates. Tensile force occurs in the convex side of a long bone undergoing bending (Fig. 4.3). Muscles also generate tensile forces within the muscle proper as the elasticity of the tissue reacts to the strain imposed by the elongation created by contraction. During shear there is internal deformation that causes the tissue to change internally. This demonstrable shear, shown in Figure 4.2, is also shown in Figure 4.4. In the latter case note that tension and compression also produce shear strain. Virtually all human tissues are subjected to shear forces. Menisci of the knee are very vulnerable and must accommodate the twisting of the femur on the tibia. Anterior or posterior displacement of the tibia on the femur would have a similar effect (6, 11, 23).

Bending, as indicated above, creates both compression and tension forces. However, at the neutral or central axis there are no stresses or strains. Moving away from the central axis the stresses increase in proportion to the distance moved (Fig. 4.3). Throughout the body bending forces are regularly produced. This bending motion is resisted by the very nature of the structure and is usually not readily discernible as gross motion. Individual bones are continually subjected to bending forces, but only in extreme cases would a fracture result.

Torsional forces, by nature of application cause shear stress distribution over the entire material. Similar to bending, stresses are increased as the distance from the axis of rotation is increased. With the application of torsional forces the maximal shear stress is on the plane perpendicular to the axis of rotation (Fig. 4.5). Also note in Figure 4.5 that the tensile and compressive stresses are on a plane diagonal to the neutral axis. These forces are commonly seen in compound fractures, classic examples being provided by the lower extremity fractures in downhill skiers. Any of these five types of forces can occur in a pure sense, but most frequently they occur in combinations (Fig. 4.1), particularly in producing pathological situations (6, 11, 23).

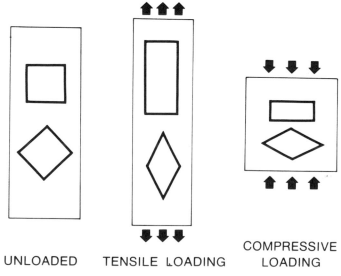

UNLOADED   TENSILE LOADING   COMPRESSIVE LOADING

Figure 4.4. A structure depicted in three different states. Refer to text for a complete description. (From Frankel VH, Nordin M: *Basic Biomechanics of the Skeletal System.* Philadelphia, Lea & Febiger, 1980, p 29.)

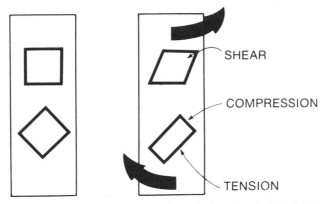

Figure 4.5. Segment of bone unloaded (*left*) and then loaded (*right*) in torsion. (From Frankel VH, Nordin M: *Basic Biomechanics of the Skeletal System*. Philadelphia, Lea & Febiger, 1980, p 35.)

Forces and Loads

Often there is confusion about the differences between forces and loads. Forces are any action that tends to change the shape, size, or state of inertia or the motion of a body (23). A load is a force or moment applied to the material. In a strict sense, loads should be considered as torsional, bending, normal, or shear. Buckling loads are sometimes also listed as a type of load. The application of muscle tension to a bone in fact applies a load to the bone. Units are total load, such as 1000 lb(f), or unit load, such as 200 psi. More typical units are newtons/m². No matter the specific classification system used, the terminology should be consistently applied in relationship to the human tissues being discussed.

In summary, then, normal forces are force components directed perpendicular to the surface upon which they act. Shear forces are force components directed parallel to the surface on which they act. Bending moments are moment components directed parallel to the surface on which they act, and torsional moments or torques are moment components directed perpendicular to the surface on which they act.

LOAD-DEFORMATION AND STRESS-STRAIN

Behavior of materials is often described by means of relating an applied load to the amount of deformation that occurs in the material or tissue. From the resulting plot shown in Figure 4.6 several key characteristics may be evaluated. One is the degree of tissue stiffness, defined as the resistance offered to external loads by a specimen or structure as it deforms. The degree of stiffness is indicated by the slope of the line of the early part of the curve. Note that if the load is increased the deformation is linearly related to the load. If the load is removed the material will be classified as being "elastic" if the material returns to original shape and dimension after removal of the load. If too great a load is applied, however, the tissue becomes permanently deformed, and the elastic limit is said to have been exceeded. Even further loading will cause the failure point (strength) of the material to be reached (6, 11).

Using standardized techniques, i.e., such as during a simple tension or compression test, the load per unit area and the amount of deformation can be

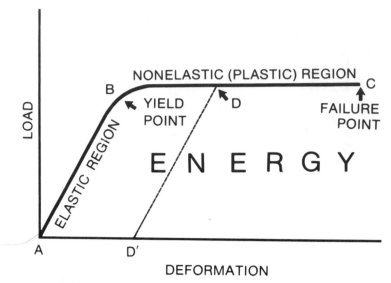

Figure 4.6. Load-deformation curve for a material considered somewhat pliable. If loading proceeds into the nonelastic region and is then released, permanent deformation results. Loading to point *D* and unloading will cause permanent deformation as shown by *A* to *D'*. Other features are included in the text. (From Frankel VH, Nordin M: *Basic Biomechanics of the Skeletal System.* Philadelphia, Lea & Febiger, 1980, p 16.)

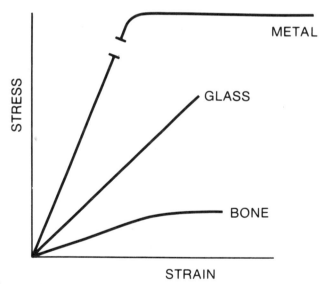

Figure 4.7. Stress-strain curves for a metal, glass, and bone. Note that bone is not linearly elastic in behavior. The soft metal, being ductile, has a long plastic region. Glass, having no plastic region, is brittle. (From Frankel VH, Nordin M: *Basic Biomechanics of the Skeletal System.* Philadelphia, Lea & Febiger, 1980, p 19.)

determined. Recognize that loading is the manner of force application and that stress is obtained by dividing the load with the cross sectional area. Thus, stress is not directly measured but rather derived. To determine strain the deformation is divided by the value of the original length of the material.

Such a test produces a curve known as the stress-strain curve. The resulting relationship represents the mechanical behavior of a material. Samples of stress-strain curves are shown in Figure 4.7, demonstrating configurations similar to those of the load-deformation curve. The differences in stiffness are readily indicated by the differences in the slopes during the portion of the curve demonstrating elasticity. That is, the slope of the linear elastic part of the stress-strain diagram (Modulus of Elasticity) varies with each of the materials. On each of the plots the yield point also occurs at a location specific to the material being tested. The yield point is defined as that point where progressive deformation occurs without increasing the load on the material (Fig. 4.6). The soft metal has a great deal of deformation, whereas glass would be considered a brittle material since there is little deformation before failure.

OTHER PROPERTIES

Other terms that may be used in describing stress-strain properties include plastic, essentially meaning nonelastic, and ductility, meaning that the material has the capacity to absorb large amounts of plastic deformation energy before failure. Two other properties of significance to normal and pathological motion are the concepts of creep and relaxation. Creep, defined as the increase in strain with time under constant load, is applicable in cases where tissue elongation is attempted. Cases of serial cast application for clubfoot or for treatment of scoliosis are excellent examples of the direct application of methods used to alter tissue properties. Principles of relaxation can also be demonstrated by means of evaluating the effects of stress on tissues. White and Panjabi, defining relaxation as the decrease in stress in a deformed structure with time when the deformation is held constant, use the stress diminution in a vertebral body as an example. Figure 4.8 adequately demonstrates the experimental conditions, showing the constant deformation with time. Concurrently the force in the specimen, as revealed by the force transducer, diminishes with time. The resulting decrease in stress with time demonstrates relaxation (23).

Resilience, damping, and viscosity are also of importance. Resilience is defined as the ability of an object to rebound from a surface or another object. Tennis balls demonstrate much greater resilience than do nylon and foamed plastic materials. Lead would be considered nonresilient. Examples of different states of resiliency are shown in Figure 4.9. Damping is the opposite of resilience. In this case the material would return to original shape slowly. Because many human tissues of interest to therapists are viscoelastic materials, hysteresis is a factor in the physiologic behavior of human tissues. By definition hysteresis is the phenomenon associated with energy loss exhibited by viscoelastic materials when subjected to loading and unloading cycles. Thus, the shaded areas in Figure 4.9 represent the hysteresis for the materials tested (6).

Each of the material properties discussed has a distinct application to pathological motion. The concepts presented in this section will be discussed further in this chapter, but the principles applied to each joint will be discussed within the respective chapter.

PROPERTIES OF HUMAN TISSUES

The properties of tissues vary, depending upon the available collagen, the amount of elastin, other constituents, and the structural arrangement and proportion of these elements. Each tissue's material properties can be examined by applying specific tests to the tissue of interest. For example, stress-strain tests applied to various structures produce the forms shown in Figure 4.10 (11).

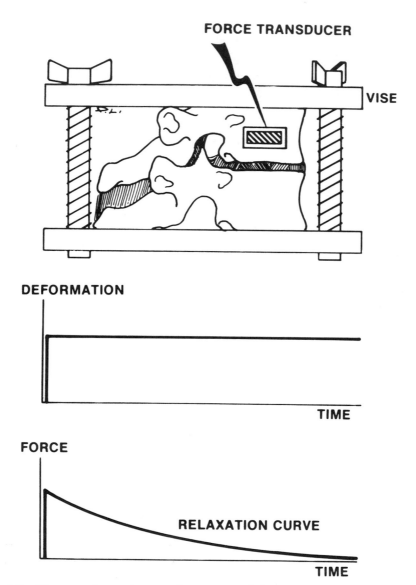

Figure 4.8.   The experimental setup, the constant deformation, and the resulting relaxation curve are shown from top to bottom. (From White AA, Panjabi MM: *Clinical Biomechanics of the Spine*. Philadelphia, JB Lippincott, 1978, p 495.)

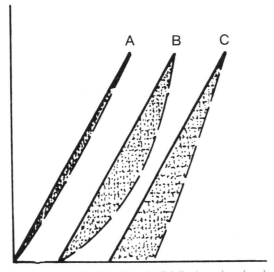

Figure 4.9. Stress-strain curves for loading (solid line) and unloading (dashed line) of a resilient (A), poorly resilient (B), and an elastic (C) material. Shading represents hysteresis. (From Frost HM: *An Introduction to Biomechanics*, 1967, p 16. Courtesy of Charles C Thomas, Springfield, IL.)

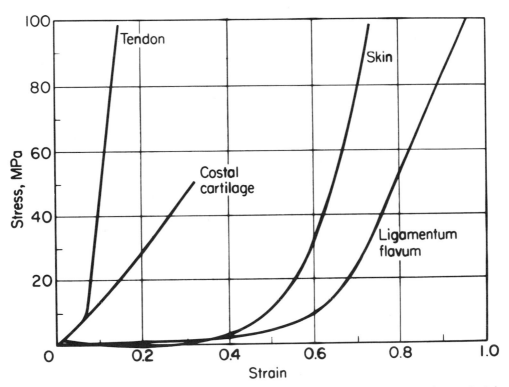

Figure 4.10. Stress-strain plots for various human connective tissues tested in uniaxial tensions. (From Barbenel JC, Evans JH, Jordan MM: Tissue mechanics. *Eng Med* 7:5, 1978.)

Bone

Bone has been frequently evaluated in order to determine material properties associated with strength and failure. Fatigue failure is also of interest, since some pathologies are directly related to stresses and strains resulting from activities requiring the performance of cyclic loading. Frost has indicated that for bone the proportional limit and rupture strength are approximately equal. Because the proportional limit is the greatest stress at which stress is still proportional to strain, bone is classified as a brittle material. Caution must be exercised, however, because strength will depend upon the loading mechanism. For example, shear strength is approximately 4,000 psi, tensile strength 12,000 psi, and compressive strength 15,000 psi (6).

As a result of existing material properties, bone is seldom deformed greater than 3%, and the tensile forces to fracture are generally less than the compressive forces. Age, sex, wetness, and other elements are also factors in influencing the material properties. Yamada provides a thorough presentation of data for a variety of mechanical tests on all types of bone under a series of different conditions (24). Numerous investigators have established that cellular structure has adjusted to accommodate for the needs of the bone to bear loads. Trabecular structure through the femoral neck is known to be configured in a pattern that will effectively resist the large bending moments. Further, that bone responds by adaptive remodeling has been shown by Churches et al (2).

Cartilage

Cartilaginous tissue is also important in pathologies because the tissue is frequently injured. Cellular makeup of articular cartilage was discussed in Chapter 3. The peripheral cellular orientation is adeptly suited to resist shear forces of articular surfaces (4). Warwick and Williams point out that hyaline, white fibro-cartilage, and yellow elastic fibrocartilage contain different proportions of certain tissue types, particularly collagen and elastin (22). Frost states that a large amount of water is contained in cartilage, up to 75% in the hyaline form (6). Thus, cartilage can respond to loads as a viscoelastic material. For almost 40 yr evidence has accumulated that articular cartilage deforms instantaneously upon application of loads. Some creep follows this elastic phase. Because the cartilage has properties of a viscoelastic material the response is time-dependent. That is, when rapidly loaded, the initial stiffness is high, followed by deformation over a longer interval of time (11).

In discussing white fibrocartilage Warwick and Williams indicate that the tissue, heavily laden with collagen, has considerable toughness and sufficient elasticity to resist long-term effects of pressure and friction (22). An example of the material-testing procedures performed on tissues is demonstrated in the work of Uezaki et al (21).

Muscle

Mechanical properties of muscle have also been determined. The features attendant to behavior of muscle have been somewhat addressed in Chapter 2. As for other tissues the specifics of the properties will depend upon the muscle evaluated and also heavily upon age. Yamada has evaluated the stress-strain features of several muscles of humans. Figure 4.11 demonstrates these features for several muscles (24). Further, since muscle is essentially a viscous structure surrounded by an elastic membrane the properties are therefore similar to other

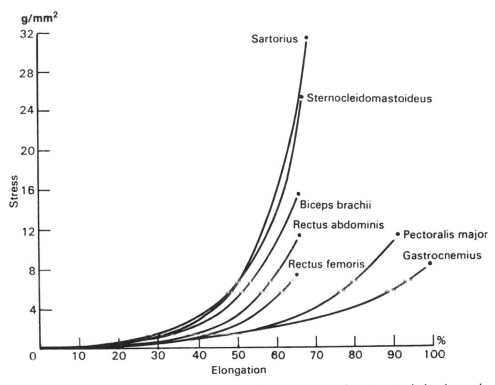

Figure 4.11. Stress-strain plots derived from the application of tension to skeletal muscle in 29-year-olds. (From Yamada H: Mechanical properties of locomotor organs and tissues. In Evans FG (ed): *Strength of Biological Materials.* Baltimore, Williams & Wilkins, 1970, p 95.)

viscoelastic materials. The difficulty in arriving at precise properties for muscle is due to the attachment of fibers to tendinous attachments at one or both ends of the muscle. Of the muscles tested the sartorius appears to have the greatest ultimate strength, while the gastrocnemius and the rectus femoris have the least. Further, ultimate strength is greater in thin muscle than in thick and also in extensor muscles as opposed to flexor muscles (24).

Collagen

Common to ligaments, tendon, and skin is collagenous tissue. Incorporated within these tissues are three types of fibers: collagen for strength, elastic for elastic properties, and reticulin for bulk. A fourth, but less important component is the ground substance.

According to Frankel and Nordin the behavior of collagen is affected by three factors. First is the fiber orientation. The organization in each of the three tissues is remarkably different (see Fig. 4.12). Because of the parallel fiber orientation the tendons are capable of bearing the highest tensile loads. The skin, with a more diverse arrangement of fibers, is more extensible for the allowance of tension, compression, and shear. Ligamentous behavior would be somewhere between tendon and skin, although certainly designed to tolerate tensile loading.

The second factor is the properties of the individual collagen and elastic fibers. These make up approximately 90% of the tissue and are also important features in determining the mechanical characteristics. Collagen is ductile, while the

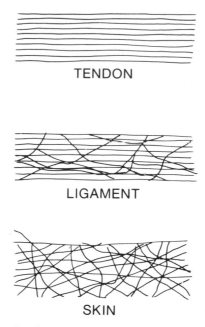

Figure 4.12.   Orientation of collagen fibers in tendon, ligament, and skin. (From Frankel VH, Nordin M: *Basic Biomechanics of the Skeletal System*, Philadelphia, Lea & Febiger, 1980, p 88.)

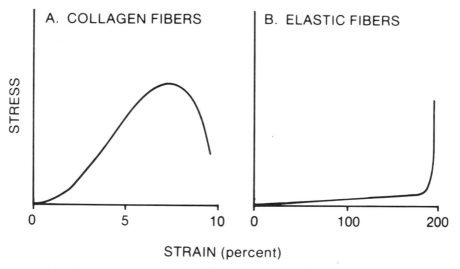

Figure 4.13.   Stress-strain curves for collagen and elastic fibers when tested to failure in tension. Note the remarkable differences in the shape of the curve and the scale of the abscissa. (From Frankel VH, Nordin M: *Basic Biomechanics of the Skeletal System*. Philadelphia, Lea & Febiger, 1980, p 91.)

elastic fibers are brittle. If the fiber behavior is shown on stress-strain plots grossly different features are demonstrated (Fig. 4.13). Note also that the percent of strain axis is of different magnitude.

The third factor that determines behavior is the relative proportion of the collagen and elastic fibers. The proportion is usually according to function. For example, tendons have virtually all collagen. Thus, great loads can be tolerated without a large degree of tendon deformation as tension is developed within the muscle. Yamada indicates that the percentage of elastic recovery in certain ligaments is as high as 99% (24). Fielding et al, as cited by Frankel and Nordin, have shown that ligaments are also mainly collagen, while the ligamentum nuchae and ligamentum flavum are made up of over 60% elastic fibers (11). As a result, ligamentous strength is directly related to the number of fibers and the thickness and width of the fibers. During testing, and probably during function and/or injury, note that the elastic limit approximately equals the ultimate strength.

Tendon

Tendon, with collagen fibers arranged largely in parallel, can tolerate high loads. For example the estimated tensile breaking strength of human calcaneal tendon is approximately 5.6 kg(f)/mm^2 (24). Frankel and Nordin cite several studies that have determined in vivo loading of tendons. Results suggest that in normal activities the tendon is subjected to less than 25% of the ultimate stress of which the tissue is capable of withstanding (11). Readily observed is that the larger muscle masses are accompanied by larger tendons that can effectively manage increased loads

Skin

The material properties of skin are often ignored, but because of their importance in manipulation of skin (resulting from surgery) and in scarring, considerable attention should be paid to the material properties. Gibson, in 1979 discussed the biomechanical aspects of plastic surgery, specifically discussing the material properties of the skin. The collagen and elastin fiber makeup accounts for the tension that normally exists in skin, mostly in retraction. Generally the crease lines parallel maximum tension, the minimum being at right angles. Therefore, wounds across tension lines produce hypertrophic scarring. He also points out four effects of increased tension:

1. Blanching and necrosis
2. Rupture of the dermis (for example, the straie in the abdomen during pregnancy)
3. Permanent stretching
4. There is no effect on surrounding normal skin (i.e., scar contractures do not induce surrounding skin to stretch) (8).

As will be further emphasized in later sections the response of skin to pressure and the tissue's natural "creep" with deformation over a period of time is an important consideration. In general, interest is being renewed in the material properties of the skin since the mid-1800 work of Langer. For example, a work by Potts et al has evaluated the dynamic in vivo properties of human skin in response to applications of shear waves over a frequency from near 0 to 1000 Hz (13). Implications for pressure sores resulting from sitting postures and prostheses and orthoses would be a natural topic for study by therapists.

APPLICATIONS TO PRACTICE

There are numerous effects of material properties of biological tissues on human performance, in injury and in treatment procedures. Physical therapists frequently treat patients with fatigue failures and fractures. The pathology has been caused by repetitive loading and unloading within the design limits. In other words, the number of cycles through which the material is loaded is critical.

For example, a glass rod, manufactured to fail at 200,000 psi will fail at 10,000 psi after a thimble full of sand grains has fallen on the rod (6). Often, material properties are modified by means of providing greater strength than actually needed to function effectively. Bone, as an example, can tolerate loads of 8,000 psi in shear parallel to the long axis but to 12,000 psi across the long axis (7).

Soft Tissue Injuries

Another area where material properties are important is in soft tissue ruptures or avulsions. These injuries can occur at virtually any site but are frequently seen as avulsion fractures. In other words, tensile strength is not sufficient to prevent the fracture.

In the area of ligamentous tissue, Tipton et al have reported that the lowest values for ligamentous strength occur in immobilized animals. The highest values appeared in trained animals. Those that are trained also have higher collagen content with increased thicknesses and diameters. Junctional strength also increased with training (20). Figure 4.14 shows a load deformation curve for the anterior cruciate ligament in the tension mode. All of these animals' ligaments were immobilized for 8 weeks. It is interesting to note the minimal effect of local exercise. That is, the tissue response postimmobilization does not appear to be the same as the reconditioned curve that included ambulation and free activity for a period of 5 months. One of the questions that yet remains to be answered is whether or not there is an increase in ligament strength, above the normal,

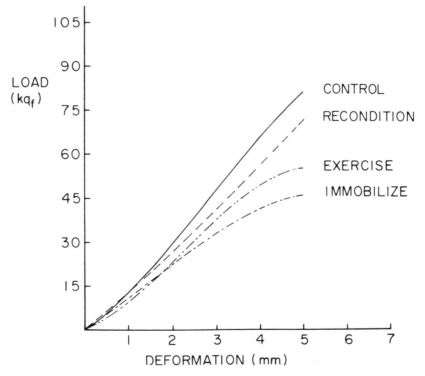

Figure 4.14. Calculated load-deformation curves for experimental groups subjected to immobilization and rehabilitation. See text for details. (From Noyes FR: Biomechanics of ligament failure. II. An analysis of immobilization, exercise, and reconditioning effects in primates. *J Bone Joint Surg [Am]* 56:1413, 1974.)

created by exercise. The study by Noyes et al would seem to lend credence to that possibility (12).

Material properties are important in plastic surgery and in the formation of scar tissue resulting from burns. Barbanel has, in fact, shown that excised skin that has undergone repeated cycling causing extension demonstrated progressive alteration of response in uniaxial tension. That is, the strain curve shifted to the right for equivocal stresses applied over different periods of time (1). The concept of creep may also become very important in treating these tissue injuries caused by burns. Further, pressure sores are the result of reaction forces at the skin and the support surface interface. The site is usually over bony prominences. Many other examples will be provided in the area of joint forces and their distribution as to how tissue properties play a role in the pathology and the rehabilitative treatment that physical therapists will provide.

Specific studies have also been completed to evaluate the strength of tendon. Investigators have found that tendons are weakest 3 to 14 days postsurgically because the collagen remains relatively soft. The ability of these tissues to resist the shearing at the suture area that occurs during tensile loading is markedly diminished (10). Although clinical experience indicates that 3 weeks of immobilization is necessary to prevent rupturing, anything greater than 3 weeks yields adhesions between the tendon and the sheath and the surrounding soft tissues. Approximately 40 to 50 weeks is necessary to regain normal strength postsurgically (11). Work by Steiner may provide the clinician with some guidelines. His study on the biomechanics of tendon healing has shown that after 4 weeks of healing of unsutured rat tendon 70% of the normal stiffness and only 40% of the normal muscle rupture strength had returned. About 25% of the normal tendon strength had returned at 4 weeks. These relatively low values indicate that high loading in the early stages of recovery must be avoided (17).

Treatment Implications

Because therapists frequently encounter different surgical techniques and apply loads on these tissues, evaluations have been completed on various surgical methods associated with tendon suturing. Interrupted sutures provide tensile load directly on the tendon ends, while the Kessler technique provides mostly tensile and some compressive force through the adjacent tendon ends. Bunnell's technique utilizes both compression and tensile forces, while the fishmouth or endweave creates some shearing at the anastamosis sites as well as compressive loads. This latter technique provides the greatest immediate strength but is relatively bulky (11).

In a review article Soderberg has detailed some of the work pertaining to alterations in the morphological and physiological features of biological tissues as a result of immobilization and treatment procedures (16). Studies have shown a rather significant decrease in the available number of sarcomeres as a result of immobilization (18, 19). These results are of significance because they indicate that elongation tension is apparently needed to facilitate the return of sarcomeres and the subsequent length-tension relationship required for normal function of the musculotendinous unit.

Other work relates to the effect of immobilization and passive motion techniques upon tendons. These investigative works have shown that mobilized animals had greater increases in strength and stiffness and more callous formation than the caged or immobilized groups (7, 15). Material properties have also been shown to be a factor in the production of soft tissue pathology. Excessive elongation, particularly at high rates, are conceded to produce either strains or complete ruptures of soft tissues. That muscle rupture is far more common than tendon rupture is substantiated by work showing the maximum stress to failure for tendon to be twice that for muscle (5).

Orthotics and Prosthetics

Properties of materials used in orthotic and prosthetic appliances are also of importance. Of main concern is that consideration be given to the material's maximum permitted stress, stiffness, weight, and fatigue life. Materials available include metals, plastics, wood, and leather. Primary support, however, needs to be offered by metals and plastics. Table 4.1 contains a contrast of the stress, stiffness, and weight (9). Redford and Licht state that of the metals, steel and aluminum alloys are most suitable for orthotic appliances (14). Henshaw discusses the use of reinforced plastics and states that although the latter have excellent tensile strength and stiffness qualities and other features, other qualities are often not satisfactory. Consider also that the materials are subjected to bending loads. Because the thin metals or alloys do not resist these loads well the materials may be unsatisfactory for use at least in certain situations (9). Further, aluminum alloys have a much higher incidence of fatigue failures than do the steels. They are also relatively corrosion-resistant and of high strength. Magnesium alloys are now appearing as a major component of wheelchair fabrication because of their light weight and amenability to welding and brazing (14).

The over 30 major families of plastics have revolutionized the practice of orthotics. Splinting has been dramatically simplified. Two major categories of plastics are thermoplastics and thermosetting plastics. Thermoplastics soften with heat and harden when cooled. They can be remolded with additional heating. Thermosetting plastics develop a permanent set when heat and pressure are applied and cannot be softened or reshaped when heated. As an example, polypropylene is a rigid material with high impact strength. The material is also

Table 4.1. Comparison of the Stress, Stiffness, and Weight of Materials[a]

Material	Maximum permissible stress (tensile)	E (stiffness)	Weight
High tensile steel	45–85 ton/inch^2 (70–130 × 10^7 N/m^2)	30 × 10^6 lb/inch^2 (2.1 × 10^{11} N/m^2)	0.283 lb/inch^3 (0.0078 kg/cm^3)
Mild steel	30 ton/inch^2 (46 × 10^7 N/m^2	30 × 10^6 lb/inch^2 (2.1 × 10^{11} N/m^2)	0.283 lb/inch^3 (0.0078 kg/cm^3)
Titanium	70 ton/inch^2 (108 × 10^7 N/m^2)	16 × 10^6 lb/inch^2 (1.10 × 10^{11} N/m^2)	0.16 lb/inch^3 (0.0044 kg/cm^3)
Plastics (unreinforced)	3–7 ton/inch^2 (5–11 × 10^7 N/m^2)	0.35 × 10^6 lb/inch^2 (approx.) 0.024 × 10^{11} N/m^2)	0.03–0.07 lb/inch^3 (0.0008–0.0019 kg/cm^3)
Plastics (carbon fiber reinforced) High strength	Up to 200 ton/inch^2 (309 × 10^7 N/m^2)	33 × 10^6 lb/inch^2 (2.3 × 10^{11} N/m^2)	0.06–0.07 lb/inch^3 (0.00166–0.00194 kg/cm^3)

[a] Modified from Henshaw JT: The design of orthotic appliances. In Murdoch G (ed): *The Advance in Orthotics.* Baltimore, Williams & Wilkins, 1976.

able to withstand several million repetitive flexures before showing signs of failure. The molecular structure of this and other plastics provide the properties necessary for functional use. Resistance to bending, impact, and fatigue, while affording the patient a lightweight structure, are thus all important considerations in orthotic materials (14).

SUMMARY

Included in this chapter has been a discussion of material properties of biological tissues. Examples of how the basic concepts of load, stress, and strain apply to humans has also been provided through representative examples. Further applications to specific tissues will be included in subsequent chapters and related to meaning in clinical practices.

References

1. Barbenel JC, Evans JH, Jordan MM: Tissue mechanics. *Eng Med* 7:5–9, 1978.
2. Churches AE, Howlett CR, Waldron KJ, Ward GW: The response of living bone to controlled time-varying loading: method and preliminary results. *J Biomech* 12:35–45, 1979.
3. Cochran GVB: *A Primer of Orthopedic Biomechanics*. New York, Churchill Livingstone, 1982.
4. Edwards CC, Chrisman OD: Articular cartilage. In Albright JA, Brand RA (eds): *The Scientific Basis of Orthopedics*. New York, Appleton-Century-Crofts, 1979.
5. Elliott DH: The biomechanical properties of tendon in relation to muscular strength. *Ann Med* 9:1–7, 1967.
6. Frost HM: *An Introduction to Biomechanics*. Springfield, IL, Charles C Thomas, 1967.
7. Gelberman RH, Woo SL-Y, Cobb N, et al: Flexor tendon healing: the effects of early passive mobilization. *Proceedings of the 27th Annual Orthopedic Research Society*. Chicago, Dependable Publishing Co., 1981, p 81.
8. Gibson T: Biomechanical aspects of plastic surgery. In Akkas N (ed): *Progress in Biomechanics*. Gravenhage, Netherlands, Sijthoff and Noordhoff, 1979.
9. Henshaw JT: The design of orthotic appliances. In Murdoch G (ed): *The Advance in Orthotics*. Baltimore, Williams & Wilkins, 1976.
10. Mason ML, Allen HS: The rate of healing of tendons: an experimental study of tensile strength. *Ann Surg* 113:424–459, 1941.
11. Nordin M, Frankel VH: Biomechanics of whole bones and bone tissue. In Frankel VH, Nordin M: *Basic Biomechanics of the Skeletal System*. Philadelphia, Lea & Febiger, 1980.
12. Noyes FR, Torvik PJ, Hyde WB, et al: Biomechanics of ligament failure. II. An analysis of immobilization, exercise, and reconditioning effects in primates. *J Bone Joint Surg [Am]* 56:1406–1418, 1974.
13. Potts RO, Chrisman DA, Buras EM: The dynamic mechanical properties of human skin in vivo. *J Biomech* 16:365–372, 1983.
14. Redford RL, Licht S: Materials for orthotics. In Licht S (ed): *Orthotics Etcetera*. New Haven, CT, E. Licht, 1980.
15. Salter RB, Bell RS: The effect of continuous passive motion on the healing of partial thickness lacerations of the patellar tendon of the rabbit. *Proceedings of the 27th Annual Orthopedic Research Society*. Chicago, Dependable Publishing Co., 1981, p 82.
16. Soderberg GL: Muscle mechanics: their clinical relevance. *Phys Ther* 63:216–220, 1983.
17. Steiner M: Biomechanics of tendon healing. *J Biomech* 15:951–958, 1982.
18. Tabary JC, Tabary C, Tardieu C, et al: Physiological and structural changes in the cat's soleus muscle due to immobilization at different lengths by plaster casts. *J Physiol (London)* 224:231–244, 1972.
19. Tabary JC, Tardieu C, Tardieu G, et al: Experimental rapid sarcomere loss with concomitant hypoextensibility. *Muscle Nerve* 4:198–203, 1981.

20. Tipton CM, James SL, Mergner W, et al: Influence of exercise on strength of medial collateral knee ligaments of dogs. *Am J Phys* 218:894–902, 1970.
21. Uezaki N, Kobayashi A, Matsushige K: The viscoelastic properties of the human semilunar cartilage. *J Biomech* 12:65–74, 1979.
22. Warwick R, Williams PL (eds): *Gray's Anatomy, ed 36.* Philadelphia, WB Saunders, 1980.
23. White AA, Panjabi MM: *Clinical Biomechanics of the Spine.* Philadelphia, JB Lippincott, 1978.
24. Yamada H: Mechanical properties of locomotor organs and tissues. In Evans FG (ed): *Strength of Biological Materials.* Baltimore, Williams & Wilkins, 1970.

5

Analysis of Normal and Pathological Motion

Kinesiologic evaluation requires skills fundamental to the collection of kinematic and kinetic information that pertains to human motion. These skills are important in initial and serial patient evaluations, whether a fundamental task of raising the arm overhead or a more complicated function such as gait is being attempted. In addition, clinicians will constantly be exposed to literature that uses motion analysis techniques. Reliable measurements, the ability to accurately record motion, are important both within and between day and across different persons making the measurements. It is essentially a precursor to validity, in other words, a necessary but not sufficient condition for validity. Validity simply means that the tool, system, or device measures what it purports to measure. Another concern in analyzing motion is objectivity. In all cases, the quantifiable measure should not suffer from prejudice. This chapter will focus on available methods used to gather objective and reliable information as related to normal and pathological motion. Emphasis will be placed on improving the ability to interpret literature and apply the information to pathological motion.

COORDINATE SYSTEMS
Clinical

Fundamental to motion analysis is the method adopted. In all circumstances the technique should be designed and tested for the purpose of adequately describing the position that the human body and individual body segments can assume. Although many methods purport to fulfill this criterion, measurement error can significantly distort the data of interest. Of import to any of the methods, either clinical or laboratory, is the adoption of some coordinate system.

As previously indicated, motion is usually described according to three planes. However, certain motions occurring within the joints, such as rolling and gliding, are not included in the triplanar analyses. Consider an example at the glenohumeral joint. First raise the arm into forward flexion of 90°. Then, direct the arm laterally for 90° before lowering the arm to the starting position at the side of the body. If conscious effort is taken to not rotate the forearm during this series of motions the hand is noticed to be in a position 90° rotated from the original position. Known as Codman's paradox the rotation is due to the geometry and the interaction of the male and female surfaces of the respective humeral head and glenoid.

Note that the clinical system would have described this sequence as motion in the three cardinal planes, ignoring the rotation that has certainly occurred. To overcome this difficulty a number of methods have been proposed, but all have suffered a lack of support, and therefore their adoption is seemingly prohibited. An example of this can be seen in the system developed by Roebuck (30). The system developed is applicable for description of total body or link motion. Included in Roebuck's method is a triplanar angular coordinate system and a notation system that completely and adequately describes motion. However, the method has not been adopted by either the clinical or research community and subsequently is nonexistent. Albert's perimeter, detailed in Steindler, is another example of a little used motion analysis system (36).

Despite the advances in technology the clinical methods and terminology used for describing and quantifying motion will not likely be replaced. Although suffering from weaknesses in reliability and objectivity the clinically applicable techniques are the most widely used. As indicated, one of the most acute limitations of the clinical system is the inability to adequately describe certain movements, therefore limiting validity. Yet, ease of application and understanding, coupled with widespread and longstanding use, indicate that clinical techniques will necessarily thrive. Perhaps as a more thorough understanding of athrokinematics becomes available the intrinsic joint movements will be able to be incorporated into the methods currently used.

Reference Frames

Spatial reference frames may be of relative or absolute form. The former method requires the anatomical coordinates to be reported relative to a fixed anatomical landmark. Thus, this method is used to describe the position of one limb relative to the other. Using the absolute system means that coordinates are located in relation to an external reference frame located in space. In this case motion is described in relation to the ground or the direction of gravity. The study of gait frequently uses this method. Use of either system is dependent on the means of data collection; either system will provide sufficient information for the determination of the kinematic data. However, note should be made that an absolute method is seldom used in the clinical setting (see Appendix B).

Cartesian

Another method frequently used for motion analysis is the cartesian coordinate system. Using this method the therapist has a choice of use of one, two, or three dimensions, depending on the type of movement being studied. Polar coordinate technique limits the analysis to one or two planes, the latter allowing the determination of three-dimensional motion. Most studies analyzing complex motions will utilize the cartesian system because virtually any movement characteristic can be derived.

KINEMATICS

Recall that kinematics is the description of motion regardless of the forces causing the movement. Inherent to this description are time and displacement parameters. In the clinic, temporal events may be estimated from the second hand on one's watch. In the laboratory, a large number of decimal places may be required to provide adequate resolution. Similar statements may be made about angular or linear displacement data. In some cases millimeters of displacement cannot satisfy the rigors necessary to comply with laboratory accuracy. Yet, in docking great ocean liners meters of displacement are satisfactory to accomplish the task at hand. Instruments are available to quantify and highly resolve these parameters if the purpose of the technique can be justified in terms of the expense and sophistication involved.

There are a wide range and types of techniques available for purposes of collecting kinematic information, but the primary determining factor usually relates to the purpose for the data gathering. Laboratory systems are frequently dependent upon computer control and/or interpretation of the data derived. And, although simple systems are available for use in the clinical settting, their use is limited by interest, expense, time, or other factors.

Kinematic data collection systems can be conveniently considered to fall into two main categories, direct and indirect. The direct form includes goniometers, accelerometers, and polgons. The indirect, or imaging methods include cinematographical forms, videotape, and optoelectronics. Each will be discussed in terms of technique and advantages and disadvantages. Examples of output form and how each can be interpreted will also be included.

Direct

The direct recording techniques include goniometers, accelerometers, and polgons. Use of clinical goniometers have been in existence and widely used for the assessment of joint motion for decades. Available in multiple sizes and shapes for the measurement of any joint they have proved to be reliable when used under controlled circumstances (7). Although suffering from various sources of error, such as interrater reliability and landmark locations, their utility will continue in the clinical setting.

Electrogoniometry

More complex forms of collecting angular displacement data have been in use for a number of years (22). In practice, the electrogoniometer is an electrical potentiometer attached to a mechanical arrangement (or exoskeleton) (Fig. 5.1). In turn, attachment is made to body segments so that displacement changes the voltage through the potentiometer. As an inexpensive means of collecting data this technique also provides an output signal in the form of relative angles. There are, however, some difficulties in fitting and accommodating the mechanical systems to wide ranges of body types. Accuracy, however, given an adequately designed system, is regarded to be good (31). Patient encumbrance may also become significant if multiple joints or multiple axis goniometers are used. An example of a multiaxis goniometer has been provided by Johnston and Smidt (19). They were able to develop a triaxial goniometer for the hip and knee and demonstrate the utility of the device when studying patterns of hip motion in patients with hip pathology (Figs. 5.2 and 5.3).

More recently Morrey et al have used a triaxial goniometer in studying elbow motion during a variety of functional activities (24). Chao has thoroughly discussed the triaxial goniometer, pointing out that although the spatial goniometer is capable of measuring both rotary and translatory motion in joints, the current system does not provide a direct joint motion measurement. He further states that the three axis Eulerian angle system is more convenient because there is a close match with the neutral position as defined clinically (9).

Electrogoniometers have also been used to produce angle-angle plots that

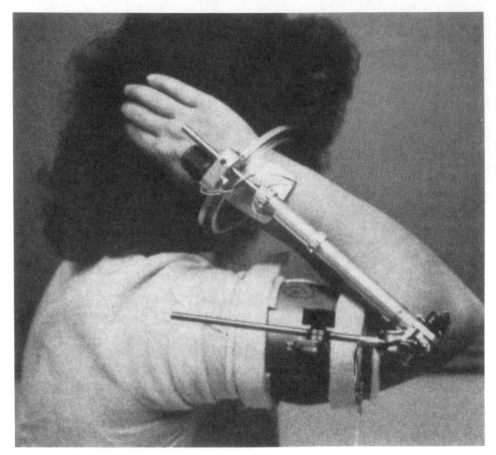

Figure 5.1.   A triaxial goniometer applied to the right elbow. (From Morrey BF, Askew LJ, An KN, et al: A biomechanical study of normal functional elbow motion. *J Bone Joint Surg* [*Am*] 63:872, 1981.)

yield useful information about the interaction of two joints (Fig. 5.4) (14). These plots, shown to be useful in providing clinically relevant data, are usually derived with the assistance of digital computers. One further interesting application of a series of planar goniometers has been suggested by Bajd et al. Their system proposes use of simple trigonometric calculations for measuring step length. The average error of 3% makes the method attractive, in spite of the need for a minicomputer (4).

Accelerometry

The use of accelerometers is another direct technique used in motion studies. These devices are relatively simple electrical circuits that measure accelerations of the segment or segments to which it is attached. Morris, in a 1973 paper, describes how the technique is used and how it may be extended to other body segments. Included is an appendix that describes how the signals from six accelerometers can be used to completely define the movement of a body in space (25).

Smidt et al had earlier demonstrated the utility of such a technique in

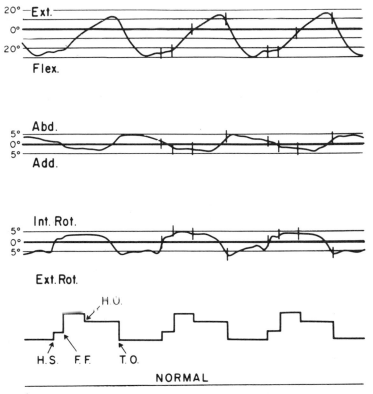

Figure 5.2. Electrogoniometric pattern for hip motion in a normal subject. Degrees of motion as shown on the scales. For the foot switch pattern shown at the bottom *H.S.* indicates heel strike, *F.F.* is flatfoot, *H.O.* is heel off, and *T.O.* is toe off. (From Johnston RC, Smidt GL: Measurement of hip joint motion during walking. *J Bone Joint Surg [Am]* 51:1087, 1969.)

discriminating among normal subjects, those using assistive devices, and those suffering from pathology. Figure 5.5 shows the accelerographic patterns for fore-aft and vertical directions for a normal and a postoperative hip surgery patient who walked with a crutch (32). Even though triaxial accelerometers are available, problems still arise because of difficulties associated with attaching the device to the body. Encumbrance also becomes a problem if a large number is used. Offsetting the disadvantage that the acceleration is relative to the position on the limb segment is the advantage that output is readily available for direct recording or additional processing. In practice accelerometers are little used. Most commonly high accuracy displacement data are desired so that acceleration and velocity can be derived. However, utilization of the acceleration data directly into the $F = M \times A$ equation is a desirable feature of this method.

Polgons

Another direct technique has used polgons (polarized light goniometers). Output data form is similar to the electrogoniometer. Although the method and application has been detailed, the technique is not widely used clinically or seen in the literature (23).

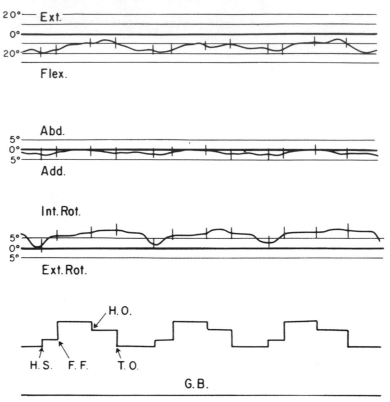

Figure 5.3. Similar recording except for a patient with degenerative arthritis of the hip and accompanying pain. Compared to Figure 5.2 note the marked limitation of motion. (From Johnston RC, Smidt GL: Measurement of hip joint motion during walking. *J Bone Joint Surg [Am]* 51:1090, 1969.)

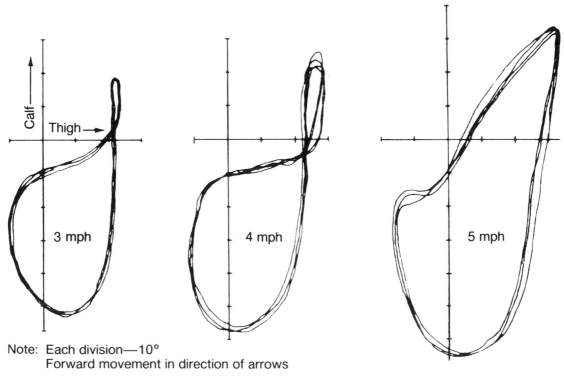

Note: Each division—10°
Forward movement in direction of arrows

Figure 5.4. Graphs of lower leg versus upper leg angle. This subject completed a number of walking cycles, shown by the multiple lines, at velocities indicated in each plot. (From Grieve DW, Miller DI, Mitchelson D, et al: *Techniques for the Analysis of Human Movement*. Princeton, NJ, Princeton Book Company, 1976, p 59.)

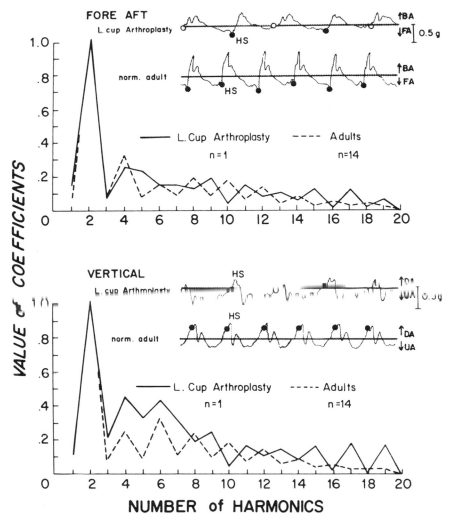

Figure 5.5. Acceleration patterns, in two directions, and corresponding harmonic analysis spectra for normal adults and a subject with arthroplastic surgery of the hip. Accelerations indicated as backwards (*BA*), forwards (*FA*), downwards (*DA*), and upwards (*UA*). *Solid circle* is heel strike of normal side and *open circle* is heel strike of affected side. (From Smidt GL, Arora JS, Johnston RC: Accelerographic analysis of several types of walking. *Am J Phys Med* 50:297, 1971. © 1971, Williams & Wilkins, Baltimore.)

Indirect

The indirect or imaging methods, the most widely used, include cinemato-graphical forms, videotape, and optoelectrics. By far the most common is the use of photography, both low and high speed. Since the early moving picture days of Muybridge, use of cinematography has expanded to great proportions (26). His works of animal and human motion are considered to be classics, particularly when considering the state of the art in the 1800s.

More recently, a strong case has been made for the use of video recording systems. Other more sophisticated devices have also been developed that promise to simplify (and increase the cost of) the technique of collecting highly accurate kinematic data. Generally these photographic techniques are moderate in cost and provide minimal encumbrance on patients and subjects. Data may also be permanently stored for later use. However, reduction time for photographic methods can be increased unless automated systems are used.

Photography

Of the cinematographical forms, 16-mm cameras are most frequently chosen because of the cost and the adequacy of the image size. A wide variety of cameras are available for filming in either the clinical or laboratory setting. Cameras with higher frame rates are necessary for the higher velocity movements used in athletic events, but for clinical and most other purposes frame rates of greater than 64 frames/sec are seldom required.

Procedures for reducing data to displacements of joints vary. Location of colored dots at joint centers has been used so that filming from the lateral view can produce sagittal plane motion data that will yield measurements from the screen on which the film is projected. The reader is referred to the texts of either Hay or Miller and Nelson for a detailed description of the technique (16, 21). Location of cameras at multiple angles provides the capability for determination of three-dimensional displacement but simultaneously requires significant methodological attention both in the collection and reduction of the data. The presentation of Sutherland and Hagy provides the details of this approach (37). In any case, displacement data can then be used in the velocity and acceleration calculations so that kinetics can be studied.

Other innovative uses of photography have been developed and utilized. The Crowninshield et al work detailed in 1978 a method using two 35-mm cameras and a system of flashing, light-emitting diodes. They were able to effectively derive displacement data that could be used, along with kinetic data in determining hip joint forces (11). Soderberg and Gabel had previously described the use of a similar system in describing sagittal plane gait kinematics for both normal and pathological subjects (35). This particular methodology essentially produces multiframe images on a single frame of film. Because the lights flash at a designated frequency temporal factors are easily determined. As explained in the above references both linear and angular displacements are readily determinable. Aptekar et al have used a similar system for both normal and cerebral palsied children, but their data are graphic and not readily quantifiable (2, 3).

The strobe light has also been used in displacement determinations. A representative example is the work of Richards and Knutsson (20, 29). In this technique reflective targets were attached to the head or neck and the extremity segments while the subject walked in a strobe-illuminated room in front of an open shutter camera. Figure 5.6 contains the recording of the pattern produced in a normal walking subject. Measurements of angular displacement can be made directly from the film and converted to acceleration and velocity. This system is relatively attractive economically but suffers from limitations associated with planar movements and the requirements for rather subdued lighting.

Another simple photographic technique is the sequence camera. This commercially available low cost camera takes a series of eight photographs in a temporal sequence that can be preset, depending on the velocity of the movement being photographed. The camera has multiple uses and provides reasonable quality photographs that may be used for descriptive purposes (Fig. 5.7) (17).

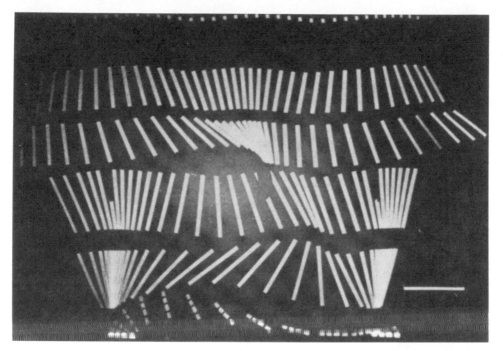

Figure 5.6. Examples of a recording of sagittal plane motion using strobographic technique. Strobe frequency was 20 Hz. The horizontal bar represents 30 cm. (From Richards C, Knutsson E: Evaluation of abnormal gait patterns by intermittent-light photography and electromyography. *Scand J Rehabil Med*, Suppl 3:63, 1974.)

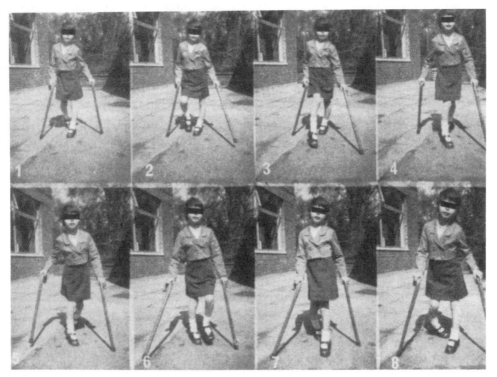

Figure 5.7. Sequential frontal view of a subject walking. A range of time intervals between photos is available so that the time between photos can be controlled. Note the distortion, i.e., the difference in subject size, as the subject approaches the camera. (From Holt KS, Jones RB, Wilson R: Gait analysis by means of a multiple sequential exposure camera. *Dev Med Child Neurol* 16:742, 1974.)

Video Recorders

Detailed descriptions for use of video recorders have been provided in the literature (13, 28, 39). Winter et al have been strong advocates of this form of kinematic analysis, citing a lack of patient encumbrance and the ability to collect multiple trials and analyze immediately as the primary advantages of this method. Although perhaps limited by the respective inherent North American and European 60 and 50 display fields/sec, the constraint is not great unless high velocity movements are under consideration. Technical advances are currently underway that will probably negate the slow rate limit.

Optoelectrics

A sophisticated system of optoelectric techniques has also been developed for purposes of gathering kinematic information. Using infrared diodes the emissions of light are identified by a special camera and focused on a special semiconductor diode surface. The method allows light source identification and location on two coordinates. Multiple light data can be processed simultaneously. With knowledge of the temporal history of the light pattern, displacement data can be generated by companion electronics. Analysis of three-dimensional motion is possible, but at this point use of this system is generally limited to the laboratory setting (38).

Event Markers

Required for analyses of human motion are event markers and or other indicators of temporal events. Many of the kinematic systems, such as the diode and certain cine procedures, have the timing events included on the film. Others need to incorporate a timer into the field of view. Footswitches and other event markers, such as voice or manual controls, are frequently helpful in determining events. Special care must be taken to synchronize the processes if multiple techniques are used simultaneously.

Each of the systems described in this section has been shown to have adequate reliability for the gathering of kinematic data. Development of the therapist's capability to analyze human motion will be primarily dependent on the purpose of the data gathered. Clinicians would be most interested in the inexpensive methods that provided immediate replay and efficient quantification. Minimal expenditures would be in the hundreds of dollars, depending on whether a videotape system existed in the health care facility in which most professionals are based. Laboratory-proven methods require substantial investments, varying from a few to thousands of dollars.

KINETICS

To completely analyze motion, that is, arrive at solutions for joint forces, muscle forces, and moments, the derivation of kinetic information is necessary. To accomplish this purpose a host of transducers designed to measure force is available. Mechanical and electrical strain guages are all widely utilized in converting forces to meaningful quantities. Essentially, all work on the principle that strain produces known deformation in materials that can then be converted to the measure of interest. In applications of kinesiologic interest force is of most interest. There are, however, many other types of transducers available for the measurement of forces derived from blood, air, and fluid flow.

Among the most frequently used devices are cable tensiometers and dynamometers. Handgrip dynamometers are frequently used to evaluate grip strength.

Other hand-held dynamometers are often used in the clinic. The device usually used measures the magnitude of compression resulting from an isometric muscle contraction (Fig. 5.8). Output of these devices, in kilogram force (kgf) or pound force (lbf), is useful because the measure can be used in the calculation of the moment being created about the joint axis. A simple measurement of the distance to the joint axis from the perpendicular application of the restraining cable or dynamometer guarantees a measurement unit, torque, that can be utilized in other comparisons. (See Chapter 2 for further details.)

An example of a force curve generated during isometric knee extension is shown in Figure 5.9. Transducers have also been developed for direct clinical application. One example is a plate that can be inserted into a shoe. By means of electronic circuitry the amount of pressure required to produce an output voltage can be varied by the clinician. The output can in turn be monitored such that audio tones can be generated, indicating the amount of pressure being exerted. A very practical application occurs when the degree of weight bearing needs to be controlled during gait. By adequately calibrating the transducer the clinician can set the level of pressure required for feedback to the patient (10).

The other most commonly used transducer for the collection of kinetic information is the force plate. Formerly using a system of electromechanical guages, plates have now been designed that use piezoresistive or piezoelectric types of transducers so that response time of the plate has been remarkably improved. Output includes the force in the vertical, medial-lateral, and fore-aft directions. Moments about the three principal axes can also be determined, as can the center of pressure. Figure 5.10 shows the three-dimensional forces from a plate for the stance phase of one extremity during gait. Shown in Figure 5.11 are the moment data generated. These ground reaction forces are then used, in

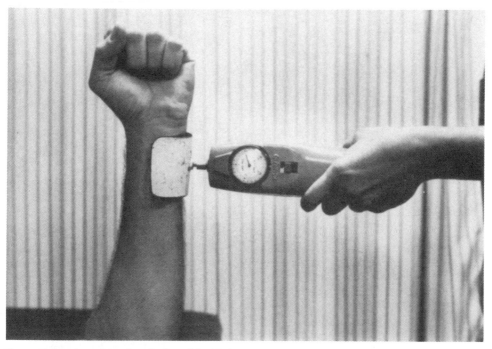

Figure 5.8.   An example of a hand-held dynamometer. In this case the isometric strength of the extensors of the elbow is being tested.

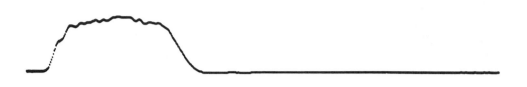

Figure 5.9. Isometric force-time curve for knee extension. This information was obtained by an on-line computer. Peak force was multiplied by distance to obtain torque for this contraction that was held about 3 sec.

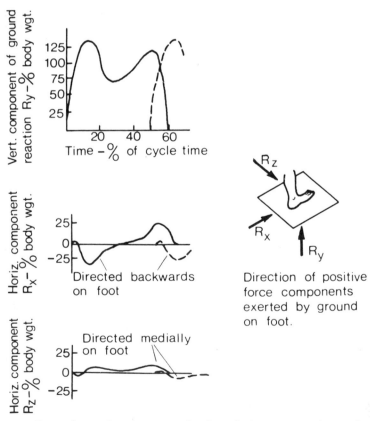

Figure 5.10. Ground reaction forces at the foot during stance phase of walking for a normal subject. (From Grieve DW, Miller DI, Mitchelson D, et al: *Techniques for the Analysis of Human Movement.* Princeton, NJ, Princeton Book Company, 1976, p 168.)

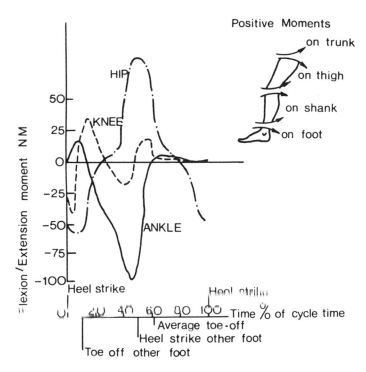

Figure 5.11. Sagittal plane moments generated during the stance phase of walking for a normal individual. (From Grieve DW, Miller DI, Mitchelson D, et al: *Techniques for the Analysis of Human Movement*. Princeton, NJ, Princeton Book Company, 1976, p 169).

concert with body segment parameter information and kinematic data in calculation of the joint forces acting at the various joints of the lower extremity (14).

That force patterns are perturbed in pathological gait has been well established. Stauffer et al have demonstrated the changes in patients with hip disease (Fig. 5.12) (33). Others have used the force plate to collect comprehensive data sets for purposes of determining forces on the femoral head during activities of daily living (8). Cook and Cozzens developed a real-time ground reaction force-line visualization technique that uses an optical beamsplitter for superimposition of a scaled vector image as an overlay on the patient image. The displayed force vector is directly proportional to the force represented, as is the orientation of the force. A sample frame is shown in Figure 5.13 (10). Other uses include similar determinations for the knee and ankle as well as for studies involving energetics. More details on the work as applied to each joint will be provided in the chapters on the lower extremity.

Other forms of electromechanical dynamometers are available for clinical use. One isokinetic dynamometer provides output in torque (foot pounds). Because of the wide range of selectable speeds this device has applicability to many evaluation and reassessment procedures commonly employed. Calibrated graphs assist with record interpretation so that data may be interpreted immediately. Because paper readouts, at known speed, are available from the constant velocity exercise, determination of the joint kinematics is easily obtained. Samples of torque curves generated at two different velocities are presented in Figure 5.14.

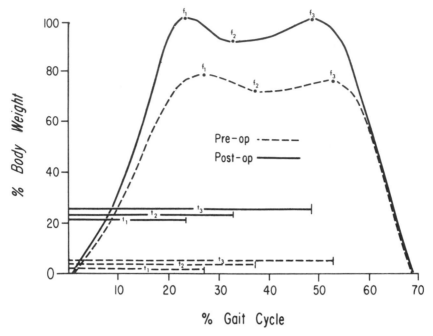

Figure 5.12. Vertical component of the floor reaction force in the hip. The *f* locates important force points, while the *t* demonstrates how the temporal aspects vary between the normal subject and the patient with hip disease. (From Stauffer RN, Smidt GL, Wadsworth JB: Clinical and biomechanical analysis of gait following Charnley total hip replacement. *Clin Orthop* 99:73, 1974.)

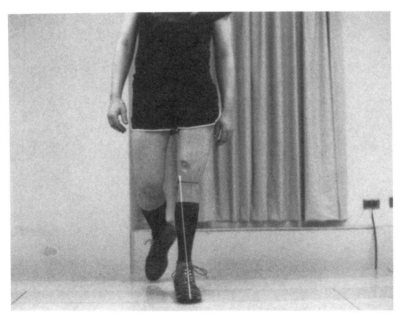

Figure 5.13. Force-line visualization technique for the sagittal plane for a normal subject. Note that the direction and magnitude of the force are both represented. (Courtesy of T. M. Cook, The University of Iowa, Iowa City, IA.)

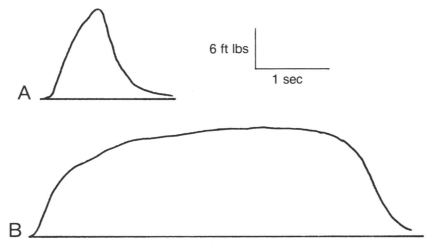

Figure 5.14. (A) Torque curve generated by knee extension at 150°/s. (B) Same conditions as in A except completed at 30°/sec. Note that the peak torque is higher at the slower velocity, consistent with explanations of Chapter 2.

THEORETICAL AND MATHEMATICAL ANALYSES

The comprehensive study of human motion, particularly dynamic activities, requires the collection and analysis of complete sets of kinematic and kinetic data. For clinical analysis therapists often use manual techniques or functional activities to determine the torque-generating capabilities of their patients. The result of these tests requires that joint forces be generated in and distributed throughout the body. Because clinical methods are limited in their ability to make determinations of generation of the joint forces and how they are distributed, comprehensive data sets can be generated and subjected to rigorous analysis. To complete such procedures both theoretical and mathematical analyses are used.

More and more studies that have used these methods are becoming available, and virtually every joint in the body has been subjected to these analytic techniques. In general, their purposes are to determine the resultant forces and torques at the joint or joints under study. The problem is complex because the sets of equations generated to perform the solution are indeterminant, i.e., they cannot be solved because the number of unknowns exceeds the number of equations.

Andrews points out that there are two basic approaches to solving the equations to determine the force and torque resultants at each joint during a given time interval. The first method of solution, using reduction, makes the equations determinant and places crude upper bound estimates for muscle forces (1). These resultants are then, in effect, distributed to bones, ligaments, and muscles based on certain "limits" set by known physiological information or based on assumptions. For example, kinematic data provide information about muscle length. Subsequently, estimates of available tension can be made. Likewise, knowledge of joint configuration provides data on ligament length that can be related to data from studies of ligament tensile strength. The other process, optimization, assumes that the body controls muscle tension in order to optimize some mechanical or biochemical process. An "objective" function, usually mathematical, is maximized or minimized in this solution process. That is, this technique attempts to model muscle tension by means of a mathematical process. In this latter case validations are frequently done with the electromyographic data derived concurrently with the kinematic and kinetic data. Recent studies that use these techniques have been described by Brand et al, Hardt, and by Patriarco et al (8, 15, 27).

ELECTROMYOGRAPHY

Since Galvani discovered in the 18th century that electrical potentials were derived from muscle, the role of electromyography (EMG) in the study of function has expanded significantly. Inman et al (1944) completed the first major comprehensive EMG study by evaluating function of the shoulder (18). Since that time there has been an exponential growth of EMG in the study of human motion. Knowledge of the rudiments of EMG and how it might be interpreted are fundamental to adequate understanding of kinesiology and pathokinesiology. Further, EMG is commonly used in analyzing motion or making inferences about the forces responsible for the motion.

Scope of Use

The uses of EMG may be placed into several broad categories. In pathologies EMG is useful in delineating the nature, scope, and prognosis of diseases involving the neuromuscular system. In a different application, pre- and post-surgical evaluations are being accomplished at several institutions throughout the world. The primary intent of using EMG in this situation is to evaluate whether or not muscles are functioning phasically during periods of time that will facilitate effective surgical results. These will be discussed more specifically in the area of the lower extremity and gait. Another area more recently developed in which EMG is becoming heavily used is myoelectrics. In this situation the action potentials derived from muscle are electronically modified in order to control some other body part, segment, prosthesis, or orthosis that has been applied to the patient. Further, great strides have been made in the utilization of EMG as a biofeedback device. Utilization has included headache control, reeducation following muscle transfers, and in rehabilitation techniques as required for the treatment of stroke. Finally, EMG has been used to study kinesiologic function of muscle. A recent review has been provided by Soderberg and Cook (34). Use of the electromyogram has clarified pure functions of muscles and furthered the understanding of the relationship between concentric and eccentric contractions. EMG is of interest to the biomechanician in order to attempt to establish a relationship between EMG and tension level.

Physiological Basis

The electromyograph records the electrical activity of a muscle, the fundamental contractile unit of which is the motor unit. By definition a motor unit is one motor neuron, its axon, and all the muscle fibers innervated by that neuron. The discharge of the motor neuron causes subsequent depolarization of the muscle fibers, and the electrical activity can be evaluated both visually and by means of the sound produced. How the potential is derived from the fibers within each unit is shown in Figure 5.15. Each motor unit has a specfic size, shape, and sound. The voltage of each unit will range from 300 μV to 5 mV. Variation is due to age and the muscle studied. The duration of the motor unit

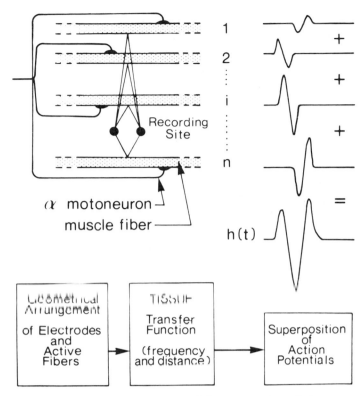

Figure 5.15. Diagrammatic representation of the generation of the motor unit action potential. Note that each fiber generates a potential that is summated to produce h(t). The summation of the temporal and voltage characteristics are responsible for the features that produce the unique shape of each motor unit. (From Basmajian JV: *Muscles Alive: Their Function Revealed by Electromyography*, p 55. © 1979, Williams & Wilkins, Baltimore.)

action potential ranges from 3 to 16 msec, with a mean time of 9 msec. Based on the literature, motor units are distributed over 12 to 26% of the cross section of a muscle, with a mean distribution of 17%. Further, Feinstein et al reported a different number of muscle fibers per motor unit depending upon the muscle (12):

Laryngeal, 2 to 3 fibers per motor unit
Lateral rectus of eye, 9
Platysma, 25
First lumbrical, 108
First dorsal interosseous, 340
Anterior tibialis, 562
Masseter, 640
Lateral head of gastrocnemius, >1000

Recording Methods

In order to record the small myoelectric potentials it is necessary to have an amplifier and a display device. An oscilloscope or light beam recorder is suggested. To record the myopotentials, surface electrodes are most frequently used. The size, shape, and configuration of the attachment of the surface electrodes are at the discretion of the user. These electrodes have advantages, i.e., they can be easily applied, the technique is standardized and is relatively pain-free. Disadvantages of using surface recording electrodes are the area recorded from is relatively large and recordings only represent superficial muscle activity.

As a result of these limitations, some have used needle or implanted fine wire electrodes. For kinesiological study needle electrodes are seldom used. Rather, implanted fine wires are the standard. They are inserted into a muscle with a needle. Then the needle is withdrawn, the wires remaining in the muscle to record the action potentials. One advantage is considered, by some, to be ease of this technique. Disadvantages include the puncture of skin required by the needle. In addition, there is a tendency for the wires to migrate within the muscle. The degree of migration is dependent upon the type of contraction and the strength of the contraction.

The first and most important feature of EMG display is to evaluate the raw signal. A sample is shown in Figure 5.16. After evaluation for quality, the signal may be electrically managed in many fashions. Some devices will produce a linear envelope after the raw EMG has been full wave rectified. Another name typically applied to these linear envelopes is averaged. In addition there are others who prefer to integrate the signal. According to Figure 5.17 several modes of integration are available. Other forms of analysis available include envelopes and "off-on" techniques. No matter which of these signal modifications is used, the user or interpreter must be cognizant of the potential for artifacts induced into the recording by such things as 60-cycle current, mechanical movement of lead wires, and other extraneous signals. Hence, the need to first evaluate the raw EMG signal.

Relationships to Muscular Tension

EMG is most frequently used to evaluate the amount of muscle activity occurring in any given muscle. Many have attempted to relate EMG activity to muscle tension. There is general acceptance that as muscle length becomes shorter, the electromyographic output increases. Although some of this may be due to increasing the number of fibers below the recording electrodes, the relationship generally holds. Figure 5.18 shows the EMG derived from three lengths of muscle. Note the changes as the length has been altered.

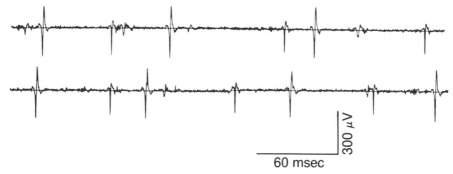

Figure 5.16. A continuous record of about 600 msec showing several motor units firing during a 5-sec maximum voluntary isometric contraction. (From Nelson RM, Soderberg GL: Laser etched bifilar fine wire electrode for skeletal muscle motor unit recording. *Electroencephalogr Clin Neurophysiol* 55:239, 1983.)

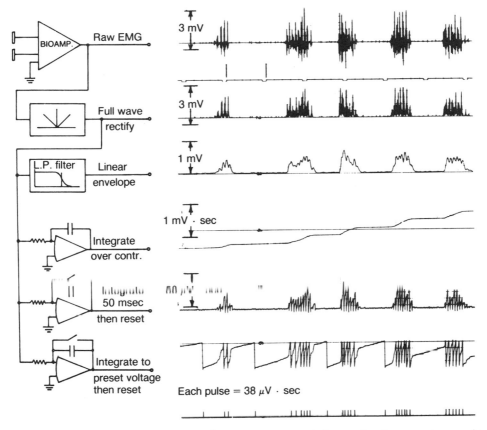

Figure 5.17. Depiction of the raw electromyogram and the mode of processing used to provide the output shown. The raw EMG used in the top line was used for all processing represented in the figure. (From Winter DA: *Biomechanics of Human Movement*, p 140. Copyright © 1979. Reprinted by permission of John Wiley & Sons, Inc.)

Because, as already introduced, the total tension increases at longer muscle lengths, it is speculated that the contractile component (and subsequent EMG) is effectively reduced in order that damage due to the generation of too much tension can potentially be avoided.

Most evaluation of the muscle tension-EMG relationship has occurred during isometric contractions. Considerable evidence supports a linear relationship between electromyography and isometric contraction. Conversely, some have shown a nonlinear relationship, depending upon the circumstances attendant to the study of isometric contractions. Representative examples, as produced in Winter, are shown in Figure 5.19 (38).

The general rule for concentric and eccentric contractions is that there will be less EMG activity in eccentric contractions. When making these comparisons it is essential to establish similar mechanical conditions. A primary reason that activity from eccentric contractions is less is that the muscle can effectively use the elastic elements in order to generate tension. Therefore, for the eccentric contraction to have the same amount of tension as concentric contractions, there needs to be less activity in the contractile component. Subsequently, the EMG activity of eccentric contractions is generally less. Others have also evaluated

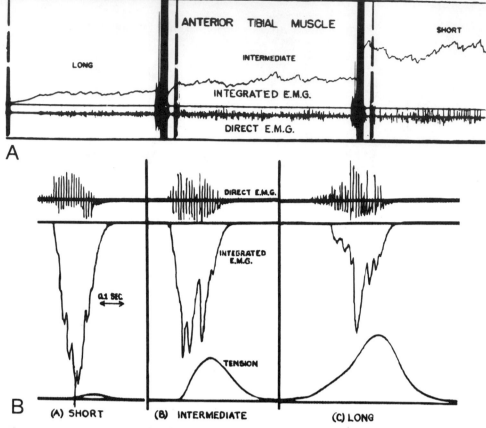

Figure 5.18. (*A*) Maximal voluntary isometric contractions for normal subject. As the muscle is tested at shorter lengths note that the EMG is dramatically increased. Note that the integrated EMG is really a linear envelope (Fig. 5.17). (*B*) The same relationship holds for the triceps muscle of the cineplastic amputee. Isometric tension is also shown. (From Inman VT, Ralston HJ, Saunders JB, et al: Relation of human electromyogram to muscular tension. *Electroencephalogr Clin Neurophysiol* 4:193, 1952.)

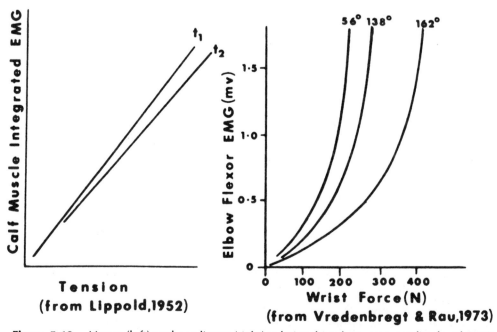

Figure 5.19. Linear (left) and nonlinear (right) relationships between amplitude of EMG and muscle tension under conditions of isometric contraction. (From Winter DA: *Biomechanics of Human Movement*, p 143. Copyright © 1979. Reprinted by permission of John Wiley & Sons, Inc.)

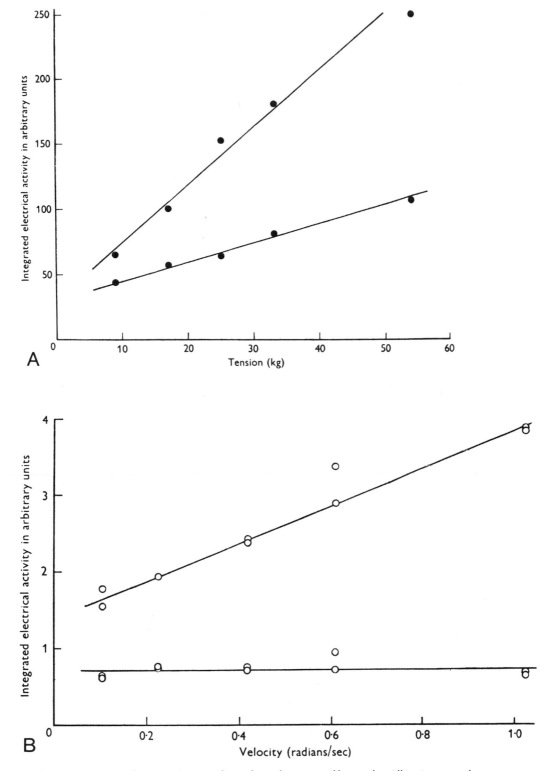

Figure 5.20. Surface EMG recordings from human calf muscle. All points are the mean of ten trials for one subject. (*A*) Integrated EMG is plotted versus tension. Concentric contraction (steeper slope) and eccentric contraction were performed at constant velocity. (*B*) Integrated EMG plotted versus shortening (above) and lengthening at the same tension. (From Bigland B, Lippold OCJ: The relation between force, velocity and integrated electrical activity in human muscles. *J Physiol* 123:218, 219, 1954.)

the relationship under conditions of constant velocity and constant tension. Figure 5.20 demonstrates those conditions (6).

Anyone interpreting EMG records or data included in either the clinic or laboratory must exercise discretion in analyses of the information. Because recordings from different muscles are influenced by the amount of subcutaneous tissue, electrode configuration, orientation of muscle fibers, and other factors, there are extreme limitations imposed on across channel comparisons. Comparisons between subjects are also dangerous, for similar reasons, unless care is taken in the technique and study methodology. A common method to allow for comparisons is the normalization process whereby the subject performs a maximum voluntary contraction while EMG is recorded. Then, data collected during subsequent trials can be related to this quantity (for example in terms of percent of activity evoked during the maximum contraction). Quantified data can then be compared across subject and muscle.

SUMMARY

In summary, all techniques of motion analysis can play a valuable role in the therapist's understanding of the normal and pathological function. Therapists should critically evaluate the techniques that appear in the literature and be able to utilize these techniques when applicable in their own clinical setting. EMG assists in helping to establish the scientific basis for both assessment procedures and treatment techniques commonly used in practice.

References

1. Andrews JG: On the relationship between resultant joint torques and muscular activity. *Med Sci Sports Exerc* 14:361–367, 1982.
2. Aptekar RG, Ford F, Bleck EE: Light patterns as a means of assessing and recording gait. I. Methods and results in normal children. *Dev Med Child Neurol* 18:31–36, 1976.
3. Aptekar RG, Ford F, Bleck EE: Light patterns as a means of assessing and recording gait. II. Results in children with cerebral palsy. *Dev Med Child Neurol* 18:37–40, 1976.
4. Bajd T, Kljajic M, Trnkoczy A, Stanic U: Electrogoniometric measurement of step length. *Scand J Rehabil Med* 6:78–80, 1974.
5. Basmajian JV: *Muscles Alive: Their Function Revealed by Electromyography.* Baltimore, Williams & Wilkins, 1979.
6. Bigland B, Lippold OCJ: The relation between force, velocity and integrated electrical activity in human muscles. *J Physiol* 123:214–224, 1954.
7. Boone DC, Azen SP, Lin C, et al: Reliability of goniometric measurements. *Phys Ther* 58:1355–1360, 1978.
8. Brand RA, Crowninshield RD, Johnston RC, et al: Forces on the femoral head during activities of daily living. *Iowa Orthop J* 2:43–49, 1982.
9. Chao EYS: Justification of triaxial goniometer for the measurement of joint rotation. *J Biomech* 13:989–1006, 1980.
10. Cook TM, Cozzens BA: The effects of heel height and ankle-foot-orthosis configuration on weight-line location: a demonstration of principles. *Orthotics Prosthet* 30:43–46, 1976.
11. Crowninshield RD, Johnston RC, Andrews JG, et al: A biomechanical investigation of the human hip. *J Biomech* 11:75–86, 1978.
12. Feinstein B, Lindegard B, Nyman E, Wohlfart G: Morphological studies of motor units in normal human muscles. *Acta Anat (Basel)* 23:127–142, 1955.
13. Foley CD, Quanbury AO, Steinke T: Kinematics of normal child locomotion—a statistical study based on tv data. *J Biomech* 12:1–6, 1979.
14. Grieve DW: Electromyography. In Grieve DW, Miller DI, Mitchelson D, Paul JP, Smith AJ: *Techniques for the Analysis of Human Movement.* Princeton, NJ, Princeton Book Co, 1976.

15. Hardt DE: Determining muscle forces in the leg during normal human walking—an application and evaluation of optimization methods. *J Biomech Eng* 100:72–78, 1978.
16. Hay JG: *Biomechanics of Sport Techniques.* Englewood Cliffs, NJ, Prentice-Hall, 1978.
17. Holt KS, Jones RB, Wilson R: Gait analysis by means of a multiple sequential exposure camera. *Dev Med Child Neurol* 16:742–745, 1974.
18. Inman VT, Ralston HJ, Saunders JB, et al: Relation of human electromyogram to muscular tension. *EEG Clin Neurophysiol* 4:187–194, 1952.
19. Johnston RC, Smidt GL: Measurement of hip-joint motion during walking. *J Bone Joint Surg [Am]* 51:1083–1094, 1969.
20. Knutsson E, Richards C: Different types of disturbed motor control in gait of hemiparetic patients. *Brain* 102:405–430, 1979.
21. Miller DI, Nelson RC: *Biomechanics of Sport.* Philadelphia, Lea & Febiger, 1973.
22. Milner M, Dall D, Ruff AL, et al: Pre and post operative angle diagrams in cases of total hip reconstruction. *Digest of the 5th Canadian Medical Biological Engineering Conference.* 1974, vol 17, p. 3a, b.
23. Mitchelson DL: An opto-electronic technique for analysis of angular movements. In Cerquiglini S (ed): *Biomechanics III.* Basel, Switzerland, Karger, 1973, pp 181–184.
24. Morrey BF, Askew LJ, An KN, et al: A biomechanical study of normal functional elbow motion. *J Bone Joint Surg [Am]* 63:872–877, 1981.
25. Morris JRW: Accelerometry—a technique for the measurement of human body movements. *J Biomech* 6:729–736, 1973.
26. Muybridge E, in Brown LS (ed): *Animals In Motion.* New York, Dover Publications, 1957.
27. Patriarco AG, Mann RW, Simons SR, et al: An evaluation of the approaches of optimization models in the prediction of muscle forces during human gait. *J Biomech* 14:513–525, 1981.
28. Pedersen E, Klemar B: Recording of physiological measurements based on video technique. *Scand J Rehabil Med* 3(Suppl):45–50, 1974.
29. Richards C, Knutsson E: Evaluation of abnormal gait patterns by intermittent-light photography and electromyography. *Scand J Rehabil Med* 3(Suppl):61–68, 1974.
30. Roebuck JA: Kinesiology in Engineering. Paper presented at the Kinesiology Council, Convention of the American Association for Health, Physical Education and Recreation, March, 1966.
31. Smidt GL: Hip motion and related factors in walking. *J Am Phys Ther Assoc* 51:9–21, 1971.
32. Smidt GL, Arora JS, Johnston RC: Accelerographic analysis of several types of walking. *Am J Phys Med* 50:285–300, 1971.
33. Stauffer RN, Smidt GL, Wadsworth JB: Clinical and biomechanical analysis of gait following Charnley total hip replacement. *Clin Orthop* 99:70–77, 1974.
34. Soderberg GL, Cook TM: Electromyography in biomechanics. *Phys Ther* 64:1813–1820, 1984.
35. Soderberg GL, Gabel R: A light emitting diode system for the analysis of gait: a method and selected clinical examples. *Phys Ther* 58:426–432, 1978.
36. Steindler A: *Kinesiology of the Human Body under Normal and Pathological Conditions.* Springfield, IL, Charles C Thomas, 1935.
37. Sutherland DH, Hagy JL: Measurement of gait movements from motion picture film. *J Bone Joint Surg [Am]* 54:787–797, 1972.
38. Winter DA: *Biomechanics of Human Movement.* New York, Wiley, 1979.
39. Winter DA, Greenlaw RK, Hobson DA: Television-computer analysis of kinematics of human gait. *Comput Biomed Res* 5:498–504, 1972.
40. Wolf SL, Binder-MacLeod SA: Use of the Krusen limb load monitor to quantify temporal and loading measurement of gait. *Phys Ther* 62:976–982, 1982.

6

Shoulder

Both clinicians and investigators have confirmed that shoulder function is a complex phenomena. The ability of man to elevate the hand over the head and assume numerous functional tasks requires great flexibility, while integrity is maintained for the multiple joints operative during normal function. At the most proximal series of joints strength must not be totally sacrificed at the expense of mobility because frequently movements that require a great deal of power are performed. In this chapter the anatomical constraints and functional relationships will be presented. The interaction of four joints as they comprise the shoulder complex will also be considered in view of explaining how effective shoulder function is carried out. Finally, selected pathologies will be discussed in terms of altered kinematics and kinetics.

MUSCULATURE

Musculature can be considered to function in isolated fashion or in collective groups. Matsen classifies the musculature as scapulohumeral and claviculohumeral, scapuloradial, scapuloulnar, thoracohumeral, thoracoscapular, and thoracoclavicular (19). A more functional classification may be to use the terms scapulohumeral, axioscapular, and axiohumeral, since all muscles can be classified in a less cumbersome fashion. No matter the system selected for classification the musculature must be thought of in functional terms.

In terms of function, importance has been attributed to the major muscles of the shoulder complex, the trapezius, serratus anterior, and deltoid (18). Of these, the trapezius has a primary role in support of the upper limb upon the axial skeleton. Bearn has shown the muscle to be electrically quiet during normal postures when no objects are simultaneously held in the hand (1). Although some activity is produced when weight is supported by the arm, most subjects were able to cease activity. The passive mechanisms utilized for support may provide some indication of the postures which lead to difficulties with the vascular and neural tree as each exits the thorax to supply the upper limb. Certainly a primary and necessary function of this muscle is to cause and/or maintain upward rotation of the scapula on the thorax.

The serratus anterior muscle, by virtue of attachment sites, is dedicated to motion of the scapula on the thorax. A primary responsibility is thought to be the motion of protraction, described to be the anterior gliding of the scapula on the wall of the thorax. The result has been the labeling of the muscle as the boxer's muscle. Another important function appears to be the action of the

109

lower portion of the serratus in effectively assisting with upward rotation of the scapula. Together then, with the trapezius upper and lower fibers, effective scapular upward rotation can be achieved as the arm is elevated over the head (17). Loss of these individual or this collective group of muscles will be specifically discussed in the section on pathokinesiology found later in this chapter.

More importantly, the trapezius and serratus anterior muscles act as an effective force couple in the accomplishment of scapular upward rotation. To understand this function, consider, as shown in Figure 6.1, the axis of rotation to be located in the center of the scapula. As the upper and most lateral fibers of the trapezius pull upwards on the distal aspect of the spine of the scapula the inferior fibers of the serratus anterior pull the inferior angle of the scapula in a lateral and anterior direction. Thus, the muscles exert torques resulting from effective utilization of the principle of force couples. Also note that the lower trapezius fibers can act with the serratus anterior, creating another force couple. In relation to this function it is interesting to note that during man's evolution the trapezius has lost, presumably due to lack of use, fibers that run parallel to the spine of the scapula. Further specialization of the serratus anterior is unanticipated, since this muscle has already been separated from the levator scapulae muscle by virtue of loss of the intermediate fibers that formerly connected these two muscles (11). The relationship between these two muscles can be demonstrated by means of study of the innervation of these two muscles. The levator, supplied by cervical roots 3, 4, and part of 5, and the C5, 6, and 7 innervation of the serratus anterior, show that these muscles were once continuous with each other (34). Similarly, the rhomboids, teres major, and latissimus dorsi form couples for purposes of lowering the arm to the side. Such action is produced during specific motions, such as pullups, or during high velocity activities such as wood chopping.

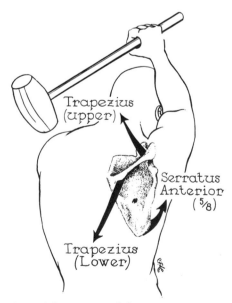

Figure 6.1.   Representation of the action of the serratus anterior and the lower fibers of the trapezius as a force couple. See text for description. (From MacConaill MA, Basmajian JV: *Muscles and Movements: A Basis for Human Kinesiology.* Baltimore, Williams & Wilkins, 1969, p. 189.)

For the pectoralis major muscle selective activity of the sternal and clavicular heads has long been conceded (26). Superficial and deep layers used to exist until differentiation took place. In fact, in most animal forms the pectoralis minor attaches to the humerus instead of to the coracoid process (11). However, in man, the coracohumeral ligament can be considered a vestige of the former humeral attachment (13). Now there is little question that this muscle is important for powerful movements of the arm across the trunk. Similar comments may be made about the latissimus dorsi when referring to glenohumeral extension and internal rotation. Together these two muscles account for considerable internal rotation torques that are little used in everyday function.

The increase in the size of the acromion is perhaps indicative of the increase in the deltoid muscle mass. Inman, in 1944, stated that the deltoid makes up approximately 41% of the mass of the human abductor group (11). Today this value would perhaps be considered very conservative. The deltoid also formerly contained a lower portion now known as the teres minor, offering a useful tool for remembering the similar axillary (C5-6) innervation of these two muscles (34).

The deltoid muscle is of interest because of the relatively large mass and the division of separate fiber groupings into anterior, middle, and posterior. This muscle provides reason to discuss the direction of the muscle's fibers in relation to the axis of rotation for the glenohumeral joint. In Chapter 1 the representation of muscle forces was discussed in relation to their capability to generate tensile loads at some given location with respect to an axis of rotation. The result, depending on the magnitude of the tensile force and the perpendicular distance from which the force is applied, determines the resultant torque. If we consider the anterior deltoid fibers while viewing the body in a frontal plane (Fig. 6.2) the fibers are clearly superior to the axis of rotation. The resulting function for this muscle for this plane is thus abduction. Considering the same muscle from the superior view the muscle essentially passes anterior to the axis of rotation, thereby producing internal rotation. Finally, in the sagittal view, the anterior location leads to the conclusion that flexion torque would result from muscle contraction. Similar diagrammatic representations for the middle deltoid would yield functions of abduction but no internal rotation or flexion, since for the latter two motions the muscle fibers pass through the instant center of rotation of the joint. Whereas available tension and the muscle "moment arm" are factors involved in producing torques (or lack of torques) about joints, a constant and continual realization of the anatomy of the joint will assist in the conceptualization of the possible and real muscular capabilities as each contributes to joint torques. Conceptualization of the muscle as an effector of three-dimensional motion will be a useful tool in understanding complex interactions as other joint functions are discussed.

In spite of relatively small individual muscle masses, the collective functions of the rotator cuff musculature become important in normal and pathological motion. The rotator cuff, composed of the supraspinatus, infraspinatus, teres minor, and subscapularis muscles, is so labeled because of its effect upon the glenohumeral joint. Slips from each of the muscles are intimately woven into the capsule of the glenohumeral joint, thereby strengthening and reinforcing the capsule. It is noteworthy that the weakest portion of the capsule is inferior, where there are few reinforcing fibers contributed by cuff musculature. Although of interest to note the evolutionary loss of some of the mass of the supraspinatus muscle, it is of more interest to study the specific function of the teres minor

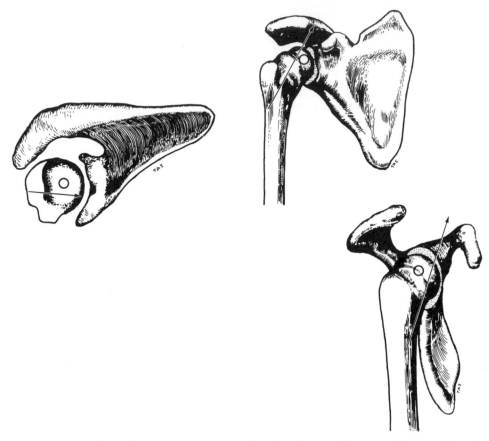

Figure 6.2.   Triplanar diagrammatic view of the glenohumeral joint, exclusive of clavicle. Anterior deltoid force represented by vectors, axis by O. See text for complete details.

muscle. Because of the attachment locations the muscle is capable of depressing the head of the humerus in the glenoid during isolated action. However, the muscle's function is probably most important as a depressor during abduction and/or forward elevation of the arm.

Using elevation of the hand directly laterally from the body as an example, one can readily see that the deltoid muscle would play an important role in the early part of the range of motion. Specifically note that when the arm is still near the body the deltoid would have the effect of elevating the humerus on the glenoid (*ftd* in Fig. 6.3) rather than producing the angular rotation required to raise the arm out to the side. Such is the case because the muscle tension will tend to move the humerus in the vertical direction. (See the section on forces in Chapter 1.) Consequently, in the early part of the range the teres minor, and perhaps the infraspinatus and supraspinatus muscles, contract to depress the head in the glenoid. Figure 6.3 shows that the net effect of the contraction of the deltoid and teres minor muscles is rotation by means of a force couple that contributes to effective elevation of the arm away from the body (19, 34).

Saha labels the muscles of the rotator cuff as "steerers," stating that these muscles are mainly responsible for the rolling of the head of the humerus in the glenoid in different positions of elevation while the prime mover raises the arm. He uses electromyographic evidence to confirm the role of the subscapularis

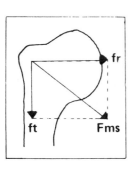

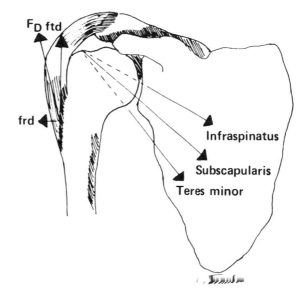

Figure 6.3. Representation of an anteroposterior view of the scapula and humerus, showing the force couple of the deltoid (F_D) and the muscles of the rotator cuff. The resultant effect (Fms) is to keep the head of the humerus in articulation with the glenoid while abduction of the humerus is accomplished. Note that the F_D vector is somewhat parallel to the Fms force. If the axis of rotation is placed between these two forces a couple can be visualized. (From Norkin CC, Levangie PK: *Joint Structure and Function: A Comprehensive Analysis.* Philadelphia, FA Davis, 1983, p. 174.)

and infraspinatus as stabilizers in the early range while demonstrating electrical activity in the infraspinatus, almost solely, in the terminal phases of arm elevation (29).

ARTHROLOGY AND ARTHROKINEMATICS

Anatomical structure and resulting functional capabilities reveal that evolutionary changes associated with the scapula and its movement on the trunk are consistent with the requirements for functional activities. Bechtol has detailed these changes (Fig. 6.4), comparing the scapula of man to other forms of primates (2). Kent also provides a discussion of the changes of the functional anatomy of the shoulder girdle. She comments that the scapula has increased in length and decreased in width, the primary changes occurring in the infraspinous fossa (Fig. 6.5) (13).

The clavicle, not present in standing animals, is present in those that use the upper limbs for holding, grasping, and climbing (25). According to Kent's citations, several functions have been attributed to the clavicle, including the provision of a bony framework for muscle attachment and for purposes of protecting the peripheral vascular and nervous systems (13). Further, the clavicle serves as the attachment mechanism for the arm to the body, being at least partially responsible for supporting the weight of the upper limb. Without maintenance of the load with this force in the superior direction the arm would be free to be pulled inferiorly by gravity, potentially resulting in impingement of the vascular and nervous elements that exit the thorax. The clavicle also maintains the scapula and humerus in a position so that the arm can be held away from the body. In the case of congenital absence, shown in Figure 6.6, interesting

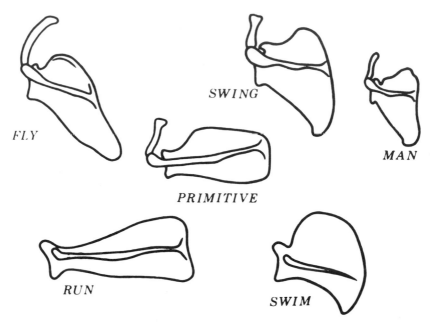

Figure 6.4. Schematic representations of the scapulae of numerous animal forms. The adaptations for running and swimming are of interest because the scapulae no longer has a clavicular attachment that serves to impede movement of the bone. The scapula is also hinged on the vertical border. (From Bechtol CO: Biomechanics of the shoulder. *Clin Orthop* 146:38, 1980.)

effects are seen (30). In addition, the clavicle has been given credit for assisting with transmission of the force of the trapezius to the scapula through the coracoclavicular ligament and facilitating or developing a mechanism for increasing the range of motion in the shoulder complex.

Bony changes have also developed in the humerus as a result of the evolutionary process. Positioning of the arm in space, as required by man's upright posture, has caused development of torsion in the humeral shaft as depicted in Figure 6.7. That is, as the scapula rotated dorsally the humerus followed, resulting in torsion in the humeral shaft that now amounts to 164°. An additional change that has occurred in the humerus is that the deltoid tubercle has migrated distally, therefore increasing the "mechanical advantage" of the deltoid muscle (11).

The scapula, clavicle, and humerus thus make up the bony framework of the shoulder complex. The proximal articulation of each, plus the articulations with each other, form four primary joints affected by the previously described musculature. Thus, specific consideration needs to be given to functions of the sternoclavicular, acromioclavicular, glenohumeral, and scapulothoracic joints. An understanding of the motion available at each joint and the interaction among the joints is critical to either normal or pathological motion of the shoulder complex.

The sternoclavicular joint is the only bone to bone attachment of the upper limb to the trunk. Within this synovial joint an intraarticular disc blends intricately with a capsule that has been identified as being loose but strong. Additional strength is provided to the joint by the sternocleidomastoid, sternohyoid, and sternothyroid muscles, even though the available ranges of motion are accomplished by other muscles of the shoulder complex. Ligaments of significance

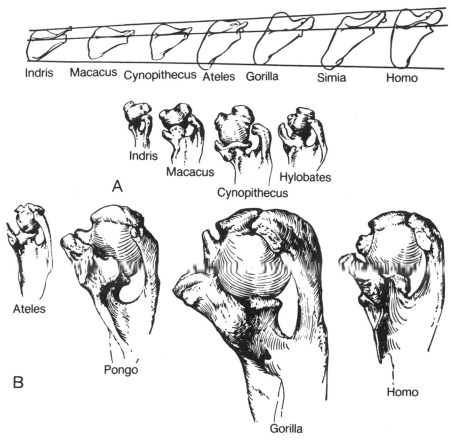

Figure 6.5. Scapular indices and alterations in the size of the acromion for different species. (From Inman V, Saunders M, Abbott LC: Observations on the function of the shoulder joint. *J Bone Joint Surg* [Am] 26:2, 3, 1944.)

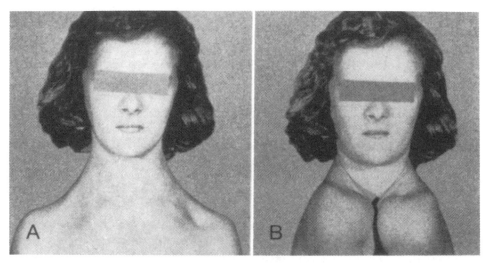

Figure 6.6. (*A*) Young girl with cleidocranial dysostosis appears normal when natural posture is assumed. (*B*) When the shoulders are brought anteriorly the absence of the clavicles allows the scapula to move anteriorly so that the glenohumeral joint is now located under the chin. (From Shands AR: *Handbook of Orthopedic Surgery*, ed 5. St. Louis, CV Mosby, 1971, p. 63.)

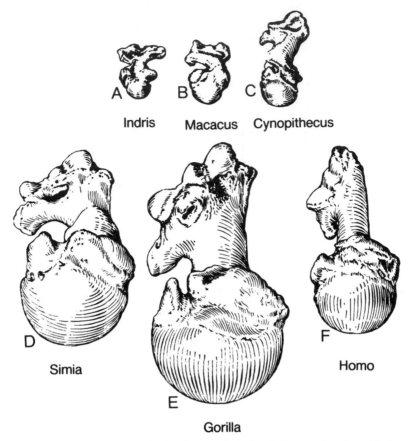

Indris   Macacus   Cynopithecus

Simia   Gorilla   Homo

Figure 6.7. Changes in torsion in the humeral shaft relative to the glenoid. (From Inman V, Saunders M, Abbott LC: Observations on the function of the shoulder joint. *J Bone Joint Surg* [Am] 26:4, 1944.)

include the interclavicular, costoclavicular, and the anterior and posterior sternoclavicular.

The acromioclavicular joint is also a synovial joint that contains an intraarticular disc. There is some disagreement as to the overall strength of the capsule, and in the case of the acromioclavicular joint, ligaments play a primary role in motion that is allowed or achieved as the arm is elevated over the head (8). The coracoacromial ligament, blended with the trapezius and deltoid muscle attachments, provides a roof over the humeral head. The coracoclavicular ligament, which runs superiorly and posteriorly from the coracoid process, contains two portions. The conoid or most medial portion is a separate entity from the more laterally directed trapezoid portion. Functionally, then, these ligaments provide for more glenohumeral joint abduction while also limiting scapular medial displacement and abduction (34).

The glenohumeral joint is also a synovial joint. The glenoid cavity, extending approximately 41 mm in length by 25 mm in width, is considered to be approximately 75% as long and 60% as wide as the humeral head. While the fibrocartilaginous labrum adds depth to the glenoid, Matsen points out that the articular radius of curvature of the surface of the glenoid (i.e., the longitudinal distance) is 35 to 50 mm (19). Further, the glenoid is, on the average, tilted 7°

posteriorly (28). In the anatomical position the shaft of the humerus forms an angle of 135° with the glenoid. Retroversion in the humerus causes the humeral head to face posteriorly by about 30° (19).

The capsule is attached to the circumference of the glenoid cavity and labrum and the anatomical neck, except for the medial aspect which is attached slightly inferiorly. Such an arrangement conveniently adds to the glenohumeral laxity required for arm raising activities. Strength is added by the rotator cuff fibers that are intimately blended with the capsule. Muscles, such as the triceps, pectoralis major, and teres major, also send slips into the capsule that reinforce its strength. Likewise, the long head of the biceps is continuous with the glenoid labrum and intricately blends with the capsule. Of primary importance are the anterior (or glenohumeral) ligaments. All segments, the superior, middle, and inferior, have been credited with strengthening the capsule. Also of significance is the anterior superior or coracohumeral ligament from the greater and lesser tuberosities to the coracoid process. Finally, the transverse humeral ligament connects the two primary tubercles located on the humerus, thereby forming a tunnel for the passage of the long head of the biceps brachii. In general, the capsule has been identified as loose for motion, primarily anteriorly and inferiorly (34).

Functionally the sternoclavicular joint operates as a mechanism simulating a ball and socket. Although generally described to have 3° of freedom, demonstrated by elevation and depression, protraction and retraction, and rotation (Fig. 6.8), it is also possible for translatory motion to exist at the sternoclavicular joint in both the anterior-posterior and superior-inferior directions. Thus, because of the additional ability to distract and compress the joint, 6° of freedom can be demonstrated. The acromioclavicular joint is also believed to have 3° of freedom, although the same general principles that apply to the sternoclavicular joint could be advocated for the acromioclavicular joint. Motion at the acromioclavicular joint exists with upward scapular rotation from 20 to 60° of arm elevation. This motion occurs around an anterior-posterior axis. Another motion often described as winging of the scapula occurs around the vertical axis. Thirty to 50° of winging can ordinarily be produced. Tilting, anterior and posterior, of approximately 30° occurs around the medial-lateral axis (13). The glenohumeral, or "ball and socket" joint, allows for large ranges of motion in flexion and extension, adduction and abduction, and in both internal and external rotation. However, constraints are placed on passive movements of all these joints.

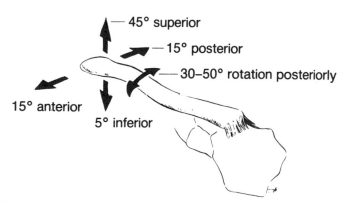

Figure 6.8.   Representation of the available ranges of motion in the sternoclavicular joint. (Courtesy of R. C. Skovly, Miami Beach, FL.)

Because some motions, such as acromioclavicular, are due to tension in ligaments, active musculature is not required. Further, extremes of ranges of motion require tightening of other ligaments. For example, while glenohumeral abduction and external rotation are allowed by the relative slack in the inferior capsule, extremes of these motions will produce tightening and eventual achievement of the close packed position (12). Note, however, the influence of the position of the joints of the scapulohumeral complex on ligamentous tension and the subsequent passive motion. To demonstrate, perform pure abduction to 70° and externally rotate the glenohumeral joint as far as possible. Then abduct an additional 40° and note the increase that has occurred, apparently in the external rotation range of movement. Perhaps the glenohumeral and coracohumeral ligaments have been placed on a relative slack, accounting for the increased motion. In essence, though, the glenohumeral joint demonstrates mobility at the sacrifice of stability.

With an understanding of the structures involved in shoulder motion and the interplay required among the tissues and joints two other aspects are important. The first is the function of the coracoacromial arch. This area, sometimes labeled as the subdeltoid joint, is important because of the contents of the area and the effect of motion on the contents. To be specific, recall that the coracoacromial ligament forms a roof over the humeral head. While serving a protective function for the superior elements from direct trauma, the unyielding nature of the structure limits the available space for the tendons of the rotator cuff muscles. As a result, pathology tends to be focused in this region, in spite of the strategic location of the subdeltoid bursa. Discussion of the pathologies related to this functional joint will be presented later in the chapter (27).

The second feature of import is the relationship of the greater tuberosity to the other structures. In the usually assumed posture with the arm resting at the side the greater tuberosity is outside of the acromion process. However, with 80° of abduction of an internally rotated glenohumeral joint, the tuberosity and the structures superior to the tuberosity are prone to impingement under the acromion process. To avoid the impingement of both the soft and bony structures external rotation of the glenohumeral joint is required. If sufficient range is available in external rotation and such is allowed to take place during abduction, the arm can be elevated completely over the head (31).

SCAPULOHUMERAL RHYTHM

Given an understanding of the joints and their available motions we can now discuss the complex interaction of the joints that occurs in elevation of the hand over the head. There is general agreement in the literature that during the first 30° of abduction, or the first 60° of forward flexion, the scapula is seeking stability on the thorax. This has been somewhat confirmed by Poppen's studies that have incorporated radiographic analysis (Fig. 6.9) (24). Freedman and Monroe, in 1966, utilized radiographic data from five positions of abduction. They demonstrated total scapular upward rotation of 65° with total glenohumeral abduction of 103°, concluding that for every 2° of scapular motion there is 3° of glenohumeral movement (9). The discrepancy between their data and that of others can be accounted for by the fact that the motion was allowed to occur in a coronal versus a scapular plane, the latter being 30 to 45° anterior to the true coronal plane. In another study, Doody et al, in 1970, demonstrated 1.74° of glenohumeral motion per degree of scapular motion. Under loaded conditions

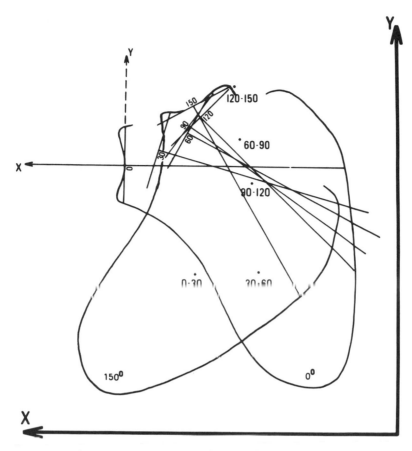

Figure 6.9. Scapular motion, in its own plane, is depicted relative to fixed axes in the body. The centers of rotation for each of five positions are located by means of the dots. The outline of the scapula is also shown for the 0 and 150° positions. (From Poppen NK, Walker PS: Normal and abnormal motion of the shoulder. *J Bone Joint Surg* [*Am*] 58:198, 1976.)

the scapular contribution was called for earlier in the range. In general, Doody et al found the ratio of 2° of glenohumeral motion to every degree of scapular movement, particularly when the total range of motion was considered (4). More recently, Poppen and Walker have demonstrated a 4:5 ratio after 30° of abduction but a 2:1 ratio for the total range of shoulder motion (24). In general, most would concede that the range of scapular motion does not exceed 60°, while that of the glenohumeral joint does not exceed 120°.

During arm raising the primary motion occurring at the sternoclavicular joint is elevation. Poppen and Walker, upon evaluating this motion by means of acromial elevation, stated that there is approximately 35 to 45° of elevation of the clavicle (24). Most of this motion occurs during the first 90° of arm elevation. Therefore, 4 to 5° of elevation occur during each 10° of the first half of arm elevation. With sternoclavicular elevation, motion also occurs at the acromioclavicular joint. Rotation of the clavicle around its own axis is due to the coracoclavicular ligaments pulling on the inferior aspect of the clavicle. This posterior rotation creates movement of the lateral clavicle on the acromion. Such motion has been more recently detailed by Dvir and Berme in a kinematic model of elevation of the shoulder complex (6). As Kent summarizes, during the first 30° and from 135° to maximum elevation, rotation of the acromioclavicular joint occurs around the longitudinal axis of the clavicle (13). The summation of these motions at sternoclavicular, glenohumeral, scapulothoracic, and acromioclavicular joints creates the ability of humans to raise the arms above their heads.

It is interesting to discover that Kapandji states that the range of motion from 0 to 90° is glenohumeral, while the motion from 90 to 150° is scapulothoracic. He cites few references throughout any of his volumes, and it is, therefore difficult to know if objective data are available to support his position. Kapandji further goes on to state that thoracic extension or contralateral flexion is needed for full flexion or abduction to be achieved to 180° (12). Observation would support this view, particularly if loads are lifted anteriorly or if unilateral abduction is attempted.

In summary, then, each of the four joints involved in motion of the shoulder complex must participate in elevating the arm over the head. Concurrently, with muscular effort of the flexors or abductors the serratus anterior and trapezius upwardly rotate the scapula, after the teres minor and deltoid have participated as a force couple. Also necessary for abduction of the arm is external rotation of the glenohumeral joint. This rotation must occur before 90° in order that the greater tuberosity of the humerus not be impinged upon the inferior surface of the acromion process. Also occurring are passive processes, such as the posterior rotation of the clavicle created by the coracoclavicular ligaments. Alterations of these normal kinematics and kinetics are produced as a result of the pathologies discussed in a later section of this chapter.

KINETICS

As a result of the complexity of motions at multiple joints, musculature must create adequate moments in order to be able to elevate the arm over the head. Poppen and Walker have provided some interesting data based on determinations of moment arms from wire sutures placed directly in muscles. Their data, shown in Figure 6.10, are for angles drawn parallel to the face of the glenoid. Evaluation of these graphs shows that the supraspinatus muscle is active throughout the abduction range of motion at a lever arm length of 20 mm. The muscle also maintains an angle with the glenoid of approximately 80°, meaning that the muscle would be effective in producing segment rotation rather than translatory motion. Muscles oriented at relatively small angles to the face of the glenoid would primarily produce shear of the joint rather than rotation. Note also that the anterior and middle deltoid increase their lever arms throughout the range of motion, while the biceps, latissimus, and the infraspinatus decrease their moment arms while maintaining a large angle with the face of the glenoid (24).

At 60° of abduction, forces generated in surrounding musculature have been calculated to be approximately ten times the weight of the limb. The muscle force required to support the limb at 90° of abduction has been calculated to be 8.2 times the weight of the limb (11). More recently, Walker and Poppen have demonstrated that the joint reaction force can equal approximately 90% of body weight, while maximum shear occurs at 60° (33). Figure 6.11 shows that the internal rotation position appears to generate greater joint compression force with some tendency to subluxate the joint. The external rotation position demonstrates greater stability.

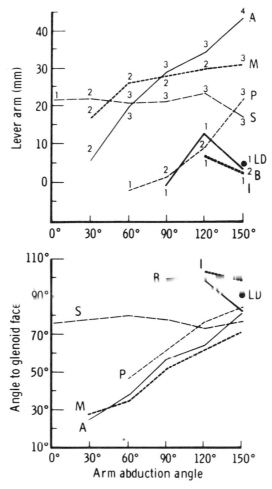

Figure 6.10. Lever arms and angles to glenoid face plotted versus the angle of arm abduction. Muscles are abbreviated as follows: *A* is anterior deltoid, *M* is middle deltoid, *P* is posterior deltoid, *S* is supraspinatus, *B* is the subscapularis, *LD* the latissimus dorsi, and *I* the infraspinatus. The numerical values are EMG activity levels on a 0 to 4 scale. (From Walker PS, Poppen NK: Biomechanics of the shoulder joint in the plane of the scapula. *Bull Hosp Joint Dis* 38:109, 110, 1977.)

Analysis of forces occurring in the shoulder complex is limited for a number of reasons. First, the motions are composed of complex interactions between multiple joints in multiple planes. Dvir and Berme have addressed these aspects, but because of the complexity of the analytic processes there may be constraints in interpreting these data in light of in vivo considerations (6). Secondly, interest in forces across the glenohumeral joint has been minimal, since the shoulder complex is not subjected to the weight-bearing forces produced in the lower limb. Further studies are needed to clarify the interactive relationships among the joints. However, some understanding of the role of the joints and the muscles can be appreciated from the study of injury or paralytic states described in the next section.

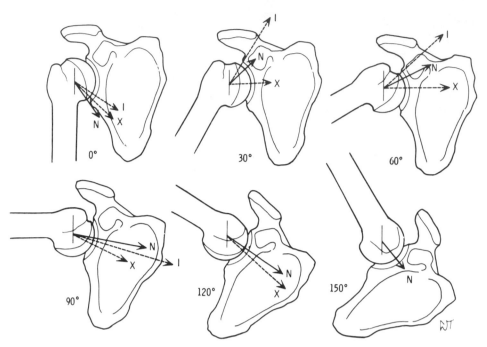

Figure 6.11. Resultant forces at the glenohumeral joint for six positions of the joint. The neutral (*N*), externally rotated (*X*), and internally rotated (*I*) positions are shown. (From Walker PS, Poppen NK: Biomechanics of the shoulder joint in the plane of the scapula. *Bull Hosp Joint Dis* 38:110, 1977.)

PATHOKINESIOLOGY

Abnormal motion of the shoulder complex is often a severe and disabling circumstance that can involve acute pain, recurrent minor episodes, or progressive dysfunction. Injuries of the soft tissues are frequently derived from work or athletic endeavors. Paralytic lesions can result from pathologies that require surgery. Further, different levels of spinal cord injury produce effects dependent on the level of injury. Each of these areas, and several other more unusual pathologies, will be discussed in this section.

Many soft tissue injuries of the shoulder complex have been identified. Common among them are anterior-inferior dislocations of the glenohumeral joint, a requisite of which is laxity but also weakness of this portion of the capsule. In most cases musculature is also weak. Saha concludes that there are several factors predisposing the glenohumeral joint to instability. Among them are decreased glenoid dimensions, anterior tilt of the glenoid, greater than normal retrotorsion in the humerus, and diminished power of the rotator cuff muscles (28).

Injury also frequently involves the rotator cuff, bursae, the bicipital tendon, and structures involved in "adhesive capsulitis" (23). In these cases there is no specific injury to tissues that should produce long-term effects on function of the shoulder complex. However, as Figure 6.12 shows, a tear of the rotator cuff can produce profound effects on the glenohumeral joint. The radiograph in (*A*) shows an anteroposterior (A-P) view of the glenohumeral joint in a patient 6 months posttear. The other radiograph, taken during maximal abduction effort, clearly shows the superior movement of the humeral head on the glenoid. Based

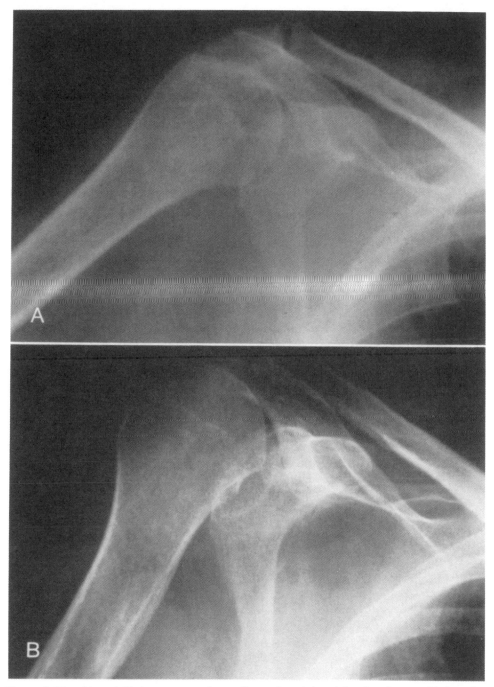

Figure 6.12. (*A* and *B*) Anteroposterior radiographs of the right glenohumeral joint of a 60-yr-old male. See text for complete description.

on what is known about glenohumeral movement there is very ineffective use of the deltoid-teres minor force couple. And, with such humeral elevation, there is likely to be impingement of subacromial structures. There is little doubt that normal kinematics must ultimately be restored in order for normal motion to occur.

Neer has discussed the impingement lesions of the shoulder and classified the problem into three stages. According to his observations the problem often occurs against the anterior edge and undersurface of the acromion, the coracoacromial ligaments, and the acromioclavicular joint itself. Further, he explains that because of the adjacency of the structures the clinician should consider that two or more structures are involved together (20). In discussing similar clinical problems in a group of 97 patients, Kessel and Watson describe the painful arc syndrome. The pain, referred to the lateral aspect of the upper arm, occurs between 60 and 120° of abduction. Although the authors point out that the syndrome can be caused by several different lesions, all result from a loss of the normal clearance between the arch formed by the coracoacromial ligament and the tuberosities below (14). Precise examination techniques are required in all cases to effectively determine which tissues are involved.

Yet, in many patients the resultant effect is, by reason of pain or discomfort, limitation of shoulder use. Subsequently, difficulties arise in putting on coats, reaching into an upper level cupboard, or simply driving a car. Concurrent with the disability comes the muscle atrophy and weakness so commonly seen in these patients. To effect early resolution of the problem, treatment of the specific cause of the lesion should restore normal arthrokinematics and osteokinematics and maintain the usual kinetics required of the muscles. Thus, rehabilitation of shoulder pathology may demand that the specific kinematics of each joint be assessed in order to determine if any joints are limiting the normal motions described in the scapulohumeral rhythm section of this chapter. For specific examples of treatments that may be necessary in these conditions use of texts such as produced by Kessler and Hertling may be necessary (15).

Although the glenohumeral joint is subject to relatively small magnitudes of forces there are occasions when total joint replacement is advised. Neer et al have recently reviewed their experience with total shoulder replacements in a consecutive series of 273 shoulders. In their series the largest numbers of patient groups were classified as 60 with old trauma, 56 with rheumatoid arthritis, and 55 with osteoarthritis. According to these authors resultant glenohumeral stability depended on the height as well as the version of the prosthetic components. Function depended on reconstruction and the rehabilitation of the rotator cuff and deltoid muscles. In emphasizing the optimum results achieved with the form of unconstrained prostheses used in these patients, the authors specified that the muscles are of critical importance to both mobility and stability (21).

One interesting musculoskeletal disorder that affects the shoulder complex is the snapping scapula syndrome. Strizak and Cowen reported a case that does not fit the classical pattern of etiology whereby subjects have performed repeated forceful actions of the shoulder. Thought to produce periosteal microtears along the medial border of the scapula, the result is a distinct thump or snapping as the scapula is moved across the thorax. One possible explanation for the syndrome is that the levator scapulae muscle has been weakened by chronic trauma or perhaps has even been avulsed (32).

Paralyses of isolated muscles of the shoulder complex are relatively rare, but when they do occur a profound disruption of scapulohumeral rhythm can occur. For example, trapezius paralysis may be an unavoidable side effect of surgical procedures in the posterior triangle of the neck (5). In these cases the scapula assumes a position of depression and protraction as the acromion droops. On occasions the sternum can be deviated to the opposite side during full elevation of the arm. The acromion cannot effectively be pulled posteriorly, and weakness in elevation of the arm is the result (Fig. 6.13).

Although not always the result of isolated or collective paralysis of muscle, poor posture or abnormal positioning can be responsible for dysfunction of the upper limb. Such has been well documented for syndromes of the thoracic outlet, where impingement of the nerve or vascular bundle will produce definitive symptoms. Often the therapist must make an accurate assessment of the posture and the arthrokinematics and arthrokinetics available to the patient before the problem can be adequately treated.

Serratus anterior paralysis can also be produced in an isolated fashion. Gregg et al have reported a case in a young athlete (10), and Fardin et al have recently reviewed a series of ten cases (7). Virtually all cases were caused by trauma from falls. On occasion the long thoracic nerve is sectioned during mastectomy. In these cases of isolated paralysis the scapula becomes winged, since there is virtually no other muscle to hold the inferior angle of the scapula against the thorax. Elevation of the arm overhead may no longer be possible (17). As for isolated paralysis of the trapezius, some difficulty can be expected with elevating the arm overhead.

When there is combined serratus anterior and trapezius paralysis there is distinct difficulty in raising the arm above the head. In these cases all motion must essentially occur at the glenohumeral joint, since effective upward rotation of the scapula has been lost. The result is, in effect, static equilibrium: as the arm reaches maximal glenohumeral abduction due to the action of the deltoid, the downward moment produced by the weight of the limb balances and prevents further scapular motion (Fig. 6.14). Further abduction of the glenohumeral joint

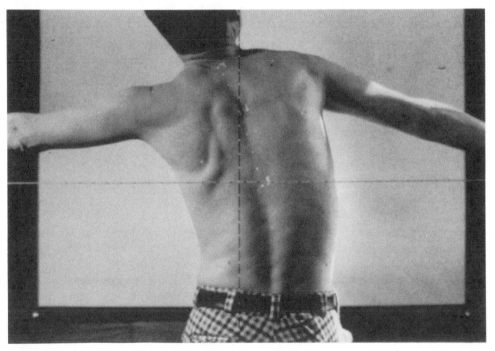

Figure 6.13.   Posterior view of bilateral abduction. Note the normal mechanics of the left side with the abnormal right side. The right glenohumeral joint appears to lack external rotation. To gain more abduction the patient leans to the contralateral side.

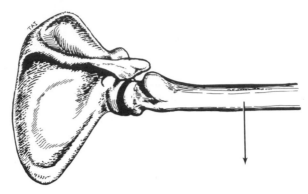

Figure 6.14. Representation of the scapulohumeral complex at the point when full abduction has been reached in the case of the paralysis of the shoulder girdle musculature. Note that the scapula assumes a position of downward rotation.

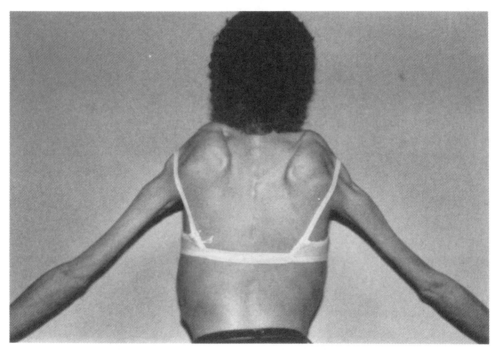

Figure 6.15. Posterior view of patient with fascioscapulohumeral muscular dystrophy. Note the downwardly rotated position of the scapulae.

is impossible because the deltoid has been sufficiently shortened so that no further tension is available. As a result, the individual can elevate the arm to approximately 60°.

Cases of facioscapulohumeral muscular dystrophy also provide useful examples of the effect of scapular stabilization upon the thorax. In these cases the scapula is winged and unable to upwardly rotate (Fig. 6.15). Comparison of the patient photo with the mechanics as diagrammed in Figure 6.14 show the similarities. To provide for better functional abilities, surgical procedures, such as those reported by Ketenjian, have been performed with results that have increased abduction by 37%, while simultaneously increasing shoulder strength and endurance (16).

Paralysis or specific involvement of either the deltoid or supraspinatus produces some weakness at the glenohumeral joint but still allows elevation of the arm over the head. Bechtol has recently suggested that the supraspinatus supplies approximately 20% of the power for arm elevation, and if this muscle is lost the individual has difficulty elevating the arm after 90° (Fig. 6.16) (2). If the deltoid and teres minor are involved as a result of injury to the axillary nerve, abduction is weak or limited because of the loss of the force couple at the glenohumeral joint. Etiologies creating this peripheral nerve involvement include subglenoid dislocations, fractures of the humeral head, crutch compression, and/or a severe blow on the shoulder.

Spinal cord injury patients provide further examples of disrupted kinetics of the shoulder complex that in turn lead to altered kinematics. The resultant loss will be directly related to the level of the lesion. For purposes of studying the shoulder the C5-6 and C6-7 lesions are of the most interest. Losses above the fifth cervical level leave incompetence of the serratus anterior (22). The results shown in Figure 6.17 are for attempted arm elevation. What results is a scapular downward rotation during a pull forward to the seated position (20). Other lower level cervical injuries that affect the remainder of the arm will be discussed in subsequent chapters.

Other neurological patients are not devoid of movement dysfunction of the shoulder complex. Hemiplegic patients have long been known to exhibit inferior subluxation of the glenohumeral joint secondary to weakness or paralysis. In postulating that subluxation is caused by brachial plexus lesions Chino indicated that 75% of the supraspinatus and deltoid muscles revealed pathological electromyographic potentials (3). If, in fact, the potential incidence is as high as these data suggest, then practitioners must give considerable attention to the glenohumeral joint. Chino suggests that the shoulder should be in a retracted position or suspended to prevent overstretching. He also cautions against overaggressive range of motion of the joint. Therapists must be reminded that indiscriminant passive stretching procedures can have deleterious effects on structures that are attempting to provide support. In addition, inert structures can have such great

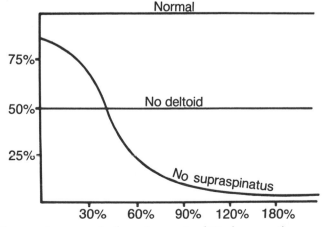

Figure 6.16. Torque, in percent of maximum, is plotted versus the range of motion in the normal shoulder. Deltoid loss would still enable abduction of the glenohumeral joint at about 50% of the torque. Loss of the supraspinatus, however, would enable 80% of the torque early in the range, falling rapidly to less than 20% by the midpoint in the range of motion. (From Bechtol CO: Biomechanics of the shoulder. *Clin Orthop* 146:39, 1980.)

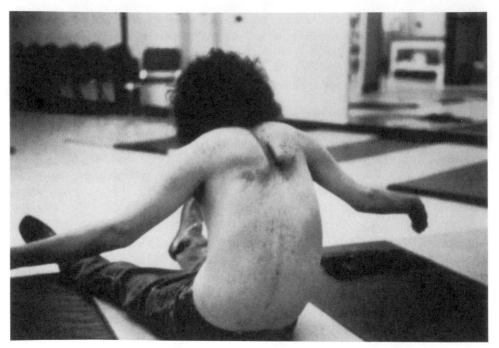

Figure 6.17.   Posterior view of attempted arm elevation for patient described in text.

tensile strength that abnormal and/or unwanted arthrokinematics may result from improperly applied therapeutic techniques. That is, motion contrary to the principles applied to joint surfaces, as established in Chapter 3, can result. To restore or maintain normal arthrokinematics a delicate balance is sought as therapeutic procedures are administered.

SUMMARY

This chapter has discussed anatomical elements in relationship to normal and abnormal motion of the shoulder complex. Fundamental principles of force representation, moments, and couples have been presented as they relate to the shoulder in both normal and pathological circumstances. Finally, various pathologies have been considered with respect to how normal motion is disrupted.

References

1. Bearn JG: An electromyographic study of the trapezius, deltoid, pectoralis major, biceps and triceps muscles, during static loading of the upper limb. *Anat Rec* 140:103–108, 1961.
2. Bechtol CO: Biomechanics of the shoulder. *Clin Orthop* 146:37–41, 1980.
3. Chino N: Electrophysiological investigation on shoulder subluxation in hemiplegics. *Scand J Rehabil Med* 13:17–21, 1981.
4. Doody SG, Freedman L, Waterland JC: Shoulder movement during abduction in the scapular plane. *Arch Phys Med Rehabil* 51:595–604, 1970.
5. Dunn AW: Trapezius paralysis after minor surgical procedures in the posterior cervical triangle. *South Med J* 67:312–315, 1974.
6. Dvir Z, Berme N: The shoulder complex in elevation of the arm: a mechanism approach. *J Biomech* 11:219–225, 1978.
7. Fardin P, Negrin P, Dainese R: The isolated paralysis of the serratus anterior muscle: clinical and electromyographical follow-up of 10 cases. *Electromyogr Clin Neurophysiol* 18:379–386, 1978.

8. Frankel VH, Nordin M: *Basic Biomechanics of the Skeletal System*. Philadelphia, Lea & Febiger, 1980.
9. Freedman L, Munro RR: Abduction of the arm in the scapular plane: scapular and glenohumeral movements. *J Bone Joint Surg [Am]* 48:1503–1510, 1966.
10. Gregg JR, Labosky D, Harty M, et al: Serratus anterior paralysis in the young athlete. *J Bone Joint Surg [Am]* 61:825–832, 1979.
11. Inman V, Saunders M, Abbott LC: Observations on the function of the shoulder joint. *J Bone Joint Surg [Am]* 26:1–30, 1944.
12. Kapandji IA: *The Physiology of the Joints*, ed 5. Edinburgh, Churchill Livingstone, 1982, vol 1.
13. Kent BE: Functional anatomy of the shoulder complex: a review. *J Am Phys Ther Assoc* 51:867–888, 1971.
14. Kessel L, Watson M: The painful arc syndrome: clinical classification as a guide to management. *J Bone Joint Surg [Br]* 59:166–172, 1977.
15. Kessler RK, Hertling D: *Management of Common Musculoskeletal Disorders*. Philadelphia, Harper & Row, 1983.
16. Ketenjian AY: Scapulocostal stabilization for scapular winging in facioscapulohumeral muscular dystrophy. *J Bone Joint Surg [Am]* 60:476–480, 1978.
17. Lehmkuhl LD, Smith LK: *Brunnstrom's Clinical Kinesiology*, ed 4. Philadelphia, FA Davis, 1983.
18. MacConaill MA, Basmajian JV. *Muscles and Movements: A Basis for Human Kinesiology*. Baltimore, Williams & Wilkins, 1969.
19. Matsen FA: Biomechanics of the shoulder. In Frankel VM, Nordin M: *Basic Biomechanics of the Skeletal System*. Philadelphia, Lea & Febiger, 1980.
20. Neer CS: Impingement lesions. *Clin Orthop* 173:70–77, 1983.
21. Neer CS, Watson KC, Stanton FJ: Recent experience in total shoulder replacement. *J Bone Joint Surg [Am]* 64:319–337, 1982.
22. Newman D: Personal communication, Iowa City, Iowa, 1983.
23. Peat M, Grahame RE: Electromyographic analysis of soft tissue lesions affecting shoulder function. *Am J Phys Med* 56:223–240, 1977.
24. Poppen NK, Walker PS: Normal and abnormal motion of the shoulder. *J Bone Joint Surg [Am]* 58:195–201, 1976.
25. Quiring DP, Boroush EL: Functional anatomy of the shoulder girdle. *Arch Phys Med* 27:90–96, 1946.
26. Rasch PJ, Burke RK: *Kinesiology and Applied Anatomy: The Science of Human Movement*, ed 6. Philadelphia, Lea & Febiger, 1978.
27. Rothman RH, Marvel JP, Heppenstall RB: Anatomic considerations in the glenohumeral joint. *Orthop Clin North Am* 6:341–352, 1975.
28. Saha AK: Dynamic stability of the glenohumeral joint. *Acta Orthop Scand* 42:491–505, 1971.
29. Saha AK: Mechanics of elevation of glenohumeral joint: its application in rehabilitation of flail shoulder in upper brachial plexus injuries and poliomyelitis and in replacement of the upper humerus by prosthesis. *Acta Orthop Scand* 44:668–678, 1973.
30. Shands AR: *Handbook of Orthopedic Surgery*, ed 5. St. Louis, CV Mosby, 1971.
31. Sohier R: *Kinesitherapy of the Shoulder*. Bristol, John Wright and Sons, 1967.
32. Strizak AM, Cowen MH: The snapping scapula syndrome. *J Bone Joint Surg [Am]* 64:941–942, 1982.
33. Walker PS, Poppen NK: Biomechanics of the shoulder joint during abduction in the plane of the scapula. *Bull Hosp Joint Dis* 38:107–111, 1977.
34. Warwick R, Williams PL (eds): *Gray's Anatomy*, ed 36. Philadelphia, WB Saunders, 1980.

7

Elbow

The joints that make up the elbow are in an important functional position in relationship to the use of the upper limb. In effect, the elbow is made up of at least three joints, each having a specific function in positioning the hand in space. In this chapter each of the joints will be discussed and their interaction described. Sections dealing with the kinematics and kinetics are included. The chapter concludes with a presentation of various pathologies as they influence the elbow.

MUSCULAR FUNCTION
Anatomical Organization

The musculature affecting the elbow is frequently described on a topographical basis. Lehmkuhl and Smith classify an above elbow group, i.e., the flexors and extensors, and a below elbow group consisting of three subgroups. The below elbow group consists of a radial group made up of the brachioradialis, extensor carpi radialis longus (ECRL), and the extensor carpi radialis brevis (ECRB). A dorsoulnar group is comprised of wrist extensor-supinator muscles. Further, the muscles originating from the medial epicondyle make up the volar medial group (19). Under other circumstances the muscles are better thought of in terms of function. Such a system would result in muscle groups of elbow flexors and extensors, supinators, and pronators. If this latter system is pursued, care must be taken to include the muscles of the hand and wrist that originate above the elbow and subsequently have a potential elbow or radioulnar joint function.

Flexor Function

There is some disagreement, and perhaps less than adequate data, regarding the function of the elbow and radioulnar joint musculature. Based on known anatomical locations, however, certain muscles have single while other muscles have multiple joint functions. A variety of studies, most of which have employed electromyography, have attempted to clarify the situation. Among the earliest was a study that evaluated the functions of the chief flexors of the elbow (5). From their data Basmajian and Latif demonstrated the biceps to be an effective flexor of the forearm only if it had been prepositioned in supine or if it were under significant load. However, the muscle played little or no role in flexion of the elbow even when a load of 2 lbs was lifted. Further, they discovered that the biceps brachii is not a supinator of the extended arm, unless supination is firmly resisted. During slow supination of the radioulnar joint little or no activity

131

is required of the biceps. Demonstration is possible by performing the lap test. With the forearm completely supported in the lap of the seated subject the fingers of the opposite hand are used to palpate the prominent tendon of the biceps muscle. Very slow supination from the initial position of pronation elicits no contraction of the biceps, but if resistance is supplied or the velocity of forearm supination increased, the biceps is felt to contract. Some have used this motion to "test" the supinator after a peripheral nerve injury. Without the supinator, no matter how slow the forearm is supinated, the biceps tenses. Generally the biceps appears to be able to generate most power for either supination or flexion when the elbow is flexed at 90°. Mechanical features identified in Chapter 2, specifically the angle of insertion, appear to be primarily responsible.

The brachialis muscle is located in an ideal position to complete elbow flexion. In their 1957 study Basmajian and Latif demonstrated that the brachialis is active during flexion "under all conditions" and generally active during most movements and postures. As a result of this study the muscle was labeled as the workhorse of the elbow joint. Note also that the length-tension relationship in this muscle does not change with pronation/supination due to the insertion on the ulna. The function of the brachioradialis muscle is less clear (5). Identified by early anatomists as the supinator longus, there is little doubt that this muscle is a flexor. Fick, as cited by Lehmkuhl and Smith, also stated that the muscle was capable of performing some pronation from the fully supinated position and some, but less, supination from the fully pronated position (19). Electromyographic data contradict these theoretical functions unless the movements are strongly resisted (5). Under these circumstances the muscle may be serving a stabilization function.

Extensor Function

Extensor muscle function is less difficult to analyze, since there are only the triceps and anconeus muscles to consider with no effect rendered on the radioulnar joint. In regard to the triceps, Kapandji has stated that the medial triceps is most active, making the muscle comparable to the workhorse status specified for the brachialis (16). Further, the lateral triceps is considered to be the strongest, while the long head is the quietest. There appear to be no data to confirm or deny these statements. On the other hand, more extensive studies have been completed on the function of the anconeus muscle. Pauly and coworkers found that this muscle was electrically active in the early phases of elbow extension. The muscle also appeared to have a stabilizing function during other upper limb motions, such as pronation and supination (25). Basmajian and Griffin have shown the anconeus to be active at levels comparable to those achieved during extension (Fig. 7.1). Activity levels of the anconeus and the triceps were judged, by these same investigators, to be comparable (Fig. 7.2). (4). The suggestion by Duchenne that the anconeus causes ulnar abduction during pronation is more likely a demonstration of a stabilization effect (8).

It is also interesting to note that the pectoralis major and anterior deltoid muscles can be effective extensors of the elbow. Such occurs when the hand is fixed or when heavy objects are pushed away from the body. Using the former case as the example, visualize the front leaning rest position assumed in the push-up. As one pushes the body up from the ground, forward flexion of the humerus onto the trunk and elbow extension occur simultaneously. However, because the hand is fixed the pectoralis major and anterior deltoid may, at least,

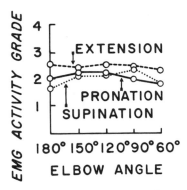

Figure 7.1. Graph of EMG activity from anconeus during supination, pronation, and extension of the elbow. (From Basmajian JV, Griffin WR: Function of anconeus muscle: an electromyographic study. *J Bone Joint Surg [Am]* 54:1713, 1972.)

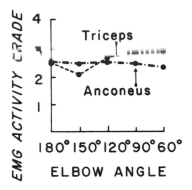

Figure 7.2. Comparison of medial head of the triceps and anconeus during elbow extension. (From Basmajian JV, Griffin WR: Function of anconeus muscle: an electromyographic study. *J Bone Joint Surg [Am]* 54:1713, 1972.)

facilitate elbow extension. This example demonstrates the concept of reversal of the origin and insertion so that muscles may perform functionally.

Supination-Pronation Function

There is relatively little information available about the function of the supinator and pronator musculature. Lehmkuhl and Smith compare the pronators quadratus and teres in terms of cross section and available shortening. They state, with assumptions, that the pronator quadratus pronates unaided by other muscles if performed slowly without resistance and active elbow flexion. The influence of elbow position upon the effective action of the pronator teres must be taken into account, since the moment arm of the muscle is significantly decreased in full elbow extension. Supination by the supinator muscle is not dependent on the degree of elbow flexion by virtue of its origination site on the ulna and lateral humeral epicondyle. Fick, according to Lehmkuhl and Smith, says that at 90° of elbow flexion, the biceps is four times as effective a supinator as the supinator muscle (19). At full elbow extension the difference diminishes to a factor of two. Repeating the lap test confirms the ability of the supinator to act alone under conditions of low load and low velocity. These findings from palpation have indeed been electromyographically confirmed earlier (5).

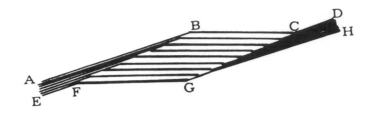

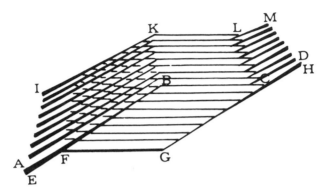

Figure 7.3. Demonstration of the parallelpipedon shape of muscle fibers. See text for complete description. (From An KN, Hui FC, Morrey BF, et al. Muscles across the elbow joint: a biomechanical analysis. *J Biomech* 14:660, 1981.)

Anatomical Influences

Recently, An et al have completed an interesting study of the muscles crossing the elbow joint. In a section describing the anatomical results they state that most muscles with "rather discrete origins and insertions" assumed the parallelepipedon form. In this configuration the muscle fibers are of uniform length, and the tendons became progressively thicker as they assumed more fibers (Fig. 7.3). Other muscles (such as the brachialis, supinator, and medial and lateral heads of the triceps) do not readily conform to the parallelepipedon shape. Further, some muscles that remained more muscular than tendinous had muscle fiber variations where longer fibers were situated farther from the joint (2). The import of these factors will be discussed in the section on kinetics found later in this chapter.

Integrated Action

Muscular actions across the elbow also should be considered from a collective viewpoint. For example, the biceps and triceps have a reciprocal relationship not only at the elbow but also at the glenohumeral joint. Recall that the biceps flexes the elbow and supinates the radioulnar joint. In addition, the muscle is anterior to the glenohumeral joint and therefore in a position to create flexion. Assume that a subject wishes to bring an object in front closer to the body. Such a functional activity requires flexion at the elbow and extension at the glenohumeral joint. Because the former motion shortens the muscle at the elbow and the latter motion lengthens the muscle at the shoulder the biceps can maintain an appropriate length so that sufficient tension can be generated throughout the range of motion. The triceps, acting in a converse fashion in pushing objects away from the body, performs similarly. Another interpretation of these events includes the concepts of links and chains as discussed in Chapter 3. If the length of the biceps and triceps is truly not changing then these muscles are adding stability to the kinetic chain but not producing the motion. Rather, single joint muscles such as the latissimus dorsi and teres major must be acting to extend, the infraspinatus and teres minor to control rotation, and the coracobrachialis to flex the glenohumeral joint. Muscles other than these are most probably involved in controlling these motions. If necessary the importance of these features should be reviewed in the length-tension section of Chapter 2 and the links and chains section in Chapter 3.

Elbow musculature also demonstrates excellent examples of synergy. Consider the case of turning doorknobs. In this activity supination of the forearm by the biceps brachii would also tend to flex the elbow, moving the hand away from the knob. In order to prevent the biceps from carrying out all its actions, the triceps muscle is activated to neutralize the flexion tendency so that effective supination can be completed. Similar results occur during the driving of a wood screw, particularly when resistance is met. Even under light manual resistance to supination triceps muscle activity can be palpated.

Also recall the differences in contraction type discussed in Chapter 2. Consider the task of simple elbow flexion combined with slight radioulnar supination, as in bringing a fork to the mouth. These motions can be completed by concentric action of the biceps brachii muscle. On return to the starting position elbow extension and radioulnar pronation ensue. However, performance of these motions is not accomplished by action of the triceps brachii muscle and prona-tors. Rather, the same muscles that performed the concentric work now perform eccentric work. That is, the muscles "let" the weight of the arm lower the segment to the table by means of a slow controlled lengthening of the biceps brachii and/or the supinator. If in fact the extensors and pronators contracted, the result would be a rapid extension of the elbow that could meet with disastrous results. This principle of controlled eccentric contraction is an important concept that must be ingrained in the therapist's technique of motion analysis. Otherwise erroneous interpretations can be applied. Virtually any time that gravity assists motion, eccentric contraction will be called into play. Primary examples include the descent to the seated position from standing, lowering the foot to the floor prior to the beginning of the stance phase in gait, and the control of one's body weight during the descent of stairs. Other examples will be provided in other chapters.

ARTHROLOGY AND ARTHROKINEMATICS

The bony structure of the elbow and radioulnar joints comprise an interesting framework around which motions occur. The spherical end of the proximal radius is unique in provision for the rotary requirements of the forearm. The ulna seems to have a cradling effect on the distal end of the humerus, perhaps for purposes of stability. Figure 7.4 shows that the joint has been likened to a ball and spool on the same axis. Note that the distal end of the humerus acts as a male surface projecting anteriorly at an angle of 45°. A similar arrangement occurs at the proximal portion of the ulna in that the olecranon and coranoid processes are also 45° offset in an anterior direction. Kapandji has likened the distal humerus to fork prongs sticking anteriorly from the axis of the humerus and the ulna. Such structure, along with the depth of the coronoid and olecranon

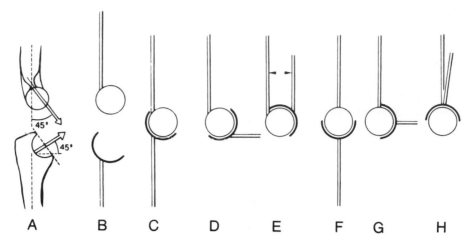

Figure 7.4. Representation of the articulation of the humerus and ulna. *A* through *E* show the normal configuration of the bony structures. If the position shown in *F* was assumed, flexion would be limited to 90° (*G*) and leave no room for muscle mass if the position shown in *H* was attempted. (From Kapandji AI: *The Physiology of the Joints*, ed 5. New York, Churchill Livingstone, 1982, p 79.)

fossae, provide for an increased range of motion for elbow flexion without creating impingement of the ulna upon the humerus. Figure 7.4 demonstrates the results if the bony offsets at 45° did not exist (16).

Asymmetry of the trochlea may also play a role in laterally angulating the ulna on the humerus. The purpose of this angulation, known as the carrying angle, is considered to be a means of keeping the arm away from the side while carrying objects. Considerable doubt as to this purpose must be expressed on the basis that objects, particularly heavy objects, are virtually always carried with the forearm in the middle of the supination-pronation range. Such a maneuver tends to negate any potential effect of the carrying angle. The angle has been found to be 10 to 15° in males and 20 to 25° in females. Steindler, in his classic treatise on kinesiology, maintained that in part due to the osteology, a gap opened on the medial side of the olecranon during extension of the elbow. Conversely, on extreme flexion the gap opened at the lateral olecranon border (27).

All of the joints at the elbow, ulnohumeral, radiohumeral, and radioulnar, are synovial joints. Reinforcement and medial-lateral constraint is provided by the medial and lateral ligaments. The medial, or ulnar, collateral ligament has anterior, intermediate, and posterior sets of fibers, of which the anterior fibers help reinforce the annular ligament of the radioulnar joint. The lateral, or radial, ligament is intimately associated with the annular ligament that surrounds the head of the radius and maintains the proximal radius in articulation with the ulna (28).

BIOMECHANICS

Only recently have comprehensive studies been completed that adequately address the kinesiology and biomechanics of the joints considered to make up the elbow complex. Most have considered the elbow to be a pure hinge joint in spite of a known mechanical influence of the radioulnar joints.

In 1978 Chao and Morrey completed a study on the three-dimensional rotation of the elbow (6). One year later Youm et al published an analysis of forearm pronation-supination and elbow flexion-extension (29). Both studies, performed on cadaver specimens, used different methodologies and provided useful information about elbow and radioulnar motion. Both studies evaluated the kinematics of the elbow and found the long axis of the elbow to rotate about 5° internally during early elbow flexion and about 5° externally during the later phases. In finding that the carrying angle varied linearly as a function of flexion, Chao and Morrey noted that the elbow proceeded from valgus in extension towards varus in flexion (6). Youm et al disagree somewhat in that four of six specimens showed a sinusoidal relationship (Fig. 7.5) rather than the linear form demonstrated in two elbows. At least part of the explanation may be that the Youm et al study demonstrated no medial-lateral movement of the proximal ulna on the humerus during the flexion extension motion (29). Both studies determined that the locus of the axis of rotation was through the trochlea, confirming the turn of the century work of Fischer as cited by Chao and Morrey (6). Figure 7.6 shows the displacement of the axis during elbow flexion. The Youm et al study further identified the radioulnar axis, specifying the location as ranging from the center of the capitulum to the distal end of the ulna (29).

In a more recent study London assessed the kinematics of elbow motion using a radiographic technique on human subjects. The results showed the instant centers of rotation to be tightly clustered in the center of the trochlea, except

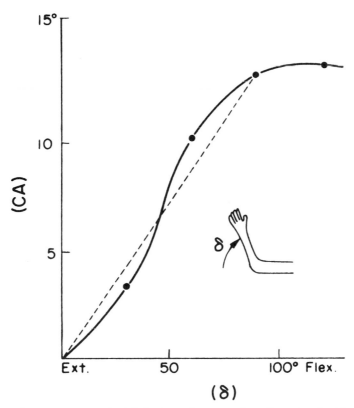

Figure 7.5. The carrying angle (*CA*) plotted versus the elbow angle. Two specimens showed a linear change, while four others demonstrated a flat sinusoidal curve up to 90°. After this point in the range of motion all of the elbows behaved similarly. (From Youm Y, Dryer RF, Thanbyrajah K, et al: Biomechanical analyses of forearm pronation-supination and elbow flexion-extension. *J Biomech* 12:254, 1979.)

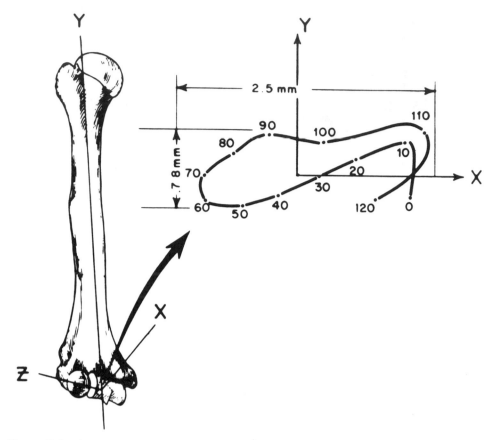

Figure 7.6. Instantaneous center of rotation for the sagittal plane for the elbow joint. (From Chao EY, Morrey BF: Three dimensional rotation of the elbow. *J Biomech* 11:67, 1978.)

during the extremes of the range of motion. For the last 5 to 10° of flexion the axis was displaced toward the coronoid fossa, while during the same extreme of extension the displacement was towards the olecranon fossa. London also studied the axis of the radiohumeral joint and found similar anterior and posterior displacements of the axes in the terminal ranges of flexion and extension (21). Location of the instant centers is of practical import, because based upon this information the osteokinematics can be described. For example, in the case of the elbow, motion of the ulnohumeral and radiohumeral joint is gliding, except at the extremes of flexion and extension. During these ranges the axis moves, indicating that gliding motion changes to rolling. The specific therapeutic import can be seen in patients with limited range. Because rolling will be important to restoration of normal kinematics required for a full range of motion, therapeutic efforts to maintain these ranges are likely to assist with positive treatment results. For specific techniques aimed at achieving these motions the reader is referred to such volumes as those by Kessler and Hertling (17).

Therapeutic consideration must also be given to maintenance or restoration of the ranges of motion required for normal function. Morrey et al have recently reconfirmed that the total range of elbow flexion is 140°. In reporting that most activities of daily living can be accomplished with 30 to 130° of flexion and from 50° of pronation to 50° of supination, they have defined limits for clinical use.

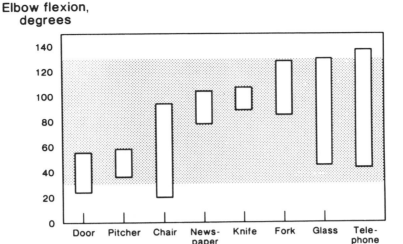

Figure 7.7. The ranges of elbow flexion required to perform various activities. (From Morrey BF, Askew LJ, An KN, et al: A biomechanical study of normal functional elbow motion. *J Bone Joint Surg* [*Am*] 63:874, 1981.)

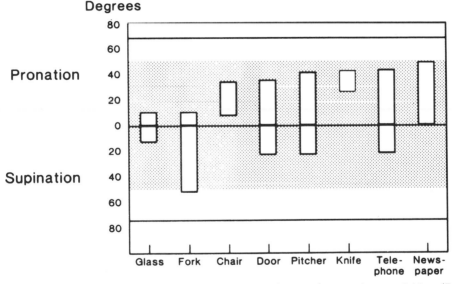

Figure 7.8. The ranges of forearm rotation required to perform various activities. (From Morrey BF, Askew LJ, An KN, et al: A biomechanical study of normal functional elbow motion. *J Bone Joint Surg* [*Am*] 63:875, 1981.)

Figures 7.7 and 7.8 represent the arcs of motion required during the activities studied (23).

KINETICS

Muscular Forces

In 1911, Fick published his well-known work on anatomy (11). According to his measurements the total cross sectional area of the elbow flexors is 26.5 cm^2, which exceeded the area of 20.3 cm^2 of the extensors. He was the first to claim that the biceps area exceeded the cross section of the brachialis muscle, by only a slight margin. Much more recently Hui et al and An et al have published results that differ (2, 15). Hui et al state that the brachialis, in terms of cross sectional area, is consistently the strongest flexor. No specific data are cited (15). The 1981 work of An et al. includes a specific analysis of all muscles that have an effect on the elbow. The cross section for both heads of the biceps muscle totaled 4.5 cm², while the brachialis was 7.0 cm². Total area for the triceps was cited to be 18.8 cm². An et al state that because the fibers of the biceps and brachioradialis muscles are relatively long the cross sectional area is relatively small (2).

Others have attempted to measure elbow flexor and extensor force. In 1966 Little and Lehmkuhl measured elbow extension force in three positions. Cable tensiometer values, with the restraining cuff positioned just proximal to the wrist, were in the range of 18.0 to 25.2 lbs (20). In another study, by Currier, extensor force was measured with the elbow in 60, 90, and 120° of flexion. Cable tensiometer values indicated that the greatest values (48.8 lbf) were reached at the 90° position. Although the 120° angle produced values only 4 lbf less, the 60° angle involved values of 35.8 lbf. That Currier used male subjects and that Little and Lehmkuhl used female subjects probably accounts for the differences in their results (7). Larson also used similar techniques in evaluating the effect of forearm positioning on flexor force. With the cuff at approximately midforearm, results showed supination force at 95 lbs, midposition at 97 lbs, and pronation at 88 lbs (18). These results are difficult to interpret because the values were not converted to torque measurements. Doing so would provide a technique for comparing within and between subjects as well as across studies.

Anatomical Considerations

As is well known, consideration of the factors determining torque include both cross section (force) and the moment arm length. The study by An et al, previously cited in this section, included a complete set of moment arm data for all musculature affecting the elbow and the radioulnar joints. Among other comments, and although various positions of supination-pronation and flexion-extension were studied, these investigators concluded that the brachioradialis, biceps, brachialis, and extensor carpi radiali were the major flexors. They provided an interesting array of diagrams that show the potential moment contribution of each muscle. One such representation is shown in Figure 7.9 (2). Hui et al say that the brachioradialis, based on moment arm, is consistently the most efficient muscle. In discussing the influence of mechanical factors, the point is made that the gain in moment production, allowed by an increasing moment arm upon elbow flexion, is not completely negated by the tension loss which ordinarily accompanies a "slackened" muscle. The net result is that a flexed elbow can resist more load than an extended elbow (15).

In an interesting sidelight of their study Andersson and Schultz calculated rough estimates of the maximum voluntary contractile strength per cross sectional area. Using estimates of shapes and area, they determined stress to be 100 N/cm². Although not of particular significance to the kinesiology or pathokinesiology of the elbow, the data offer some explanation as to the potential for muscle rupture (3). The mechanisms that pertain to the biceps brachii muscle will be discussed in the section on pathokinesiology.

Torques

Provins and Salter published work on the torque generated about the elbow. It is of interest because the radioulnar joint position was altered as both flexion

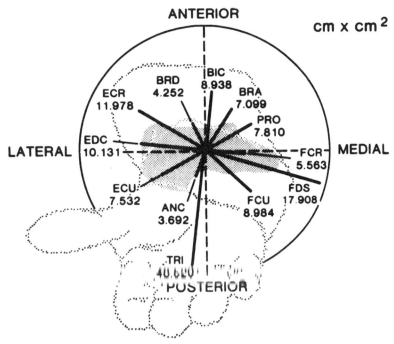

Figure 7.9. The contribution to flexion-extension and varus-valgus rotation about the joint center for the extended-supinated position of the elbow. The moment contribution of each muscle was estimated by multiplying the moment arm (cm) by its physiological cross sectional area (cm²). (From An KN, Hui FC, Morrey BF, et al: Muscles across the elbow joint: a biomechanical analysis. *J. Biomech* 14:668, 1981.)

and extension were studied. Their data are represented in Figure 7.10. Note that the elbow flexion torque was about 50% greater than the extension torque in all positions (26). Also note that for purposes of comparison the data of Elkins et al are included in the figure (10). Summarizing the results, the midposition of pronation-supination produced the greatest torque for flexors and extensors. This same finding for extension is interesting in view of the fact that hypothetically there should be no differences. The results are perhaps explainable on the bases of moment arm and muscle length. These authors completed an analysis of the length and "mechanical advantage" of the elbow flexors (Fig. 7.11). Thus, in terms of function, therapists should readily recognize that because of mechanics, the length-tension relationship, and anatomical factors, muscles may have varying roles as the joint proceeds through a dynamic range of motion. Andersson and Schultz tested healthy male subjects that generated 48 to 50 Nm of flexion torque at an elbow angle of 15°. The same subjects produced 82 to 83 Nm of torque at 90° of flexion. Their suggestion that different assisting maneuvers would increase the torque produced was not substantiated (3).

Functional Capacity

Kapandji's first volume on the physiology of joints includes a discussion of function in man as relates to "efficiency" of the flexor and extensor muscles. In discussing how the "power" of the muscle groups varies with the position of the shoulder he maintains that once the arm is stretched vertically above the shoulder, 43 kg(f) can be exerted during further attempted extension of the arm overhead. However, with the arm stretched above the shoulder and attempting

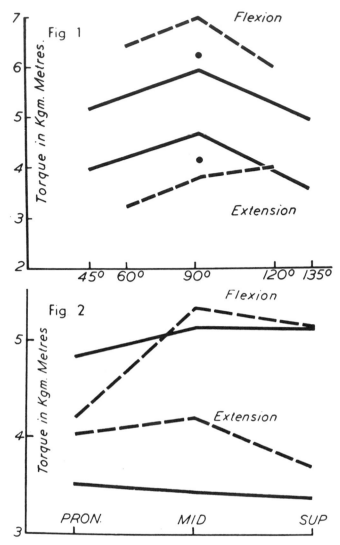

Figure 7.10. Top figure (*1*) shows the effect of elbow angle upon the maximum torque. *Dashed* and *solid lines* and *points* represent three different data sets. Bottom figure (*2*) shows the effect of forearm position on maximum torque for flexion and extension for two data sets. (From Provins KA, Salter N: Maximum torque exerted about the elbow joint. *J Appl Physiol* 7:395, 1955.)

to pull oneself upward the force is equivalent to 83 kg(f). Further, flexion forces, i.e., in rowing, are almost twice as great as forces available for pushing heavy loads forward. Thus, at least in the upper limb, man is well adapted for climbing (16).

Joint Forces

Many clinicians and basic scientists have discounted the importance of resultant joint forces at the elbow because the upper limb is non-weight-bearing. Hui et al discount this argument and show that maximal isometric flexion in the extended position yields joint contact forces equivalent to twice body weight. Shear forces in the specimens studied, although somewhat difficult to interpret

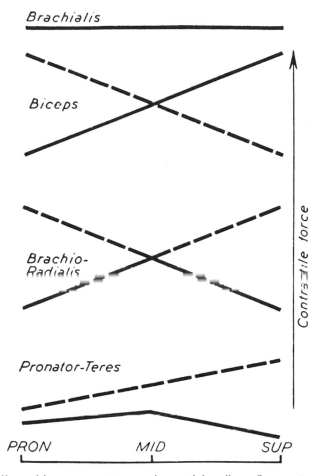

Figure 7.11. Effect of forearm position on force of the elbow flexors. Force increases on the vertical axis as shown by the vector. *Dashed line* represents length, and the *solid line* represents mechanical advantage. (From Provins KA, Salter N: Maximum torque exerted about the elbow joint. *J Appl Physiol* 7:397, 1955.)

from the data, also appeared to be considerable (15). In a very comprehensive analysis of elbow joint forces, Amis et al analyzed forearm abduction and adduction as well as elbow flexion and extension. The forces produced at the humeroulnar and humeroradial joints are shown in Figure 7.12 for flexion with triceps antagonism, and for extension with biceps antagonism in Figure 7.13. How these forces are distributed across the joint is an important factor in most circumstances where prostheses have been implanted (1). During more functional activities, Nicol, as cited by Matsen, found that dressing and eating create joint reaction forces of 300 newtons. Activities requiring pulling of heavy objects or assisting standing from sitting produce peak forces up to 1700 newtons (22).

PATHOKINESIOLOGY

Injuries affecting the joints of the elbow are usually not as disabling as those that affect either the shoulder or the wrist and hand. In neurological cases the result is frequently satisfactory in terms of kinesiological considerations because of the differing innervations of the muscles serving the elbow and radioulnar

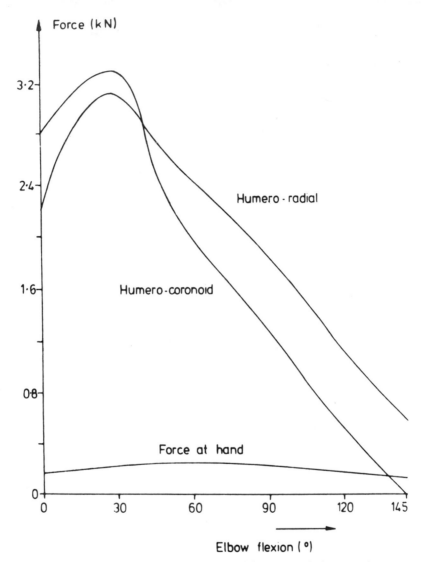

Figure 7.12. Forces at the humerocoronoid and humeroradial joints during isometric contractions with triceps antagonism. (From Amis AA, Dowson D, Wright V: Elbow joint force predictions for some strenuous isometric actions. *J Biomech* 13:772, 1980.)

joints. However, other pathologies can be acute, chronic, or require extensive surgery or immobilization. In this section the more common pathologies will be discussed by means of applying the information included in previous sections.

Neurological Injuries

Unless a patient suffers massive injury to the brachial plexus, the functional abilities associated with elbow and radioulnar joint motions are usually preserved. However, in blast injuries, as occasionally occur due to gunshot wounds or high pressure air hose explosions, limitations of the entire distal limb can be extremely debilitating. It is fortunate that the biceps and brachialis are innervated by the musculocutaneous nerve, since in rare injuries of this well protected nerve, the brachioradialis (radial nerve) and pronator teres (median nerve) muscles are

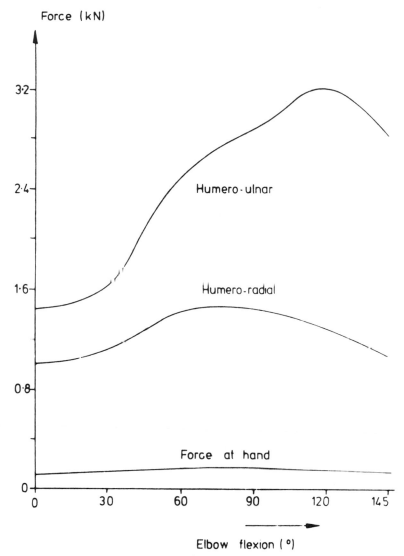

Figure 7.13. Same as Figure 7.12 except for extension with biceps brachii antagonism. (From Amis AA, Dowson D, Wright V: Elbow joint force predictions for some strenuous isometric actions. *J Biomech* 13:773, 1980.)

spared. Rarely, such as in postpoliomyelitis patients, are all elbow flexors lost. In such cases, patients have been known to flex the elbow with the ECRL and the ECRB. The point is that as long as an adequate moment arm and tension are available, a movement can be accomplished, even by a substitution.

The supination function can be carried out reasonably well by the supinator alone. However, heavy load manipulation can prove to be difficult in these injuries. Elbow flexion will be obviously weak. Injury to the radial nerve causes loss of the extensors and supinator, severely limiting the ability to extend the elbow. Du Toit and Levy have suggested the transposition of the latissimus dorsi to substitute for such a loss (9). Because the musculocutaneous nerve and the biceps muscle are still intact, the supination function is within normal limits. Finally, loss of the median nerve affects only pronation in the forearm, though its loss is disastrous to the thumb. However, because both pronator muscles are eliminated, effective pronation is lost.

Spinal cord-injured patients also show demonstrable examples of altered muscle function. For example, consider the C6 patient with no triceps available for elbow extension. However, if the hand is fixed on a surface, such as in push-ups from the seated position, the clavicular portion of the pectoralis major can serve to assist elbow extension by pulling the upper arm across the chest. Often, the torque-producing capability of this arrangement is enough to allow successful completion of the maneuver.

Soft Tissue Injuries

Soft tissue injuries are a common occurrence at the elbow. The capsule, ligaments, or tendons can be involved in inflammatory processes, sprains, or acute ruptures. Lateral epicondylitis has been related to involvement of numerous tissues, among them bursa, ligaments, and tears of the originations of the extensor musculature. Produced by overuse and often related to tennis playing the syndrome is felt by some to be a microscopic rupture and poor resulting natural repair of the origin of the extensor carpi radialis brevis (24). On the other side of the elbow, medial epicondylitis, sometimes known as "little league elbow," has been biomechanically analyzed. Hang et al hypothesized that throwing breaking pitches generates higher medial loading (14). Gainor et al determined torques and kinetic energy in the arm and also cited overloading as predisposing the humeral condylar changes that produce the symptoms frequently seen in the clinic. Several interesting cases, including a spiral fracture of the humerus, are included in their paper (13).

Inability of the soft tissues to adequately constrain motion occasionally results in the pulled radial head encountered in children. In these and other soft tissue injuries treatment is directed towards care of the symptoms, but some attention must be paid to the osteokinematics described in earlier sections. A key factor in effective treatment appears to be temporal elements as associated with periods of immobilization. Frequently the long-term results of elbow dislocations are unsatisfactory because of the inability of the patient to achieve a complete range of motion in either flexion or extension. Some of the effects of immobilization discussed in Chapter 2 may explain the difficulty in achieving the treatment goals. Although sufficient time for healing must be allowed, ultimate mobility cannot be sacrificed. More direct evidence for the advantages of early mobilization of tendons and joints will be more specifically discussed in Chapters 8 (wrist and hand) and 10 (knee).

One injury of reasonable frequency that affects the elbow is rupture of the biceps brachii muscle. Occurring more frequently in the long head of the muscle in middle aged persons, the result is immediate and permanent unless surgery is performed. Numerous causes have been postulated. Weakness in the tissue can be produced by degenerative changes, so that relatively inconsequential movements result in tensions that exceed the rupture strength of the musculotendinous unit. Also recall that the biceps brachii is a multiple joint muscle, in that joints affected are the radioulnar, elbow, and glenohumeral. As An et al. have shown, the fibers are relatively long (2). So, in sum and substance, the pronated elbow, accompanied by elbow and glenohumeral extension, could put considerable stretch on the biceps brachii muscle. Then, if additional force is added to the muscle by means of either contraction or quick stretch, the rupture point

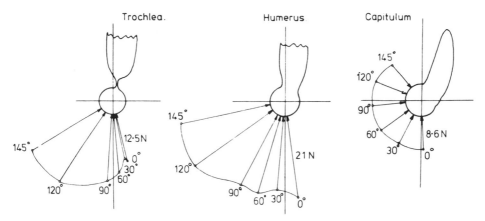

Figure 7.14. Location and magnitude of the forces at the articular surface of the humerus during extension. Forces are per unit of force at the hand. (From Amis AA, Dowson D, Wright V: Elbow joint force predictions for some strenuous isometric actions. *J Biomech* 13:773, 1980.)

may be reached, resulting in avulsion of the long head of the muscle from the glenoid labrum. Thus, since the muscle cannot produce any effective tension across the joint as intended, weakness results. Discomfort obviously results in the more acute stages, but muscles not repaired function quite adequately in the long term.

Joint Replacement

Much of the motivation for the study of the kinematics and kinetics of the elbow has been due to the more recent interest in total elbow prostheses. Based upon the data of Chao and Morrey (6), Youm et al (29), and London (21) a uniaxial hinged prosthesis has been recommended. However, caution must be exercised because either the ulnar rotation or the change in joint motion from sliding to rolling at the terminal phases of the range may be cause for loosening of the prosthetic components (6). London has also postulated that the axis of the device may not be aligned with the true axis, thus producing another potential cause of loosening (21). Amis includes a good review of the prosthetic problem and shows the forces on various components at different angles of elbow extension (Fig. 7.14). In continuing their discussion the suggestion is made that designers consider the inclusion of a flange on the lateral aspect of the olecranon for purposes of distributing shear forces (1). As other data become available certainly other suggestions for components will surface. Further discussion of the problems of prosthesis loosening will be included in Chapter 9 on the hip.

SUMMARY

This chapter has presented a discussion of the muscular contributions to the motions available in the multijoint elbow. Kinematics and kinetics were described in relation to their contribution to normal motion and possible role in pathological circumstances. Although considered a pure hinge joint, information that is surfacing is confirming that this approach is an oversimplification of the real conditions required for normal motion.

References

1. Amis AA, Dowson D, Wright V: Elbow joint force predictions for some strenuous isometric actions. *J Biomech* 13:765–775, 1980.
2. An KN, Hui FC, Morrey BF, Linscheid RL, Chao EY: Muscles across the elbow joint: a biomechanical analysis. *J. Biomech* 14:659–669, 1981.
3. Andersson GBJ, Schultz AB: Transmission of moments across the elbow joint and the lumbar spine. *J. Biomech* 12:747–756, 1979.
4. Basmajian JV, Griffin WR: Function of anconeus muscle: an electromographic study. *J Bone Joint Surg [Am]* 54:1712–1714, 1972.
5. Basmajian JV, Latif A: Integrated actions and functions of the chief flexors of the elbow: a detailed electromyographic analysis. *J Bone Joint Surg [Am]* 39:1106–1118, 1957.
6. Chao EY, Morrey BF: Three dimensional rotation of the elbow. *J Biomech* 11:57–73, 1978.
7. Currier DP: Maximal isometric tension of the elbow extensors at varied positions. *Phys Ther* 52:1043–1049, 1972.
8. Duchenne GBA: *Physiology of Motion Demonstrated by Means of Electrical Stimulation and Clinical Observation and Applied to the Study of Paralysis and Deformities.* Paris, 1855. (Translated and edited by Kaplan EB) Philadelphia, JB Lippincott, 1949, pp 98–105.
9. Du Toit GT, Levy SJ: Transposition of latissimus dorsi for paralysis of triceps brachii. *J Bone Joint Surg [Br]* 49:135–137, 1967.
10. Elkins EC, Leden UM, Wakim KG: Objective recording of the strength of normal muscles. *Arch Phys Med* 32:639–647, 1951.
11. Fick, R: *Anatomie und Mechanik der Gelenke.* Teil III, Spezielle Gelenk und MuskelMechanik. Jena, Switzerland, 1911.
12. Fischer, O: Zur kinematik der gelenke vom typus des humeroradial gelenkes. *Abh Math-Phys Cl Sk K Sachs Ges* 32:3–77, 1909.
13. Gainor BJ, Piotrowski G, Puhl J, et al: The throw: biomechanics and acute injury. *Am J Sports Med* 8:114–118, 1980.
14. Hang YS, Lippert FG, Spolek GA, Frankel VH, Harrington RM: Biomechanical study of the pitching elbow. *Int Orthop* 3:217–223, 1979.
15. Hui FC, Chao EY, An KN: Muscle and joint forces at the elbow during isometric lifting. *Abstracts of 24th Annual Orthopedic Research Society,* Dallas, Texas, February, 1978, p 167.
16. Kapandji AI: *The Physiology of the Joints,* ed 5. New York, Churchill Livingstone, 1982.
17. Kessler R, Hertling D: *Management of Common Musculoskeletal Disorders.* New York, Harper & Row, 1983.
18. Larson RF: Forearm positioning on maximal elbow-flexor force. *J Am Phys Ther Assoc* 49:748–756, 1969.
19. Lehmkuhl LD, Smith LK: *Brunnstrom's Clinical Kinesiology,* ed 4, Philadelphia, FA Davis, 1983.
20. Little AD, Lehmkuhl D: Elbow extension force measured in three positions. *J Am Phys Ther Assoc* 46:7–17, 1966.
21. London JT: Kinematics of the elbow. *J Bone Joint Surg [Am]* 63:529–535, 1981.
22. Matsen FA: Biomechanics of the elbow. In Frankel VM, Nordin M (eds): *Basic Biomechanics of the Skeletal System.* Philadelphia, Lea & Febiger, 1980.
23. Morrey BF, Askew LJ, An KN, et al: A biomechanical study of normal functional elbow motion. *J Bone Joint Surg [Am]* 63:872–877, 1981.
24. Nirschl RP, Pettrone FA: Tennis elbow: the surgical treatment of lateral epicondylitis. *J Bone Joint Surg [Am]* 61:832–839, 1979.
25. Pauly JE, Rushing JL, Scheving LE: An electromyographic study of some muscles crossing the elbow joint. *Anat Rec* 159:47–53, 1967.
26. Provins KA, Salter N: Maximum torque exerted about the elbow joint. *J Appl Phys* 7:393–398, 1955.
27. Steindler A: *Kinesiology of the Human Body under Normal and Pathological Conditions.* Springfield, IL, Charles C Thomas, 1955.
28. Warwick R, Williams PL (eds): *Gray's Anatomy,* ed 36. Philadelphia, WB Saunders, 1980.
29. Youm Y, Dryer RF, Thambyajah K, et al: Biomechanical analyses of forearm pronation-supination and elbow flexion-extension. *J Biomech* 12:245–255, 1979.

8

Wrist and Hand

The wrist and hand provide a series of joints that dictate the functional capabilities unique to man. The importance of the hand is manifested by the large area of the central nervous system devoted to control of the distal segments of the upper extremity. Capable of extremely fine movements such as required during the threading of a needle, the wrist and hand must also regularly perform gross tasks requiring considerable force. Discussed in this chapter are the arthrology and arthrokinematics, biomechanics, and kinetics associated with both normal and pathological motion of the wrist and hand.

MUSCULAR ACTIONS
Wrist

The musculature at the wrist may be conveniently considered on the basis of function as related to the four primary motions of flexion, extension, and radial and ulnar deviation. Of these motions the most important are extension and flexion, because they are crucial to effective hand function. The three primary extensors, carpi radialis longus and brevis and carpi ulnaris, are all dedicated to control of the wrist. The other tendons passing distally across the wrist must be considered to assist control of wrist extension. Included within this assistive group are extensors digitorum, digiti minimi, pollicis longus, and indicis proprius. Of some interest is that all of the extensor muscles are innervated by the radial nerve. This is of practical significance because effective hand function is ultimately dependent upon positioning of the wrist in extension.

Flexion is the responsibility of two muscles: flexors carpi radialis and ulnaris. Another muscle, the palmaris longus, may play a role in wrist flexion, but the import of this muscle is probably minimal. In fact, the muscle is often absent uni- or bilaterally. However, presence may provide a "spare" tendon for potential surgical transfer. Certainly strong assistive function is possible by use of the flexors digitorum superficialis and profundus, but only if the muscles are not being used simultaneously for flexion of the digits. Finally, the flexor pollicis longus may assist wrist flexion.

Radial and ulnar deviation at the wrist is the result of synergistic contraction of muscles whose primary action is either extension or flexion of the wrist. For example, radial deviation (RD) is carried out by the simultaneous action of the flexor and extensor carpi radialis muscles. Assistance during powerful movements may be obtained from the musculature arising from the forearm and passing to the thumb. Conversely, ulnar deviation (UD) is accomplished by contraction of

149

the flexor and extensor carpi ulnaris muscles. Furthermore, all muscles can be cyclicly contracted to perform circumduction (circling) of the wrist. Because of the location of the wrist extensors and flexors, numerous examples of antagonistic and synergistic contraction may be cited. Study of a cross section taken through the wrist confirms the actions of these muscles (Fig. 8.1). Note that the moment arms vary considerably and that many combinations of tension (synergistic action) could produce the desired result.

The radial and ulnar carpi muscles function synergistically in providing wrist positions for various hand functions. However, these same muscles act as antagonists in radial and ulnar deviation. Kauer, in an attempt to determine the role of musculature in wrist stability, recorded EMG activity in several wrist muscles during flexion-extension and radioulnar deviation with the forearm in pronated and supinated positions. Results showed that the extensor carpi ulnaris, the abductor pollicis longus, and the extensor pollicis brevis were active during both flexion and extension. Differences in activity were recorded when the supinated position was compared with the pronated position. Because minimal displacements of the tendons were noted during flexion of the wrist, Kauer concluded that these three muscles could be considered an adjustable collateral system that provides support at the wrist (14).

In another study, wrist muscle activity was evaluated during grasping motions of the normal hand. Extensor activity was observed primarily in the extensor carpi radialis brevis. Increased gripping efforts resulted in increased activity seen first in the extensor carpi ulnaris and then the extensor carpi radialis longus (22). Other cases of synergistic action are included in later sections of this chapter.

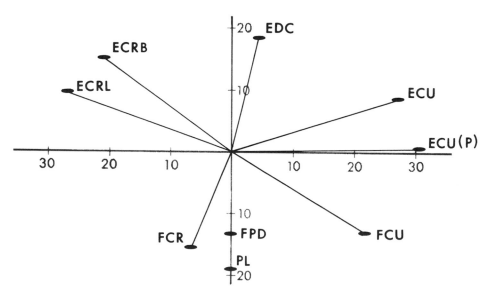

Figure 8.1.   The location of the muscles that cross the wrist are shown in terms of location from the axis of motion. All distances are in millimeters. Muscles are abbreviated as follows: *ECRL,* extensor carpi radialis longus; *ECRB,* extensor carpi radialis brevis; *EDC,* extensor digitorum; *ECU* and *ECU(P),* extensor carpi ulnaris with forearm supinated and pronated, respectively; *FCU,* flexor carpi ulnaris; *FPR,* flexor digitorum profundus; *PL,* palmaris longus; *FCR,* flexor carpi radialis. (From Brand PW: Biomechanics of tendon transfer. *Orthop Clin North Am* 5:205–230, 1984.)

Hand

Musculature of the hand is complex. A comprehensive discussion of hand anatomy is contained in classic works such as that by Landsmeer (16). Anatomic relationships are confounded by the presence of two special digits, the thumb and index finger, and because of the muscles controlling the digits arise from the forearm. That these muscles also cross the wrist means that wrist position and dynamic function will influence the activity of musculature as control of the digits is attempted.

The thumb has a complex arrangement of muscles, with four intrinsic to the hand and four extrinsic from the forearm (31). The four muscles arising from the forearm include only one brevis (the extensor pollicis) and three pollicis longi: the flexor, abductor, and extensor. Those intrinsic to the hand include two pollicis brevi (the flexor and abductor) along with the opponens and adductor pollicis. This arrangement allows one to draw the thumb across the hand and to oppose the pad of the thumb with the medial aspect of the hand or little finger. Without such capability, the function of the hand would be severely compromised.

The index, long, and ring fingers have a common muscular arrangement. Extension of all phalangeal joints is directly produced or influenced by the extensor digitorum (19). Some consider the extensor digitorum to extend only the metacarpophalangeal (MP) joints, with full extension of the proximal and distal interphalangeal joints (PIP and DIP) by the intrinsics via the dorsal hood. Warwick and Williams state that the intrinsics place tension on the dorsal hood, allowing the extensor digitorum to extend the IP joints (32). In addition, both the interossei and lumbricals flex the MP joints of their respective fingers, while the interossei are able to abduct or adduct the digit to which they are attached (Fig. 8.2). The lumbricals are unique in that they are capable of relaxing their own antagonist via their proximal attachment to the flexor digitorum profundus tendons. As they contract, the distal portions of the profundus tendons are slackened, allowing more complete interphalangeal extension while the lumbricals also tighten the extensor expansion.

Extensive study of the extensor expansion has been undertaken because of the importance of this apparatus for normal hand function. As pointed out by Smith, fiber expansions of the interossei and extensor digitorum essentially serve to assist both IP extension and MP flexion. This is accomplished via insertion of the interosseus tendons into the transverse fibers of the expansion, producing MP flexion. In addition, the remainder of the insertion goes to the extensor expansion for IP extension. Note should also be made of the use of the sagittal bands for effective MP joint extension (Fig. 8.3) (25). Other detailed accounts of the anatomy of the expansion are contained in both anatomy texts and journal articles (15, 31, 32).

Comprehensive accounts of the anatomy of the intrinsic musculature are contained in such works as those by Flatt (11). Flexion of the MP joint is produced by both the flexors digitorum superficialis and profundus. As these muscles project distally, however, the superficialis divides and sends slips to the base of the middle phalanx, allowing the profundus to pass to the base of the distal phalanx.

The little finger has anatomical features common to fingers index, long, and ring, but also has special features related to functional requirements. Abduction

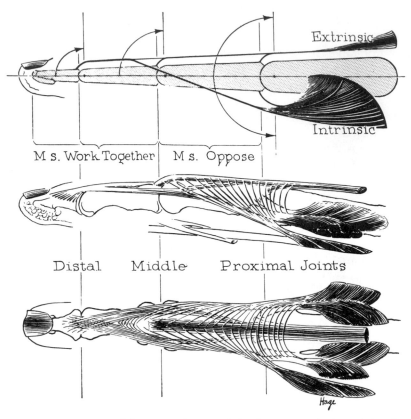

Figure 8.2. Three views of the musculature of the fingers, exclusive of the thumb. The top two are lateral views, the lowest a view of the dorsal surface. (From Flatt AE: *The Care of Minor Hand Injuries.* St. Louis, CV Mosby, 1959, p 27.)

is produced by the abductor digiti minimi muscle, in a manner similar to the first dorsal interosseus muscle and in contrast to those of the third and fourth digits. Hollowing of the palm, such as when attempting to hold water in the palm of the hand or when grasping a cylinder, is facilitated by the opponens digiti minimi. Finally, the MP joint has an additional flexor; the digiti minimi brevis. Table 8.1 provides a summary of the motions and the responsible musculature.

Combined Motions

Resulting from these anatomical arrangements is a meaningful and coordinated pattern of movement. Effective function is due to the provision of power by the extrinsic musculature, while fine control is left to the intrinsic musculature of the hand. Effective motion is created by interaction of the various segments as a particular task is accomplished. For example, extension of the interphalangeal joints is accomplished by the intrinsic muscles when the MP joint is concurrently being extended by the extensor digitorum muscle. Conversely, flexion of the MP joint is completed by the intrinsics as the extensor digitorum extends the IP joints. Furthermore, the long finger flexors can affect motion of the proximal finger and wrist joints if the more distal joints are stabilized. Or, if the proximal joints are stabilized the long flexors can effectively function through their attachments at the distal joints. The interaction of these muscles allows for motions

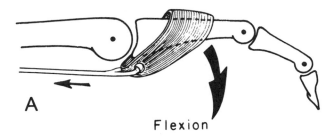

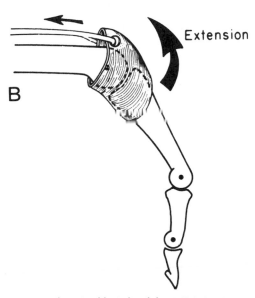

Figure 8.3.   The transverse and sagittal bands of the MP joint. In *A* note that the transverse fibers of the interosseus facilitate MP joint flexion. In *B*, the sagittal bands of the extensor tendon insert into the volar plate, acting as an extensor. (From Smith RJ: Balance and kinetics of the fingers under normal and pathological conditions. *Clin Orthop* 104:92–111, 1974.)

such as simultaneous flexion of the IP joints and extension of the MP joints by respective action of the long finger flexors and the extensor digitorum. Or, all joints of the fingers may simultaneously extend or flex, with the former by action of both the extensor digitorum and the intrinsics. Other combinations are possible, but the above include the most important combinations required for functional activities (32).

In order to effectively perform the functions just described the wrist must be held in a position that will allow the musculature to develop or maintain the required tension. Chapter Two of this volume discussed the length-tension relationship for human muscle. Because many of the muscles that affect finger motion originate in the forearm and pass across the wrist, the length of these muscles can be significantly influenced by altering the position of the wrist. Consider the case where the wrist is placed in full flexion. In this configuration, as may be the case in radial nerve injuries, the long finger flexor musculature has simultaneously been shortened. Because significantly less tension is available

Table 8.1.   Wrist and Hand Muscle Actions[a,b]

Muscle	Wrist Flexion	Wrist Extension	Wrist Abduction	Wrist Adduction	MP Flexion	MP Extension	MP Abduction	MP Adduction	PIP 1st Flexion	PIP 1st Extension	DIP 2nd Flexion	DIP 2nd Extension	CMC Flexion	CMC Extension	CMC Abduction	CMC Adduction	CMC Opposition
Flexor carpi radialis	P		S														
Flexor carpi ulnaris	P			S													
Palmaris longus	P																
Extensor carpi radialis longus		P	S														
Extensor carpi radialis brevis		P	S														
Extensor carpi ulnaris		P		S													
Flexor digitorum profundus	S				S						P						
Flexor digitorum superficialis	S				S				P								
Extensor digitorum		S				P				P		P					
Extensor indicis		S				P				P		P					
Extensor digiti minimi		S				P	S			P		P					
Lumbricals					P					P		P					
Dorsal interossei					P		P			P		P					
2nd, 3rd, and 4th palmar interossei					P			P		P		P					
Abductor digiti minimi							P										
Flexor digiti minimi brevis					P												
Opponens digiti minimi					P												
Extensor pollicis longus		S	S							P						S	
Extensor pollicis brevis			S			P									S		
Abductor pollicis longus	S		S											S	P		
Abductor pollicis brevis														S	P		
Flexor pollicis longus	S				S				P							S	S
Flexor pollicis brevis													P				S
Opponens pollicis													P			S	P
Adductor pollicis																P	

[a] From Favill J: *Outline of the Spinal Nerves.* Springfield, IL, Charles C Thomas, 1946.
[b] Abduction-adduction at MP joints is relative to line located along long axis of long finger. For thumb muscles PIP is equivalent to IP joint. Abbreviations used are: MP, metacarpophalangeal joint; PIP, proximal interphalangeal joint; DIP, distal interphalangeal joint; CMC, carpometacarpal joint of thumb; P, primary function; S, secondary function.

when the muscle is extremely shortened, only limited tension is available in the flexor digitorum superficialis and profundus. As a result, little grip strength can be achieved with the wrist in full flexion. Full and forceful wrist flexion may even cause an assailant to lose an effective grip on an intended weapon. Consequently, the optimal position for hand function is probably at 20 to 30° of wrist extension. Similar effects upon extension of the fingers can be seen if the wrist is completely extended. In this case the extensor digitorum muscle is slackened, preventing sufficient extension torques to be generated at the MP and IP joints.

There are mechanical implications arising from these anatomic features. The arrangement of the flexor digitorum profundus and superficialis muscles provides an example. Because the profundus tendon passes deep to the superficialis at a point near the proximal IP joint, the profundus can act to elevate the superficialis tendon and increase its angle of insertion into the base of the middle phalanx. Another example arises from considerations associated with the lumbrical and interosseous muscles. Although the interossei have twice the cross sectional area, the lumbrical muscles have a longer possible excursion. However, the lumbricals have a better mechanical advantage because their line of action is farther from the joint axis. Therefore, they are considered to have an overall advantage for creating joint torque during grasping.

Synergistic actions can also be readily demonstrated in the wrist and hand. Warwick and Williams, among others, cite one interesting case. When the abductor digiti minimi muscle contracts to abduct the fifth finger at the MP joint the flexor carpi ulnaris can be palpated to contract, exerting a countertraction on the pisiform bone from which the abductor originates. To prevent the flexor carpi ulnaris from producing ulnar deviation and wrist flexion, the abductor pollicis longus contracts to neutralize both motions (32). Many other complex events such as typing, piano playing, and object manipulations require serial synergistic events. The remarkable coordination demonstrated occasionally leaves us in awe of our own abilities.

Much of the functional capability of the hand is derived from the special abilities of the thumb. In particular, opposition of the thumb to the other digits provides a great variety of postures that the hand can assume in carrying out activities. Opposition is usually thought of as pulp-to-pulp (pad-to-pad) contact of the thumb with any of the other digits. In addition, the thumb can assume other relationships with the fingers, accounting for many other hand postures. Many classifications of hand function have been developed. Kapandji states that there are six modes of prehension, of which four require the thumb. One example is terminal opposition, which is considered the most precise mode of prehension. In this case a fine object is held between the thumb and index finger. Another mode is prehension by subterminal opposition, probably the most commonly used manipulative technique. An example of this mode is the grasp of a pencil or a piece of paper between the thumb and index finger (13).

Some of the other modes specified by Kapandji are similar to a more commonly accepted classification described by Flatt: tip, palmar, and lateral. Tip grip utilizes PIP joint flexion as the very tips of the digits oppose each other. The palmar grip uses more of a pad-to-pad opposition. The third type, lateral or key grip, uses the thumb against the side of the finger, usually the radial side of the first PIP of the index finger. Palmar grip is the most frequently used mechanism, especially for holding or picking up objects (11).

ARTHROLOGY AND ARTHROKINEMATICS

As for other joints in the body, the bony framework and configuration is responsible for the resulting kinematics. The close interrelationship between the hand and wrist must be kept in mind, despite the fact that they will be considered separately in this section.

Wrist

Because of the numerous bones comprising the "wrist," the analysis of motion is complex. Most sources distinguish a proximal and a distal row of carpals. Volz et al state that the two rows of carpals operate nearly as separate segments, yet with an integrated relationship (30). Kauer offers a very detailed account of carpal motion while stressing that the wrist operates as a link system. From a cineradiographic analysis, simultaneous movement was observed to occur in the radiocarpal joint and the midcarpal joints. Reference is made to the action of the scaphoid and the lunate upon each other and upon other bones. The import of the scaphoid is brought out because this bone contacts the capitate, lunate, radius, trapezium, and trapezoid. In general, carpal morphology creates a functional system composed of three parallel longitudinal chains that require simultaneous movements at multiple joints in order to achieve normal function (14).

MacConaill states that in accomplishing complete extension (the close-packed position), the carpus rotates toward supination (18). This rotary movement occurs at the junction of the scaphoid and the radius, because the other articulations have already achieved their respective close-packed positions. Kessler and Hertling have also provided a detailed account of specific kinematics. Upon flexion-extension, the scaphoid moves more with respect to the forearm than do the lunate and triquetrum. This asymmetrical motion produces tension in the joint capsules and ligaments during extension, resulting in the close-packed position. Other rotations occur during radial and ulnar deviation, with the former producing the close-packed position of the midcarpal (intercarpal) joint (15). A recent analysis of wrist kinematics modelled the normal wrist after a tight, universal joint in that little or no longitudinal rotation is allowed between one segment (hand) and the other (forearm) (2).

Specific components of wrist movement have been studied by a number of investigators. In 1977, the Sarrafian group studied flexion and extension by means of a roentgenographic analysis of 55 normal wrists. Average measurements demonstrated that 40%, or 26°, of flexion occurred at the radiocarpal joint. The remaining 60% occurred during the 40° of motion at the midcarpal joint. Conversely, the radiocarpal joint involved two-thirds of the extension in comparison with one-third at the midcarpal joint. A summary of these findings is shown in Figure 8.4. The functional significance of this study was the conclusion that the scaphoid belongs to the second row of carpals during extension and to the first row during flexion (24).

The center of rotation of the wrist during flexion, extension, radial deviation, and ulnar deviation has been identified. During these motions, the center is located at the base of the capitate bone, being slightly more proximal during flexion-extension than radial-ulnar deviation (Fig. 8.5) (34). Youm and coworkers also found that for passive radial deviation from neutral to 20° motion was minimal in the proximal row. However, for passive ulnar deviation up to 37° of motion occurred at both the radiocarpal and midcarpal joints.

Note should also be made that the articulation of the metacarpals with the carpals varies from the radial to the ulnar side of the hand. The joints are limited in range for the index and long fingers, but for the ring and little there is increased motion. Observation of this effort can be made by viewing the dorsal surface of the hand while proceeding from a light to a strong grip. The increased motion apparently allows for more effective grip and cupping of the hand.

Hand

The MP and IP joints have also been examined from an arthrokinematic viewpoint. Flatt noted that the narrow metacarpal head allows for lateral movement at the MP joint in full extension. However, upon full flexion, the collateral ligaments tighten due to the shape of the head of the metacarpals (11). Youm et

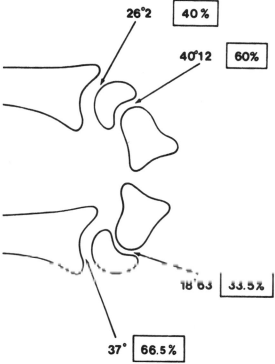

Figure 8.4. Representation of motion in the wrist. Flexion is shown in the upper view and extension in the lower. Both actual motion and percentages are shown for the radiocarpal and midcarpal motions. (From Sarrafian SH, Melamed JL, Goshgarian GM: Study of wrist motion in flexion and extension. *Clin Orthop* 126:153–159, 1977.)

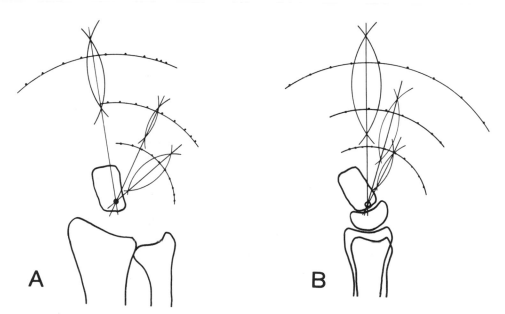

Figure 8.5. Centers of rotation during radial-ulnar deviation (*A*) and flexion and extension (*B*) for the wrist, indicated by the circle in the proximal capitate. (From Youm Y, McMurtry RY, Flatt AE, Gillespie TE: Kinematics of the wrist. *J Bone Joint Surg* [*Am*] 60:423–431, 1978.)

al, in a companion work to their efforts on the wrist, studied the kinematic behavior of the MP joint and quantified radial-ulnar deviation at the joint during various positions of MP flexion and extension. They measured 40° of radial-ulnar deviation in neutral, only 10° in full flexion, and 25° at a position 30° past full extension. They found the center of rotation of the MP joint to be fixed on the midline of the metacarpal, at a point proximal to the joint line by one-tenth the metacarpal length (33).

The DIP and PIP joints lack a collateral ligament tightening mechanism. In fact, Flatt states that the collateral ligaments are tight in all positions of the IP joints (11). Study of the distal IP joints demonstrates some of the unique features associated with joint surfaces. Asymmetries of the metacarpal head are the rule, causing an incomplete fit and ensuing accessory motions. Furthermore, because the condyles of the phalanges do not extend distally to the same amount, the long axes of the ring and middle finger deviate toward the long finger (12). The resultant effect is that upon flexion, the fingers rotate toward the thumb, helping to maximize the function of the hand.

Special consideration should be given to the thumb, because of the import of this digit to effective hand function. In fact, some consider the thumb to be 40% or greater of the hand's functional value (31). Techniques of wire fixation, goniometry, and cineradiography have been used to study the function of the carpometacarpal (CMC) joint. Cooney et al, however, have presented quantitatively derived, in vivo data. With respect to a reference system associated with the third metacarpal, the CMC joint had 53° of flexion-extension, 42° of adduction-abduction, and 17° of rotation. A key finding was that the 17° occurs in conjunction with the four primary movements of flexion, extension, abduction, and adduction. The motions of the CMC and the MP joint of the thumb, which together are responsible for opposition, are a result of joint surface geometry, muscle action, and limitations imposed by ligamentous structures (9).

BIOMECHANICS

Published information relating to the biomechanics of the wrist and hand has usually been specific to either kinematics or kinetics. More global studies are limited by the complexity of the series of articulations, therefore making comprehensive studies difficult or impossible on the grounds that all of the many variables cannot be controlled. In spite of these problems, the anatomy and applied mechanics of the hand provide the opportunity to further our knowledge of the significance of altering mechanics by injury or through surgical repair. For example, the results of tendon transfer are directly related to altering the "mechanical advantage" (moment arm) and/or the excursion capability of the transferred muscle. Because the clinician and the patient assess effectiveness of tendon transfers in terms of function and because the long finger muscles are frequently used in transfers, most of the current information concerns these muscles.

As can be anticipated from knowledge of the extensor mechanism, the moment arm of the extensor tendons remains virtually constant throughout the range of flexion and extension. Conversely, as the MP joint moves from extension to full flexion the moment arm of the flexors increases about 50% (33). An et al studied the influence of excursions of the index finger joints and confirmed previous work. Figure 8.6 shows relatively constant moment arms for the extensors and minor changes produced in the radial and ulnar interossei muscles during MP

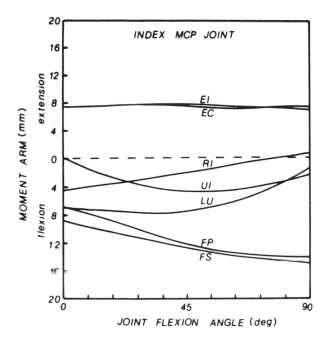

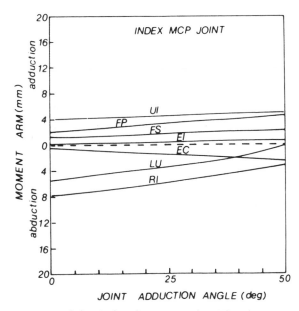

Figure 8.6. Moment arms of the index finger muscles. The determinations were made at the MP joint for flexion and extension (above) and abduction and adduction (below). Muscles abbreviations are: *FS*, flexor digitorus superficialis; *FP*, flexor digitorum profundus; *EC*, extensor digitorus communis; *EI*, extensor indicis; *RI*, radial interosseous; *LU*, lumbrical; and *UI*, ulnar interosseous. (From An KN, Ubea Y, Chao EY, Cooney WP, Linscheid RL: Tendon excursion and moment arm of index finger muscles. *J Biomech* 16:419–425, 1983.)

joint flexion. Note, however, the increase for the long flexors produced by MP joint flexion, but little effect produced by MP abduction-adduction (1).

Another method was used by Brand et al in evaluating muscles of the forearm and hand. Extensive dissection and calculations were completed to determine mean fiber length and "physiological" cross section of various muscles. Based on data for all the muscles in the forearm a "tension fraction" was calculated for each muscle, yielding a determination of its "tension" relative to all other muscles in the forearm and hand. Their data are valuable because excursion values, one determinant of function, are also included in their analysis (5). Others, including Youm et al and An et al, have also studied tendon excursion in the hand. The former group determined that tendon excursions of the long flexors generally exceeded 20 mm when the MP joint was moved from 30° of extension to 90° of flexion. Little change in tendon excursion occurred in the interossei during MP flexion-extension, and only slightly more was noted upon finger abduction-adduction. These investigators also pointed out that MP joint stability is dependent on the action of the intrinsic muscles in the neutral position (33).

An et al displaced all joints of the index finger in evaluating tendon excursion. A representative result is shown in Figure 8.7. Negative values indicate shortening, while positive values demonstrate elongation. Note the essentially linear changes in the long flexors and extensors and the tendency for the intrinsic muscles to reach their peak change at midrange. Excursions for the IP joints and the MP joint in adduction-abduction were of relatively small magnitude when considered in relationship to the changes produced by MP flexion (1).

KINETICS

Forces delivered to the various joints of the thumb, hand, and wrist are critical to the function of the hand. The balance of forces is carefully regulated within the normal hand by phenomena that are not precisely known. When an imbalance is created by injury or disease, restoration of function is contingent on generating sufficient tension in the correct temporal sequence. However, little is known about the true forces exerted by the musculature in the forearm and hand.

Tension generated in muscles can be estimated from the cross sectional area of the individual muscles. Care must be taken as to the fiber direction in order to make a precise determination of the available tension, i.e., cross sectional areas must be taken perpendicular to the fiber direction. Studies specifying the cross section have been completed, but the work of Brand and coworkers is the first to actually calculate "tension fractions" based on the individual muscle's contribution to the total mass of the forearm and hand (5). (See earlier section.)

Theoretical work has also been completed on the static forces in the thumb. Results showed tendon forces that varied from 0.9 to 3.52 kg for the tip grip and from 1.29 to 5.61 kg for the lateral grip. During grasp, tendon forces reached over 50 kg in the abductor pollicis longus muscle (8).

Joint forces have not been studied frequently in the upper limb because of its nonweight-bearing role and the few pathological changes created by its relatively low compression forces. In a study completed by Cooney, shear, rotation, bending, and compression forces were determined for all of the joints in the thumb. Generally, the magnitudes of these joint forces were 2 kg or less at all joints for 1 kg of tip or key grip force. Joint compressive force, however, reached

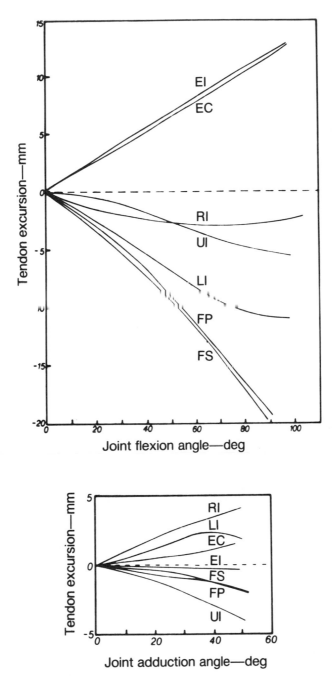

Figure 8.7. Tendon excursion plotted versus joint angle at the MP joint. Positive values are elongations (distal) displacements, negative are shortening (retraction) movements of the tendons. Flexion and adduction are shown in the respective graphs. Muscle abbreviations are: *FS*, flexor digitorum superficialis; *FP*, flexor digitorum profundus; *EC*, extensor digitorum communis; *EI*, extensor indicis; *RI*, radial interosseous; *LI*, lumbrical; and *UI*, ulnar interosseous. (From An KN, Ubea Y, Chao EY, Cooney WP, Linscheid RL: Tendon excursion and moment arm of index finger muscles. *J Biomech* 16:419–425, 1983.)

as much as 120 kg at the CMC joint during strong grasp (8). Volz et al showed that small compressive loads are transmitted through the scaphoid, lunate, and distal radius. As the load is increased, compressive load is also transmitted through the distal radioulnar fibrocartilage surfaces (30).

Thus, significant forces do occur in the tissues of the wrist and hand. The requirements during functional activities have been assessed on a limited basis, and more information is needed in this regard (7). Disruption of kinetics resulting from pathologies, such as arthritis or trauma, or from surgical procedures may lead to deformity and dysfunction. How such disruptions in kinematics and kinetics are manifested is discussed in the next section.

PATHOKINESIOLOGY

Located at the distal portion of the limb made free by the assumption of the upright posture, the wrist and hand are essential to the function of man. Gross positioning of the limb in space is essentially ineffective if objects or functions cannot be carried out by a dextrous hand. Simple experiences with hands that have become extremely cold are demonstration enough of the loss of abilities upon which humans so depend. Subsequently, any loss created by neurological or musculoskeletal injury has the potential to be devastating. The remainder of this chapter will discuss how commonly encountered pathologies affect function of the wrist and hand.

Nerve Injuries

The effects of peripheral nerve injury are well established. Individual or collective loss of the radial, median, and ulnar nerves have differing effects, the magnitude of which depends upon the degree and site of injury.

Ulnar nerve injuries that are proximal, i.e., above the innervation site for the flexor digitorum profundus muscle, will cause loss of abduction and adduction of all the fingers. Flexion power will also be decreased, particularly in the ring and little fingers. Typically, the hand assumes a posture similar to that assumed for purposes of clawing at some object. More distal injury to the ulnar nerve leaves the flexor profundus and flexor superficialis muscles intact; thus, the effects on gripping are not as pronounced. Loss of the lumbricals for the ring and little finger, in combination with the loss of the interossei and thumb adduction, produce significant changes (Fig. 8.8). The ring and little fingers are unable to flex at the MP joints or extend at the IP joints, resulting in the ulnar "claw hand" (Fig. 8.9). A further implication is that the long finger flexors cause IP flexion, preventing opposition to the thumb. Sensory changes are apparent over the ulnar two fingers and the ulnar surface of the hand. The ulnar one-half of the long finger may also demonstrate loss in some patients.

Median nerve injury affects the thumb, in severe cases so much so that the thumb remains extended. The thenar eminence is markedly flattened (Fig. 8.10). Because of the effect on the index and long fingers (superficialis and profundus), the hand assumes the posture of a brachiating ape. Sensory changes predominate over the palmar surface of the hand on the radial side, including the thenar eminence.

Combined high median and ulnar nerve losses will paralyze all interossei and lumbricals, superficialis and profundus, thus causing total loss of all finger-flexing ability. Combined paralysis of distal (forearm) ulnar and median nerves produces a hand in which no intrinsic (lumbricals and interossei) muscles are functional. The result is the intrinsic minus hand in which the MP joint is hyperextended

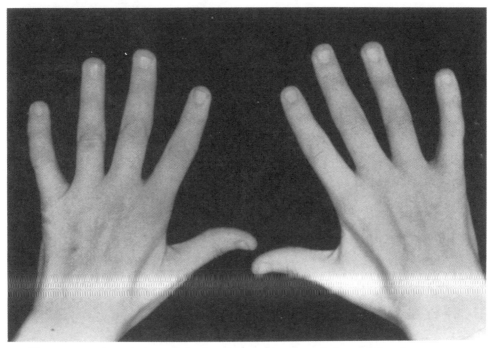

Figure 8.8.   Dorsal view of the hands, resulting from lesions of the ulnar nerves.

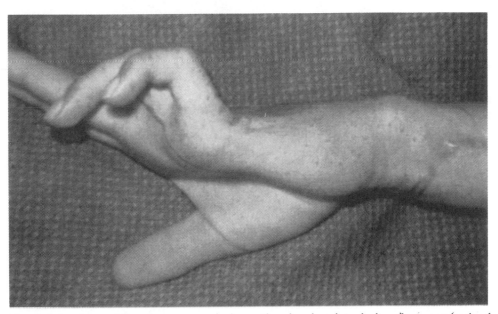

Figure 8.9.   Loss of the ulnar nerve produces the claw hand, including flexion at both of the IP joints of the ring and little fingers. (From Conolly WB: *Color Atlas of Hand Conditions.* Chicago, Year Book Medical Publishers, 1980, p 89.)

and the IP joints are flexed (Figs. 8.11 to 8.13). To study the effects, Srinivasan evaluated movement patterns of the MP and IP joints in 141 fingers. The conclusion was that the long flexors and extensors produced simultaneous rather than successive MP flexion and PIP extension. Although equal range of motion

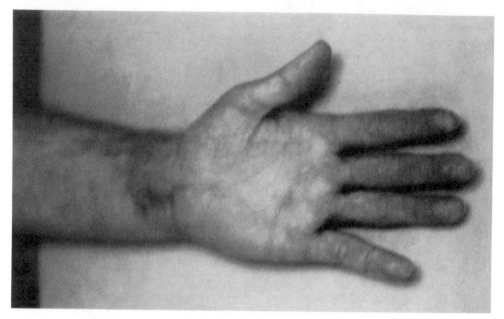

Figure 8.10.   Typical appearance of the hand following long-term injury to the median nerve. Note specifically the flattening of the thenar eminence.

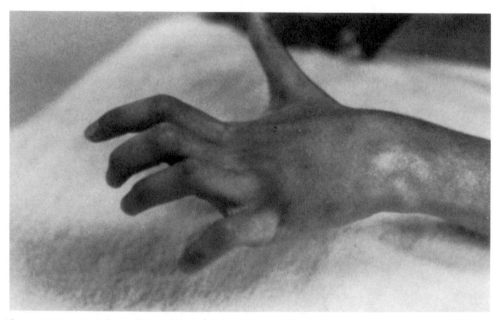

Figure 8.11.   Combined loss of the distal portion of the median and ulnar nerves produces loss of both the lumbricals and the interossei. The posture of the hand is shown.

was achieved at MP and PIP joints the latter was achieved without excessive motion at the PIP joint. In extension PIP movement lagged behind MP extension, so much so that full extension was not achieved even when the MP joint was maximally extended (27).

Radial nerve palsies may result from humeral fractures, shoulder dislocations, and other causes. Resultant loss of wrist extension, called "wrist drop," prevents

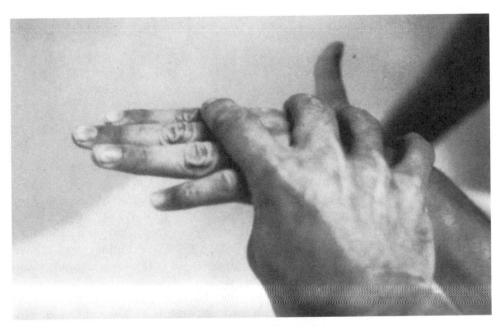

Figure 8.12. Same hand is shown as in Figure 8.11. In this view the MP joint is stabilized, allowing extension of the IP joints by the extensor digitorum.

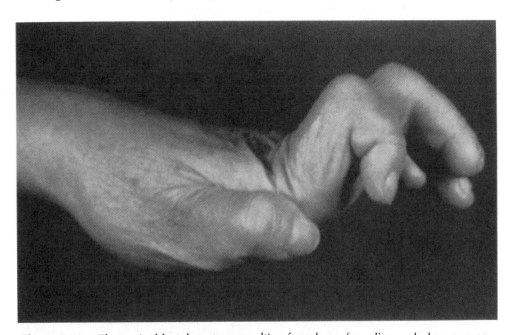

Figure 8.13. The typical hand posture resulting from loss of median and ulnar nerves.

effective grip because the long finger flexors do not have a stabilized wrist across which flexion of the fingers can occur. This is due to the fact that as the flexors attempt to close the fingers they also act to flex the wrist because the wrist extensor muscles have been lost. Due to the simultaneous flexion at the MP, IP, and wrist, effective tension is unavailable because the muscles have undergone significant shortening. Additional losses resulting from radial nerve injury include extension of the MP joints by the extensor digitorum and extension of the thumb (25).

In some spinal cord-injured patients some benefit may be derived from a flexor tenodesis, a procedure that removes a length of the flexor tendon(s). As a result, passive tension is created in the flexors as stretch is applied when maximal wrist extension is achieved. Subsequently, more effective hand function can be assumed because some grip with the fingers is restored.

Rheumatoid Arthritis

The hand of the rheumatoid arthritic provides an interesting clinical example of hand pathology. Because of the nature of the pathology, anatomical factors, and existing forces, a number of reasons for the resulting deformity and disability have been advanced. Among the reasons for ulnar drift at the MP joints are the smaller ulnar condyles of the intercarpals, the larger ulnar collateral ligaments, and the larger muscle mass associated with the little finger. Other forces known to facilitate ulnar drift include gravity, thumb pressure in the ulnar direction, and ulnar deviation associated with the power grip. These anatomic and force elements are coupled with factors associated with rheumatoid changes, such as decreased stability of the proximal phalanx. In addition, flexor and extensor tendons are displaced in the ulnar direction, facilitating ulnar deviation of the MP joint concurrently with medial deviation of the wrist (Fig. 8.14).

Hand postures are also frequently altered as a result of pathological changes. One example is a condition known as "swan-neck" deformity, involving flexion

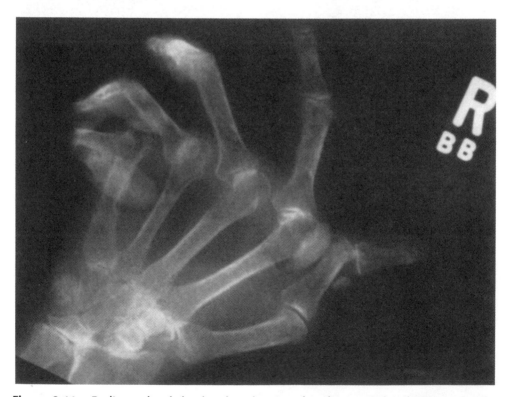

Figure 8.14. Radiograph of the hand and wrist of a rheumatoid arthritic. Note the deformity, particularly at the MP joints where ulnar drift is obvious. The wrist is also deviated, except in a radial direction.

of the MP and distal IP joints and hyperextension of the proximal IP joint (Figs. 8.15 and 8.16). This "intrinsic plus" condition significantly disturbs kinetic balance. Although multiple explanations have been proposed as the cause of the deformity, there is some agreement that tightness of the intrinsics produce the flexion deformity of the MP joint. Laxity of the proximal IP joint secondary to the disease facilitates hyperextension of this joint, again by tightness of the intrinsics. The net result of MP flexion and IP hyperextension is tension in the flexor profundus tendon, resulting in a flexion deformity at the distal IP joint and completing the clinical "swan-neck" picture (28).

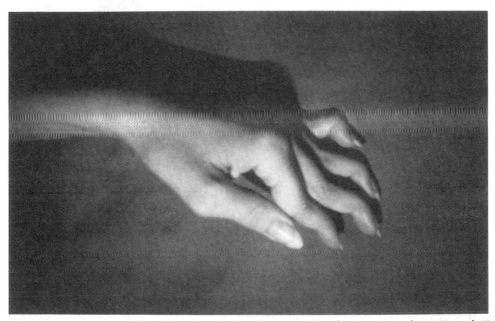

Figure 8.15. Swan-neck deformity in the rheumatoid arthritic. Note the MP and IP positions described in the text.

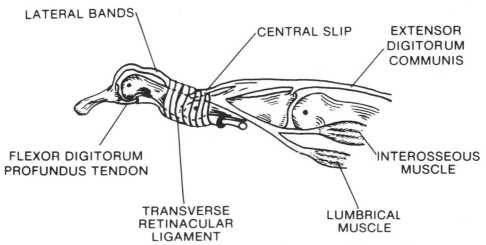

Figure 8.16. Anatomic correlate of the swan-neck deformity with laxity of the transverse retinacular ligament. (From Wadsworth CT: Clinical anatomy and mechanics of the wrist and hand. *J Orthop Sports Phys Ther* 4:206–216, 1983.)

Observing the gross deformities that can occur in rheumatoid hands demands considerable attention to the loss of functional abilities (Fig. 8.17). The advent of joint replacement procedures has greatly facilitated the rehabilitation process associated with advanced stages of the pathology (26) (Figs. 8.18 and 8.19).

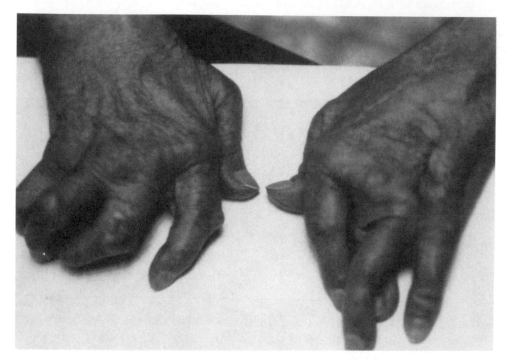

Figure 8.17.   Posture of the rheumatoid hand that impairs many of the common positions required for normal function.

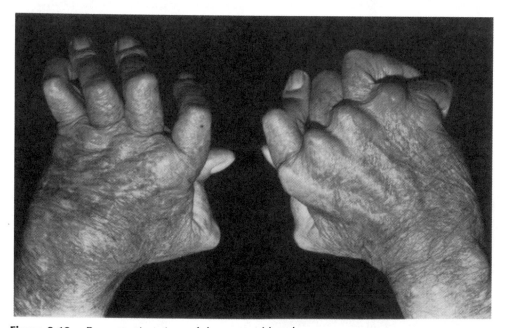

Figure 8.18.   Preoperative view of rheumatoid hands.

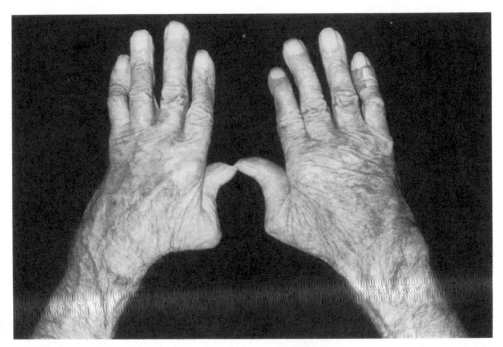

Figure 8.19. Postoperative view of the same hands as in Figure 8.18 after total joint replacement of the MP joints of the fingers, exclusive of the thumb.

Total finger joint replacements, such as the Flatt, Niebauer, Swanson, and Steffee, have been used frequently but with varied success. What success they have enjoyed is probably because the MP and IP joints are essentially nonweight-bearing and operate nearly as hinges. Prostheses are, however, subject to breakage, loosening, and difficulty in achieving sufficient joint movement. A sample of these results has been provided by Opitz and Linscheid who conducted studies on patients with MP replacements necessitated by rheumatoid arthritis (17, 21). Performance of tip prehension and grasp were improved, while power grip, pinch force, and lateral prehension remained unchanged. The effects shown in the latter group were explained on the basis of prosthetic looseness.

Comprehensive results of MP joint arthroplasties have also been presented by Blair and coworkers. In separate studies, silastic and metallic hinge prostheses were evaluated in long-term follow-ups on a large number of patients. Although some ulnar deviation recurred and some failure existed, functional ranges of motion were retained. This latter finding, coupled with high patient satisfaction, apparently establishes the worth of the procedure (3, 4). Unfortunately, 20% of the replacements eventually fractured (21). Now, Volz has provided promising results for total wrist replacement. There is, however, evidence that arthritics have a loss of volitional control of their wrist extensors during closing motions of the hand. If the mechanism is one of inhibition due to pain, reeducation procedures for the wrist extensors may need to be instituted for these patients (29).

Soft Tissue and Trauma

The hand is subject to a number of soft tissue pathologies due to traumatic events. Numerous conditions could be discussed in this section, but only a few relatively common problems that produce pathological motion are included.

One soft tissue anomaly related to rheumatoid arthritis is the boutonniere or buttonhole deformity. In this case, the central slip of the extensor tendon is avulsed, or sufficiently stretched, from the base of the middle phalanx to allow the lateral bands of the extensor hood to pass to the volar surface of the proximal IP joint. Subsequently, the PIP joint projects through the lateral bands as a button would pop through a hole (28) (Figs. 8.20 and 8.21).

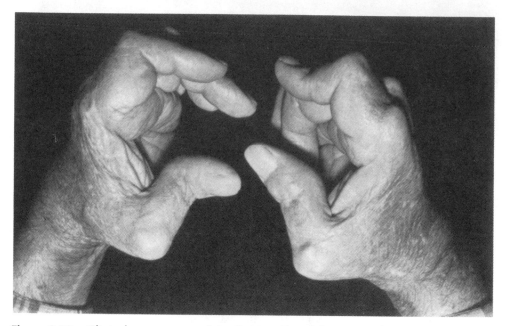

Figure 8.20.   Clinical appearance of the Boutonnière deformity as described in the text. The condition is evident in the index finger of the right hand.

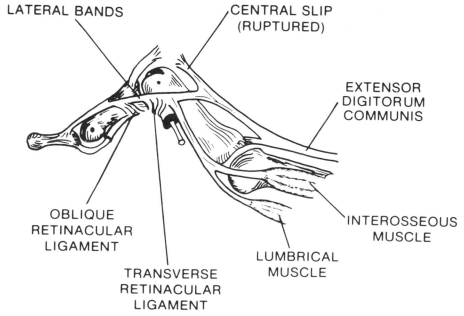

Figure 8.21.   Anatomic view of the Boutonnière deformity. (From Wadsworth CT: Clinical anatomy and mechanics of the wrist and hand. *J Orthop Sports Phys Ther* 4:206–216, 1983.)

Trigger finger is a condition that can affect any of the long finger flexors. An increase in the connective tissue of the tendon may cause a thickening or even a nodule. As the tendon attempts to pass through the flexor sheath located in the vicinity of the MP joint, the thickening or nodule catches on the small diameter opening and hinders smooth passage. Increased tension, however, may cause the thickening to squeeze through the opening, resulting in a fast flexion of the finger and resulting in a snapping movement (23). Similar findings occur when passive tension is created during finger extension.

Another pathological condition indirectly affecting the tendons is Dupuytren's contracture. Proliferation of fibrous tissue of the palm, usually more pronounced on the medial aspect, causes the ring and little fingers to be drawn toward the palm of the hand (Fig. 8.22). This progressive degenerative disease ultimately prevents the fingers from extending (23).

Because tendons are subject to trauma, high tensile loads, and degenerative processes, repairs are often necessary. As a result of the surgical procedures, care must be taken with mobilization of tendons, because tensile loads that are too great can lead to rupture at the repair site. Although some disagreement exists as to the proper duration of immobilization and aggressiveness of treatment, about 6 weeks is generally regarded as the minimum time necessary for at least some repair strength to develop. Allowing too much time before encouraging motion can lead to adhesions between the tendon and its surrounding tissues. Nordin and Frankel note that human tendon does not regain normal strength until 40 to 50 weeks postsurgery. A summary of several surgical procedures used for repair are compared in their text (20). Therapists should note that the tensile strength of individual flexor tendons may be reduced by as much as 66% as compared to losses of only 26% in hand grip strength (10). This fact

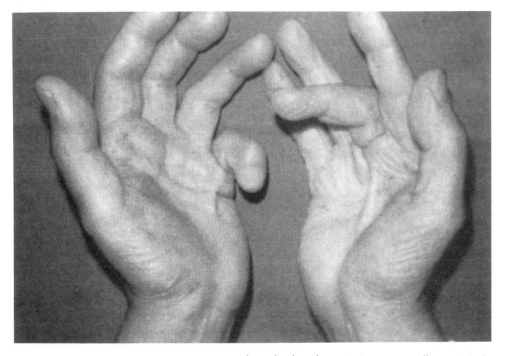

Figure 8.22.   Dupuytren's contracture as described in the text. (From Conolly WB: *Color Atlas of Hand Conditions.* Chicago, Year Book Medical Publishers, 1980, p 281.)

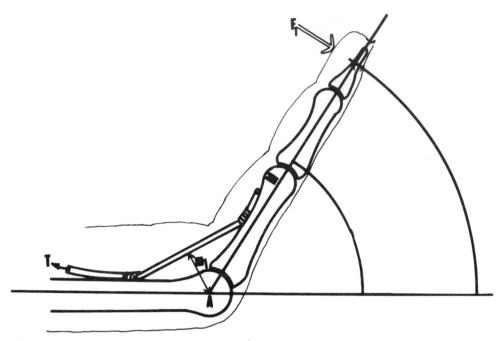

Figure 8.23.   The mechanical effects of "bow-stringing" of the flexor tendons across the MP joint are apparent. The moment arm is obviously increased, but the shortening of the muscle significantly affects the patient's ability to generate effective moments at the distal joints. (From Brand PW, Cranor KC, Ellis JC: Tendon and pulleys at the metacarpophalangeal joint of a finger. *J Bone Joint Surg* [*Am*] 57:779–784, 1975.)

reinforces the need to respect even small deficits in grip strength as possibly indicating quite remarkable weakness in the individual tendons.

Other effects on finger function occur as a result of changes within the flexor sheaths. Trauma, complications of surgery, or arthritis can create bow-stringing of the flexor tendons across the volar surface of the MP joint (Fig. 8.23). Although bow-stringing creates a better moment arm for flexion of the MP joint, it has been known to seriously weaken the IP joint flexors due to muscle shortening. In fact, Brand et al have stated that this loss in grip strength is equivalent to that created by 40° of wrist flexion. These authors also point out that the surgical procedure known as pulley advance is advocated for intrinsic paralysis, even though it does not increase the mechanical advantage when the MP joint is in full extension or hyperextension (6). This case points out the necessity of appropriate mechanical evaluation prior to instituting surgical procedures. Thus, in order to restore finger function, kinetic balance must be evaluated and monitored.

SUMMARY

The anatomy and functional biomechanics of the hand are complex, complicating the ability of kinesiologists to understand both normal and pathological motion. As more sophisticated repair techniques become available, therapists will continue to be called upon not only to comprehensively evaluate pathological motion but also to apply biomechanical principles to treatment regimens. Our patients depend on our understanding of hand function, and ultimately the critical role of the hand in mankind's development challenges us toward further understanding.

References

1. An KN, Ueba Y, Chao EY, Cooney WP, Linscheid RL: Tendon excursion and moment arm of index finger muscles. *J Biomech* 16:419–426, 1983.
2. Andrews JG, Youm Y: A biomechanical investigation of wrist kinematics. *J Biomech* 12:83–93, 1979.
3. Blair WF, Shurr DG, Buckwalter JA: Metacarpophalangeal joint implant arthroplasty with a silastic spacer. *J Bone Joint Surg [Am]* 66:365–370, 1984.
4. Blair WF, Shurr DG, Buckwalter JA: Metacarpophalangeal joint arthroplasty with a metallic hinged prosthesis. *Clin Orthop* 184:156–163, 1984.
5. Brand PW, Beach RB, Thompson DE: Relative tension and potential excursion of muscles in the forearm and hand. *J Hand Surg* 6:209–219, 1981.
6. Brand PW, Cranor KC, Ellis JC: Tendon and pulleys at the metacarpophalangeal joint of a finger. *J Bone Joint Surg [Am]* 57:779–784, 1975.
7. Brumfield RH, Champoux JA: A biomechanical study of normal functional wrist motion. *Clin Orthop* 187:23–25, 1984.
8. Cooney WP, Chao EYS: Biomechanical analysis of static forces of the thumb during hand function. *J Bone Joint Surg [Am]* 59:27–36, 1977.
9. Cooney WP, Lucca MJ, Chao EYS, Linscheid RL: The kinesiology of the thumb trapeziometacarpal joint. *J Bone Joint Surg [Am]* 63:1371–1381, 1981.
10. Ejeskar A: Finger flexion force and hand grip strength after tendon repair. *J Hand Surg* 7:61–65, 1982.
11. Flatt AE: *Kinesiology of the Hand.* American Academy of Orthopaedic Surgery Instructional Course Lectures XVIII. St Louis, CV Mosby, 1961.
12. Gigis PI, Kuczynski K: The distal interphalangeal joints of human fingers. *J Hand Surg* 7:176–182, 1982.
13. Kapandji AI: *The Physiology of Joints,* ed 5. New York, Churchill Livingstone, 1982.
14. Kauer JMG: Functional anatomy of the wrist. *Clin Orthop* 149:9–20, 1980.
15. Kessler R, Hertling D: *Management of Common Musculoskeletal Disorders.* New York, Harper & Row, 1983.
16. Landsmeer JMF: Anatomical and functional investigations on the articulation of the human fingers. *Acta Anat (Basel)* 25, Suppl 24, 1955.
17. Linscheid RL, Dobyns JH: Total joint arthroplasty: the hand. *Mayo Clin Proc* 54:516–526, 1979.
18. MacConaill MA: Mechanical anatomy of the carpus and its bearing on surgical problems. *J Anat* 75:166–175, 1941.
19. MacConaill MA, Basmajian JV: *Muscles and Movements: A Basis for Human Kinesiology.* Baltimore, Williams & Wilkins, 1969.
20. Nordin M, Frankel VH: Biomechanics of collagenous tissue. In Frankel VH, Nordin M (eds): *Basic Biomechanics of the Skeletal System.* Philadelphia, Lea & Febiger, 1980.
21. Opitz JL, Linscheid RL: Hand function after metacarpophalangeal joint replacement in rheumatoid arthritis. *Arch Phys Med Rehabil* 59:160–165, 1978.
22. Radonjic D, Long CL: II. Kinesiology of the wrist. *Am J Phys Med* 50:57–71, 1971
23. Ramamurti CP: *Orthopaedics in Primary Care.* Baltimore, Williams & Wilkins, 1979.
24. Sarrafian SK, Melamed JL, Goshgarian GM: Study of wrist motion in flexion and extension. *Clin Orthop* 126:153–159, 1977.
25. Smith RJ: Balance and kinetics of the fingers under normal and pathological conditions. *Clin Orthop* 104:92–111, 1974.
26. Smith RJ, Kaplan EB: Rheumatoid deformities at the metacarpophalangeal joints of the fingers. *J Bone Joint Surg [Am]* 49:31–47, 1967.
27. Srinivasan H: Patterns of movement of totally intrinsic-minus fingers. *J Bone Joint Surg [Am]* 58:777–785, 1976.
28. Swezey RL: Dynamic factors in deformity of the rheumatoid arthritic hand. *Bull Rheum Dis* 22:649–656, 1971–72.
29. Volz RG: Total wrist arthroplasty. *Clin Orthop* 187:112–120, 1984.

30. Volz RG, Lieb M, Benjamin J: Biomechanics of the wrist. *Clin Orthop* 149:112–117, 1980.
31. Wadsworth CT: Clinical anatomy and mechanics of the wrist and hand. *J Orthop Sports Phys Ther* 4:206–216, 1983.
32. Warwick R, Williams PL (eds): *Gray's Anatomy*, ed 35. Philadelphia, WB Saunders, 1973.
33. Youm Y, Gillespie TE, Flatt AE, Sprague BL: Kinematic investigation of normal MCP joint. *J Biomech* 11:109–118, 1978.
34. Youm Y, McMurtry RY, Flatt AE, Gillespie TE: Kinematics of the wrist: I. An experimental study of radial-ulnar deviation and flexion-extension. *J Bone Joint Surg* [Am] 60:423–431, 1978.

9

Hip

The mechanics and control of the hip joint present an interesting complex for the student of kinesiology and biomechanics. As the most proximal joint of the lower limb, the hip provides stability and gross control in space for the remainder of the leg. Activities such as stair climbing and lifting require that hip muscles exert large forces for generating appropriate moments. Anatomic structure reflects functional requirements in providing the features necessary to perform effectively. Joint pathology is rather common, mostly because of large and/or repetitive loading that occurs in the joints of the lower limb. This chapter will present kinesiology and biomechanics as related to the hip and then discuss some of the pathologies that disrupt the normal kinematics and kinetics.

MUSCULAR ACTIONS
Extensors

Action of the muscles about the hip can be categorized according to six primary motions of flexion-extension, abduction-adduction, or internal-external rotation. The extensor group, composed of the gluteus maximus and the hamstrings, is supplemented in action by muscles with different primary functions, such as the gemelli, the obturator internus, and the adductor magnus. When considered as a whole, and according to listings of data from Fick, the extensors comprise a powerful group with a physiologic cross section of over 150 cm^2 (21). If accessory muscles of the hip are excluded, a cross sectional area of over 113 cm^2 remains. Specific functions in which these accessory muscles are particularly useful include rising from a chair, stair climbing, powering the prosthesis of the above knee amputee, and propulsive activities such as running.

Fischer and Houtz analyzed individual hip extensors with the use of electromyography. A number of activities requiring hip extension were performed in different positions in order to assess the level of contraction of the gluteus maximus. Analysis revealed that the greatest activity occurred during isometric muscle setting and during maximal contractions in a position of hyperextension, external rotation, and abduction. The authors commented that extension of the flexed thigh was accomplished by the hamstrings muscles. Some caution should be exercised in deriving conclusions from these data, however, because recorder response characteristics were limited to less than the optimal suggested for EMG signals (9).

Flexors

Musculature responsible for flexion includes two primary muscles, the psoas major and the iliacus. By virtue of attachment to the lumbar spine, the psoas has potentially profound effects on the hip and spine, the latter to be discussed thoroughly in Chapter 12, "Trunk." In any case, the combined contraction of the psoas major and the iliacus accounts for powerful although infrequent hip flexion movements. Secondary hip flexors include the tensor fasciae latae, rectus femoris, sartorius, and the adductors. Other muscles, such as the gracilis and quadratus femoris, assist with flexion in only a tertiary fashion (8).

Abductors-Adductors

In comparison to the hip abductor musculature the adductor group has been believed to be of minor importance. Because large cross section is inconsistent with the need for adduction torque, perhaps secondary functions may actually be of greater importance. For example, the adductors regularly contract early in the swing phase of the gait cycle. That these muscles also participate in hip rotation and extension, depending upon the position of the thigh, is further evidence of their role as accessory muscles.

The abductor group serves an important function, particularly during weight bearing. A specific discussion of this mechanism is contained in the section on Biomechanics. In addition to the gluteus medius and minimus, the tensor fasciae latae and piriformis appear to play some role in abduction. Years ago, Inman made theoretical calculations showing the ratio of the average muscle masses relative to each other: medius, 4; minimus, 2; tensor fascia latae, 1 (14).

Merchant also completed a study that analyzed the abductor muscle force required as the superincumbent body weight varied from 20 to 60 lbs. By altering the position of the femur and pelvis this investigator noted that the tension in the abductors varied considerably. For example, with the femur externally rotated 30° while the pelvis was maintained in neutral, the tensor accounted for more than 50% of the tension required to keep the model in equilibrium. Conversely, with the femur rotated internally and the pelvis neutral no tension existed in the tensor (23).

Rotation

The rotator musculature of the hip has been relegated a position of much less importance than the rotators of the glenohumeral joint. Although internal rotation may be accomplished by as many as nine muscles, Favill considers the anterior fibers of the gluteus medius and gluteus minimus to be the primary movers. External rotation appears to be a dedicated function of the obturator externus and quadratus femoris, but portions of the adductor magnus, gluteus minimus, and long head of the biceps femoris have also been credited with contributing. The gemelli, obturator internus, and piriformis externally rotate when the hip is in extension (8). The mass of the rotators and other muscles is considerable. Kapandji states that the power of the medial rotators is only about one-third that of the lateral rotators (18). Certainly the relatively low amount of force the former are required to generate bears witness to their seeming lack of importance.

Geometry and Function

Some of the multiple actions of which the hip musculature is capable have been addressed earlier in this chapter. These actions result from the known geometric relationships that the muscles have with the hip joint. Still to be considered, however, is the relationship of the muscles to the joint as the hip is moved through a range of motion. Dostal has done extensive work in modeling the hip and has provided a complete set of data for 27 muscles at the hip. In his analysis, the hip was moved through ranges of motion while the effect on the moment arm vector component was determined. An exemplary result is provided in Figure 9.1 for the fibers representing the anterior portion of the gluteus medius muscle. From his data it is possible to determine the effect of any hip position upon the potential action of any of the muscles included in the analysis. The effects of the ranges of motions studied are shown in Table 9.1 (6, 7). Therapists may find such a description of the changes in muscle function with joint position useful is assessing and treating patients. Certainly such changes occur at all joints, and once objectively measured, they will offer the same application to patient care.

Other information available about the function of the hip musculature, as shown by Soderberg and Dostal, indicates that the gluteus medius can be divided into at least three segments. In their work, fine wire EMG was used to simultaneously record from anterior, middle, and posterior segments of the muscle during a variety of functional activities. Results definitively showed that subjects selectively activated different segments of the muscle during some of these activities. For example, during forward leaning from the standing position the anterior portion of muscle becomes relatively quiet, while the posterior segment increases in activity as the lean increases (36). Pare et al have more recently demonstrated that the anteromedial and posterolateral fibers of the tensor fasciae latae muscle also produce different EMG output during gait and other selected

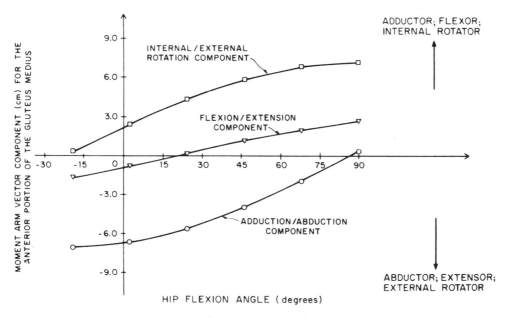

Figure 9.1. Graphic description of the changes in the moment arm vector component of the anterior portion of the gluteus medius for the motion of hip flexion. Motions in the respective planes are given at the far right. See text and Table 9.1 for further description. (From Dostal WF, Andrews JG: A three dimensional biomechanical model of hip musculature. *J Biomech* 14:803–812, 1981.)

Table 9.1. Classification of Muscles[a] According to Action at 0, 40, and 90 Degrees of Hip Flexion

Degrees	Action[b]					
	Ext.	Flex.	Add.	Abd.	Ir.	Er.
All	Bi. fem. Semiten. Semimem. Ad. post. Ad. mid.[a]	RF Sar. I/P TFL[e]	ADB ADL Ad. mi. Ad. mid.[c,d] Gra. Pec.[e]	TFL[c,d] Pir.[e]		Quad. fem.[d,e]
0 and 40 only		Pec.[c]	Ob. ex.	G. med. ant.[c] G. med. mid. G. med. post. G. min. ant.[c] G. min. mid. G. min. post.		Gem. sup. Ob. in. Gem. inf.
0 and 90 only			Ad. post.[d,e]	Sar.[d,e] RF[d,e]		
40 and 90 only	Quad. fem.[c]			Gem. sup.[c]	G. med. ant. G. min. ant. G. med. mid.[c] G. min. mid.[c]	Ob. ex.[c]
0 only	G. max.[f]		ADL[d] Quad. fem.			Pir. G. med. post.[e]
40 only						
90 only	Gra.[d] Ad. mi.[d] ADB[d] ADL[d]			Ob. in.	G. med. post. G. min. post. Pir.[d]	

[a] Muscles are abbreviated as Ad. post., adductor magnus (posterior); Ad. mid., adductor magnus (middle); Ad. mi., adductor minimus; ADB, adductor brevis; ADL, adductor longus; RF, rectus femoris; I/P, iliopsoas; TFL, tensor fascia lata; G. med. ant., gluteus medius (anterior); G. med. mid., gluteus medius (middle); G. med. post., gluteus medius (posterior); G. min. ant., gluteus minimus (anterior); G. min. mid., gluteus minimus (middle); G. min. post., gluteus minimus (posterior).
[b] Actions are abbreviated as Ext., extension; Flex., flexion; Add., adduction; Abd., abduction; Ir., internal rotation; Er., external rotation.
[c] Secondary action at 40°.
[d] Secondary action at 90°.
[e] Secondary action at 0°.
[f] Model not valid for flexed configurations.

activities (28). Considering that the tensor can act at the knee joint via the iliotibial band, these findings may have implication for control of the knee deficient of ligaments, particularly the anterior cruciate.

Specific functional roles of different muscle segments make possible fine control over the magnitude and direction of joint torque. Consequently therapists must be aware that specific training procedures may need to be implemented, assuring that specific segments of muscles are active instead of a gross contraction of a whole muscle.

A number of the biarticular muscles about the hip have effects upon several joints. Included in this category are the muscles psoas major, rectus femoris, tensor fasciae latae, gracilis, sartorius, biceps femoris, semitendinosus, and semimembranosus. Special note should be made that motion at one joint alters muscle length which then affects the muscle's function at adjacent joints. Length-tension relationships again become important if we are to effectively consider function. A discussion of the interactive effects of hip and knee joint musculature is included in the next chapter.

ARTHROLOGY AND ARTHROKINEMATICS

Anatomical characteristics of the hip joint are somewhat different from upper limb joints. The primary reason for the differences is the necessity for the joints of the lower limb to bear the superincumbent body weight. An additional reason is that the lower limb contains more massive musculature necessary to meet larger torque requirements. This section of the chapter presents a summary of the relevant anatomy and discusses the influence of these anatomical features on function.

In general the hip is considered to be a ball-and-socket joint whose center is located approximately 1 cm inferior to the midposition of the inguinal ligament (38). According to Radin both the acetabular and femoral components are mainly trabecular bone (30). The acetabulum faces somewhat anteriorly, laterally, and inferiorly and is encircled by a labrum that serves to deepen the socket (20). The functional articular surface is the portion known as the lunate surface. Shown in Figure 9.2 this ring is covered by articular cartilage that is thickest superiorly and absent inferiorly (38).

The femoral head, forming about two-thirds of a sphere, is regarded by most to be symmetrical (20). Rydell, however, indicates this is not true, because the head is slightly compressed in the anterior-posterior direction (35). Hoaglund and Low provide a summary that corroborates this position on the basis of radii and intersubject variability (13). The head is completely covered with articular cartilage except in the location of the fovea, tapering to a "neck" that joins the femoral head and shaft. In turn the neck joins the femoral shaft at an angle of approximately 135° (38). Study of the architecture of the femoral neck is important, because this section of the femur is frequently involved in pathologies.

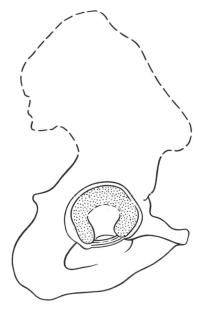

Figure 9.2.   Representation of the acetabulum. (From Radin EL: Biomechanics of the human hip. *Clin Orthop* 152:28–34, 1980.)

Studies have shown that the cross section of the neck is virtually symmetric near the femoral head and elliptical near the trochanters. This fact may account for some traumatic pathology as well as provide clues as to why some surgical repairs fail (1). Furthermore, the axis of the elliptical segment is not aligned with the long axis of the femoral shaft, thus producing further potential difficulties in load bearing (35). These issues will be discussed in the section on pathokinesiology.

One other anatomic feature that can influence hip mechanics is torsion in the femoral shaft. Antetorsion (anteversion) means that the shaft of the femur has been rotated such that the femoral neck forms a larger than usual angle with the transverse axis of the femoral condyles, as measured in a horizontal plane. Retrotorsion is the converse: a smaller than usual angle. Thought to begin in fetal life, antetorsion amounts to about 35° in the "average" newborn. During growth, however, the angle diminishes to only 14° in the typical adult (35). The significance of this factor will be discussed in the section on biomechanics.

Trabecular patterns in the proximal femur and pelvis have also been considered to be of import. Virtually any article on the biomechanics of the hip will discuss this issue in detail (18, 20, 35). Although stating that trabeculae have been overemphasized from a mechanical point of view, Rydell describes medial, lateral, and arcuate trabecular systems (Fig. 9.3) (35). The lateral portion has been given credit for resisting tensile forces applied by the abductor mechanism, while the medial group resists compressive forces through the head of the femur. The arcuate portion of the trabeculae is responsible for resisting the bending moment through the femoral neck. Note also that areas of pattern intersection have greater strength than those areas where none exists (20).

Ligaments and the extensive joint capsule also are integral aspects of the functional biomechanics of the hip joint. Three strong ligaments are of special significance. The iliofemoral, or ligament of Bigelow, simulates an inverted Y as the fibers originating from the pelvis spiral anteriorly and inferiorly to insert along the anterior intertrochanteric line (Fig. 9.4). Note how the fibers attach along the entire length of the line. Two important ligaments arise posteriorly (Fig. 9.4). The

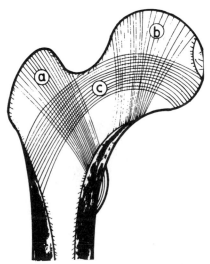

Figure 9.3.   The three main networks of trabeculae. The lateral is a, the medial is b, and the arcuate c. (From Rydell N: Biomechanics of the hip joint. *Clin Orthop* 92:6–15, 1973.)

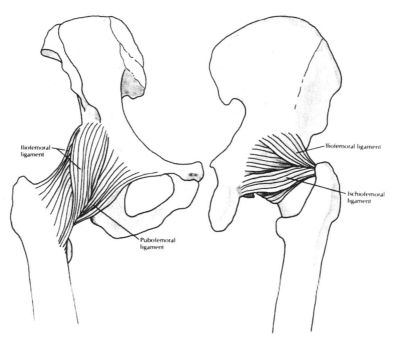

Figure 9.4. The anterior (*left*) and posterior (*right*) views of the capsule of the hip joint. See text for description. (From Kessler R, Hertling D: *Management of Common Musculo-skeletal Disorders.* New York, Harper & Row, 1983.)

pubofemoral ligament, in a more inferior location, is stretched most significantly on abduction. The ischiofemoral ligament, which also lies posteriorly, resists hip extension and internal rotation as does the anteriorly located iliofemoral ligament (20). These major ligaments blend with and strengthen the expansive capsule. Other ligaments are of little functional importance. The capsule is strongest anteriorly and superiorly, because substantial resistance to hip extension is required during postures commonly assumed. That the fibers of the capsule adopt both a circular and longitudinal orientation has no apparent mechanical significance (38). The bursae found around the joint also have no remarkable features, even though involvement is not uncommon in various pathologies.

As for any joint, the anatomical structures influence arthrokinematics. A deep acetabulum, receiving much of the femoral head, provides for maximal stability. Further support is provided by ligamentous and capsular structures. Surface joint movement occurs according to the principles of motion as described in Chapter 3. In the lower limb, however, compression due to body weight and consequent muscle contraction increases the shear forces between the joint surfaces.

BIOMECHANICS
Joint Congruence

The hip joint is an interesting joint to study because of the arthrology and myology associated with the requirements for stability while bearing relatively large loads. However, large ranges of motion exist in the three primary movements. Joint congruence, an important aspect of hip arthrology, has been detailed by Kapandji (18). Simple observation of the human skeleton confirms that, in the upright posture, the femoral head is not covered by the anterior-superior rim of the acetabulum. This finding results from a different planar orientation of the acetabulum relative to the head of the femur. Full congruence can be achieved either by moving the pelvis on the femur or moving the femur on the pelvis. In either case, maximal congruence can be achieved at about 90° of flexion and small amounts of abduction and lateral rotation. Achieving this hip position while weight bearing through the limbs leads one to a quadruped position. Thus, assumption of the upright posture has occurred in spite of decreased articular congruence at the hip positions involved in bipedal posture and movement. Confusion may arise as to the difference between congruence achieved in the quadruped position and the close-packed position involving hip extension, abduction, and internal rotation. Recall that a requirement for achieving the close-packed position is tension in the ligaments and joint capsule, a condition only satisfied when the hip is in extension. Paraplegics and amputees usually assume standing postures that cause the line of gravity to fall posterior to the hip joint. In this circumstance, the force that limits hip hyperextension and allows a relaxed standing posture is supplied by the anterior ligaments.

Bony Configuration

Anatomical features decidedly influence hip biomechanics. One is the angle of inclination, or the angle in a frontal plane made by the neck and shaft of the femur. Considerable variation in this angle across the human population has been well documented. Figure 9.5 shows two structural deviations of the hip known as coxa vara and valga. In the varus hip note that the angle between the shaft and neck is less than that of the normal 135° configuration. Such a position markedly increases the bending moment occurring in the proximal femur, because the force transmitted along the long axis of the femur has a larger moment arm in respect to the hip joint. Pauwels has included these analyses in his volume on the hip and has demonstrated that the magnitude of tensile and compressive forces produced by the bending moment vary depending upon the angle of inclination of the hip (29). These mechanical considerations affect the design of hip prostheses, in particular the selection of prosthetic materials that can bear anticipated bending moments without fracture. Examples of these problems will be presented in the section in this chapter on pathokinesiology. Conversely, the position of valgus minimizes the bending moment because the load along the shaft of the femur can be transmitted more directly into the joint.

Other influences stem from the angle of inclination, the position and mass of the greater trochanter, and the degree of antetorsion in the femur. Radin has commented that a decreased angle of inclination (i.e., greater varus) results in greater mechanical advantage of the gluteus medius muscle for controlling contralateral depression of the pelvis (described in following section). Since compared to the lever arm of body weight the lever arm of the abductors is quite small (perhaps 2 to 1), any advantage that can be provided to the abductor musculature is probably beneficial (30). Also remember that considerable hip joint compression is due to contraction of the muscles spanning the joint. Therefore, a beneficial therapeutic approach would be one that decreased the muscular forces required to generate or control the moments at the hip. This may be the mechanism for surgical procedures performed with the intent of decreasing pain or alleviating hip joint dysfunction. Radin also suggests that increased antetorsion leads to an increased moment arm for the gluteus maximus, and consequently lengthening of the muscle, together increasing the advantage for this muscle (30). Should this hypothesis be proven true, then two factors may

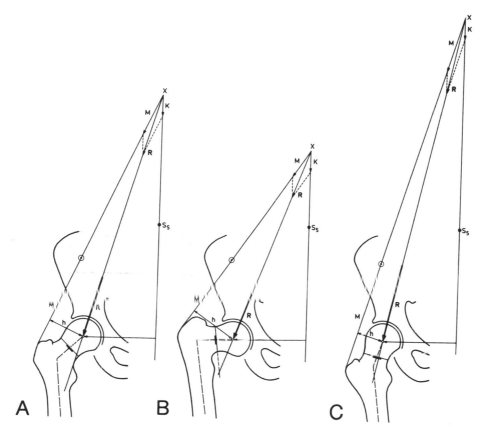

Figure 9.5. Mechanical affects of the position of the hip. The normal hip is shown in *A*. In *B* the hip is in varus, while valgus is represented in *C*. Abductor muscle force is designated with an *M* and the moment arm relative to the center of the hip with *h*. The resultant force at the joint is *R*. Point *X* is the intersection of the muscle line of insertion with the line of action of the partial body weight *K*. (From Pauwels F: *Biomechanics of the Normal and Diseased Hip*. Berlin, Springer-Verlag, 1976.)

account for increased gluteus maximus mechanical advantage with femoral antetorsion: the increased moment arm and increased muscular tension available due to the length-tension relationship.

Abductor Mechanism

Virtually any analysis of hip mechanics requires discussion of the role of the abductor mechanism. To best understand the function of this muscle consider the origin and the insertion of the gluteus medius and minimus muscles to be reversed from the classical anatomical description. Thus, when standing on one leg, the gluteus medius and minimus will be capable of pulling the rim of the pelvis towards the greater trochanter of the femur rather than performing pure abduction of the hip. This function is important for several reasons. As one walks, swinging a leg forward requires that balance be momentarily maintained over the leg remaining in contact with the ground. For purposes of maintaining balance and allowing the foot of the swinging leg to clear the ground, the abductors of the stance leg must contract in order to prevent the pelvis from dropping on the opposite side. This potential drop is caused by the weight of the trunk and swinging leg. Figure 9.6 shows the free body diagram, with body weight acting to create a moment about the center of the hip. The force and moment arm of the gluteus medius and minimus have also been added to demonstrate that the system is in equilibrium. Without this balance of moments, the system would not be in equilibrium, resulting in rotation in the direction of the greatest moment. The equation representing this free body diagram would be stated as BW $\times$ D 1 = GM $\times$ D. To explain the influence of altered mechanics Johnston has listed factors that favor instability or stability. A decrease in abductor force or moment

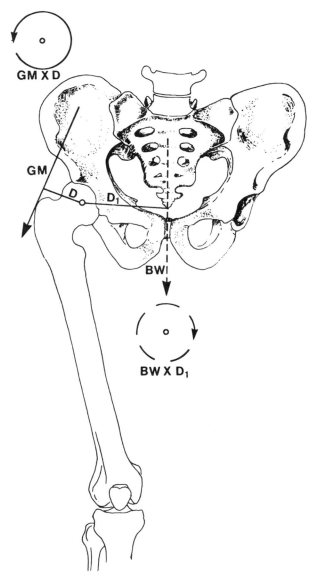

Figure 9.6.   Mechanical representation of the hip describing the function of the abductor mechanism. Moments are taken about the center of the hip. For balance and equilibrium to occur the product of body weight *BW* and D_1 must equal the product of the tension in the gluteus medius (*GM*) and *D*. (From Neumann DA, Cook TM: The effect of load and carry position on the electromyographic activity of the gluteus medius during walking. *Phys Ther* 65:305–311, 1985.)

arm would favor instability. Instability would also be more likely to occur with either an increase in body weight or an increase in the moment arm through which the weight acts relative to the center of the hip joint. Thus, mechanics indicate the reason why patients with hip joint disease or pain may be advised to lose weight, i.e., to reduce the abductor muscle requirement and diminish compressive load across the hip (16). How patients compensate as a result of pathology will be discussed in the section on pathokinesiology.

KINETICS

Large muscles are required to generate the torques necessary to function, particularly under conditions involving large loads. In producing these large torques, however, muscles also create compression of the joints they span. The magnitude of compression produced by a muscle is dependent not only upon the tension generated but also upon the direction of the muscle pull relative to the joint surface. Specifically, the greatest compression of the joint surface will occur on a plane perpendicular to the muscle's direction of pull, regardless of the degree of curvature in the convex and concave surfaces. Further, note that muscles that are parallel with the joint surface produce greater shear at the joint. This section will discuss muscle forces, torques, and joint forces.

Torques

Numerous studies have been completed on the tension generated in the hip musculature. For example, Jarvis evaluated "strength" of the hip rotators while apparently imposing a force gauge between the leg tested and the manual resistance applied by the examiner. She included a left-to-right comparison of the subjects' legs in various test positions. She noted that the internal rotators generated greater tension than external when the hip was in flexion. However, upon placing the hip in extension, the external rotators were found to exert greater tension than the internal. This reversal was not because they gained mechanical advantage in extension, but because the internal rotators lost mechanical advantage while that of the external rotators remained unchanged (15). Haley subsequently completed a similar study that addressed the issue of rotator muscle length. Although finding no correlation between joint range and joint torque, the study noted difference in torques in the sitting versus the supine testing position. For example, sitting position torques were 23 and 5% greater than supine for internal and external rotation, respectively (11).

The findings of these and other studies point to the importance of standardizing the method and the position across trials and therapists. Chapter 1 pointed out that the correct method for equating "strength" data across subjects and therapists is to use torque directly or convert force units to torque. Because many hip functions are influenced by altering the position of at least one of the joints crossed by a two-joint muscle, Nemeth et al studied the effect of knee position on isometric hip extension moment. These investigators determined that knee angle did not influence maximal hip extension torque. The moment values produced, however, progressively decreased as the hip angle progressed from 90° of flexion to full extension. Torques combined across all male and female subjects were at a maximum of 245 Nm at 90° and diminished to 55% of this value at full hip extension. Certainly the loss of torque results from the shortening of the muscles. In all cases, when the hip extensor moment was tested at knee angles 0, 30, 60, and 90°, the hip extensor torque decreased by approximately equal magnitudes (Fig. 9.7) (26).

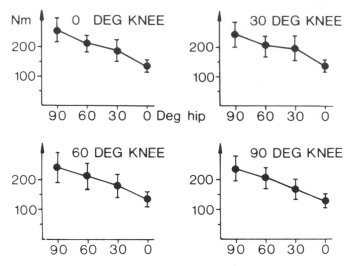

Figure 9.7.   Mean maximum hip extensor muscular moments at four different angles of the knee shown for various hip angles. Ten subjects are included with the confidence intervals at 0.05. (From Nemeth G, Ekholm J, Arborelius UP, et al: Influence of knee flexion on isometric hip extensor strength. *Scand J Rehabil Med* 15:97–101, 1983.)

Torques produced by the abductor musculature have been of longstanding interest because of their role in controlling lateral motion of the trunk during gait. As early as 1947, Inman calculated theoretical abductor torques and then measured peak values of between 1000 and 1100 kg-cm in the standing position (14). Almost 20 yr later Murray and Sepic studied both abductor and adductor torques at neutral and at 25° of abduction. Although values for both positions tested ranged from 749 to 1390 kg-cm for middle-aged females and young males, respectively, their grand mean value of 1067 agreed quite closely with the Inman data. When the test was completed at 25° of abduction the abductor torque fell to around 60% of the value produced at the neutral position. As expected, adductor torques increased from 1140 kg-cm in neutral to 1287 kg-cm at 25° of abduction (25). These changes further document the influence of muscle length upon the ability of muscle to generate torque.

Dynamic hip abduction torques have also been studied. Using the supine position Olson and coworkers produced torque values that were slightly less than 1000 kg-cm. Their data, shown in Figure 9.8, further confirm aspects of functional muscle mechanics. Concentric contractions at a constant velocity of approximately 13°/sec produced lower torques than isometric trials. Conversely, eccentric contractions performed under similar conditions and compared at similar points in the range of motion produced higher values than did isometric trials (27). All data are in strong agreement with the force-velocity relationship for shortening and lengthening contractions, with the exception of the terminal phase of the eccentric range of motion.

Joint Forces

Other forces in the hip joint and proximal end of the femur will potentially alter the condition of the joint surfaces or alter the bone because of the stress and strain produced through loading. The area of contact in the hip is about 25 to 30 cm². However, much of the load through the hip joint is transmitted

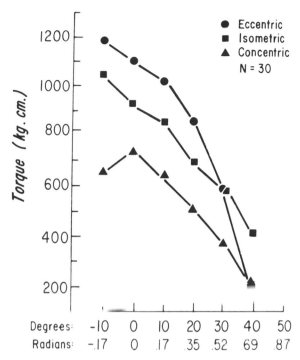

Figure 9.8. Torque curves for hip abduction for eccentric, isometric, and concentric contractions. See text for further description. (From Olson VL, Smidt GL, Johnston RC: The maximum torque generated by the eccentric, isometric, and concentric contractions of the hip abductor muscles. *Phys Ther* 52:149–157, 1972.)

superiorly and somewhat medially into the acetabulum. Concentration of the load in these areas explains the pattern of wear commonly seen in degenerative joint disease. Radin remarks that the spongy composition of the head of the femur and the acetabulum provides a degree of elasticity. Such elastic compliance serves to decrease the force per unit area since spreading occurs. Because joint congruity is less than maximal in the unloaded condition but increased under loading lends further evidence to the structure's ability to adjust for increased joint forces. Thus, flattening of the subchondral bone increases surface area, thereby keeping the loads within tolerable limits (30).

As indicated in earlier sections of this chapter, joint forces at the hip are primarily the result of two factors: body weight and muscular contraction. Considering only the effect of body weight, hip joint force in erect posture would be one-half of body weight minus the weight of the legs. However, the typical force across the joint occurring during the single limb support phase of gait ranges from two and one-half to four times body weight (16). Years ago Rydell implanted a prosthesis instrumented with strain gauges, allowing direct measurement of joint forces. Single limb standing produced forces of about two and one-half times body weight. Although stance phase forces were not as large as expected, the swing phase forces were larger than expected. Forces of four and one-half to five times body weight occurred during running (35).

Besides the direct method via the instrumented prosthesis, indirect techniques can be used in arriving at the joint forces. Brand et al have presented an example of indirect measurement of forces on the femoral head in three orthogonal

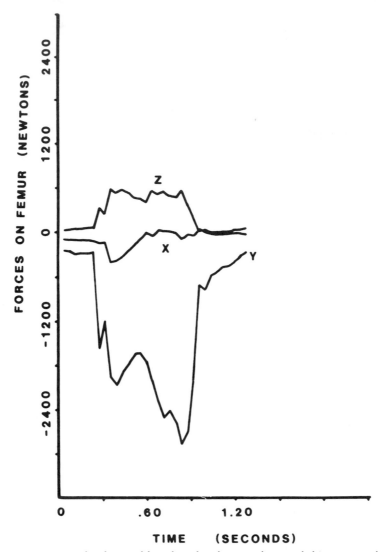

Figure 9.9. Forces on the femoral head in the three orthogonal directions. The component of greatest magnitude is in the vertical direction (Y). (From Brand RA, Crowninshield RD, Johnston RC, Pedersen DR: Forces on the femoral head during activities of daily living. *Iowa Orthop J* 2:43–49, 1982.)

directions. Notice in Figure 9.9 that the force on the femoral head exceeds 2400 newtons. Stair climbing caused forces exceeding 3500 N, equivalent to approximately 6 times body weight. Body weight itself contributes only a small portion of this total force; the majority of these relatively high values is due to muscle contraction across the joint (2). That muscle contraction plays a significant role in creating joint compression is further evidenced by Rydell's determination that straight leg raising from the supine position created a hip joint force of one and one-half times body weight (35). Even tightening of the capsule can lead to increased joint force. Such tightening may occur during less than full extension in the stance phase of the gait cycle if the capsule is shortened due to pathology in the hip.

Since many therapeutic interventions for hip pathologies ultimately are designed to decrease joint forces, therapists and others treating these patients need to be aware of the mechanics of the surgical and supportive therapy discussed in the next section.

PATHOKINESIOLOGY

Many pathologic conditions are manifested in the hip joint. The reasons for these pathologies are the frequency, magnitude, and mechanism for transmission of hip loads. The presentation of the pathologies in this section will emphasize principles of mechanics related to the condition and to principles of potentially effective treatment.

Painful Hip

Regardless of etiology pain is a symptom common to most hip pathologies, and in itself can affect hip mechanics. In such a circumstance patients assume postures that diminish the force through the hip joint. During normal standing the magnitudes of the forces are low and are usually tolerable. However, single limb stance during gait significantly increases the joint force due to the abductor muscle force required to keep the pelvis from dropping on the opposite side. To avoid these joint forces the patient has several alternatives available. The section on biomechanics explained that these alternatives are limited, since major changes in body weight are difficult to achieve. Therefore the patient must resort to mechanical means. Often, the method selected is an alteration in the line of gravity associated with body weight. This is accomplished by a lateral lean of the body weight towards the side of the stance limb, effectively diminishing the moment arm of the the body weight relative to the center of rotation at the hip. This can be seen in Figure 9.6 by locating the line of force through the body weight closer to the center of rotation of the hip about which moments are being considered. This clinical picture is described as an abductor or gluteus medius lurch. Similar mechanics occur with weakness in the abductor mechanism, because balance of the trunk over the hip is less difficult to accomplish with a decreased moment arm.

Another alternative is to instruct the patient in the use of an assistive device. Two crutches, for example, allow the patient to bear minimal weight on the involved limb, therefore decreasing the resultant joint force. A cane, held in the opposite hand, also significantly reduces the force necessary in the abductor musculature and diminishes the resultant hip joint force. This reduction is possible due to a large moment arm through which the force on the cane is applied (Fig. 9.10), necessitating only a moderate force on the cane. Using the cane on the ipsilateral side of the pathology is not as effective in decreasing joint force and generally is not recommended. In addition, use of the cane in the same hand as the diseased hip narrows the patient's base of support and alters the gait pattern by not allowing for contralateral arm swing.

Congenital Dislocation

Somewhat analogous circumstances arise in congenital dislocation of the hip. In this situation the hip does not form a fixed fulcrum or center of rotation about which moments may be generated. In addition, because of the lack of a specific location for joint forces, there is incomplete development of the acetabulum and loss of the spherical shape of the femoral head. A further complication is

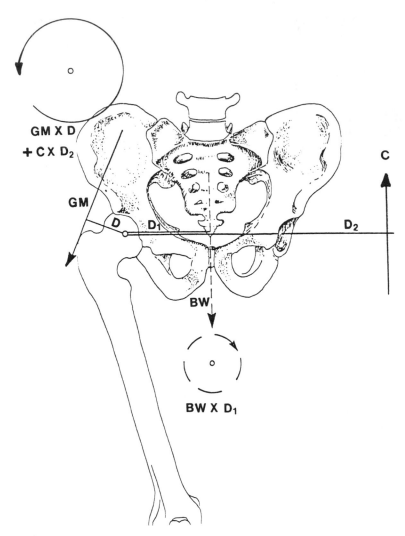

Figure 9.10. Similar mechanical representation of the hip as in Figure 9.6, except in this instance the product of the cane force (*C*) and the distance D_2 is added to the moment for the gluteus medius. To balance the moments, gluteus medius (*GM*) force can be reduced, which will lower the force at the hip. (From Neumann DA, Cook TM: The effect of load and carry position on the electromyographic activity of the gluteus medius during walking. *Phys Ther* 65:305–311, 1985.)

that the head of the femur is located superiorly and posteriorly to the usual location within the acetabulum, markedly affecting the length of the abductor musculature and diminishing its tension-generating abilities. Diminished tension on the greater trochanter results in lower vertical compressive forces that in turn lead to the tendency for a diminished angle of inclination (valgus deformity) of the femoral neck. Treatment is virtually always directed toward correcting the altered mechanics (Fig. 9.11).

Closed reduction is frequently elected because treatment goals can be accomplished by nonsurgical means, such as casting or splinting. These procedures can place the hip in abduction so that adductor and abductor forces are redirected into the acetabulum, increasing their compressive shear components. Thus, the

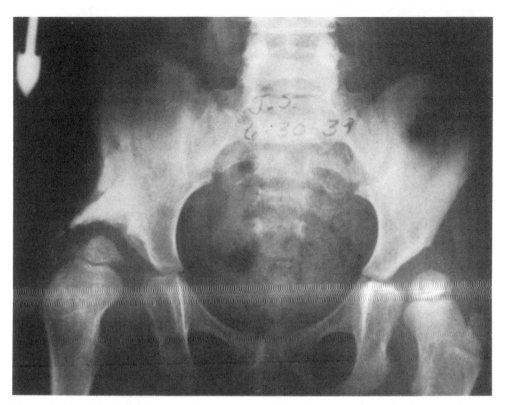

Figure 9.11. Bilateral congenital dislocation of the hips. In the right hip stability is provided by means of the surgically constructed bony shelf.

acetabulum and head of femur are stimulated to mold to each other, decreasing the tendency toward subluxation. In cases of inadequate bony development, surgical creation of a bony shelf may be necessary to provide a stable hip. In other situations varus or valgus osteotomies may be necessary. These procedures will be discussed more thoroughly under the category of degenerative joint disease (31).

The origin of congenital hip dislocation may be traced to faulty hip development in utero. Studies of neonates permit extrapolation to the developing fetus and have demonstrated that hip positions at the extremes of the range of motion create more articular cartilage deformation than do more moderate positions. Frequency and mechanism of loading have been the focus of considerable attention in both the painful and dislocated hip (12). Special note should be made, however, that the time factor of loading is also important. In many cases one can readily observe the patient avoiding sudden (impulsive) loading in favor of a long time interval in order to avoid pain in the joint.

Muscular Losses

Muscular control of the hip is provided by many massive muscles that are capable of producing large torques. Examples of these torques were cited in earlier sections of this chapter. Much less is known about hip torques under pathological situations. Often, clinicians can only estimate the torque production of their patients from knowledge of normal function. Only recently has work been done that adds to the kinesiologist's and the clinician's understanding of hip function. The data reported by Markhede and Stener are valuable, because the 46 patients studied had undergone excision of various hip and thigh musculature as a result of tumor development. In their series the hip was tested both isometrically and isokinetically, so that derived torques could be compared to the opposite limb. The loss of the gluteus maximus created only a slight decrease in extension torque, but the loss of all hamstrings produced significant reductions. For flexion, iliopsoas loss in two patients was apparently responsible for weakness only at the extreme of flexion. Rectus femoris loss in six subjects accounted for a 37% loss in flexion torque and a 17% loss in isokinetic torque. Interesting findings also were produced by the series of eight patients who lost a major portion of the abductor musculature. Even with those suffering extensive loss, the available torque ranged from just under 50% to 80% of the opposite limb. Functional losses were also evaluated, and although some changes such as a positive Trendelenburg sign were noted, the general pattern showed little impairment. Thus, remaining musculature must undergo hypertrophy to offset the losses created by the surgical procedures. The torques required may well result from forces generated in other muscles that are less mechanically advantaged to perform the functional activity (22).

Muscular power also plays a substantial role in treatment of the pathological hip. The Mustard procedure, using the iliopsoas, and the Thomas method, using the external oblique, are examples of tendon transfer techniques that often provide positive results in stabilizing the hips of young patients. In these procedures, the respective muscles are removed from their attachment and relocated onto the greater trochanter of the femur, usually by passing the muscle through an opening created in the wing of the ilium. Cabaud et al, in a retrospective study, provide evidence that these transfer procedures were effective for 23 of 38 patients in improving stability and pain. Success was thought to be primarily due to the redirection of forces. Specifically, an iliopsoas transfer converts a flexion and adduction force to an abduction force. The fact that 37 brace-dependent patients were able to function independently of their braces establishes the value of primary muscular support of the hip (3).

Degenerative Joint Disease

A complication to the normal kinesiology of the hip joint is degenerative joint disease, or osteoarthritis. As the most common disease of axial and peripheral joints, the condition is characterized by deterioration and diminution of articular cartilage (33). The problem is found most frequently in the hip, knee, and hand, but other joints are often involved. Much work has been done on the pathogenesis of the disease; certainly the primary effects are manifest at the articular cartilage. In earlier sections of this chapter, the mechanisms available for articular cartilage to absorb loads were presented. Since deformation of the cartilage is possible because of the viscoelastic properties of the tissue and its contents, loss of the cartilage severely impedes normal joint kinematics and kinetics. Radin, in discussing joint degeneration, states that cracking and tearing begin in the surface layer due to tensile stress. Stresses continue to be propagated into the remaining tissues, even though they are specifically designed to dissipate load to adjacent structures. Subsequent to these degenerative changes the joint's smooth articular surface is lost, in some cases in its entirety. Because the joint no longer possesses low friction surfaces, movement frequently becomes painful.

A practical method of dealing with degenerative joint disease is to diminish the loading through the hip. Some mechanisms have been presented earlier, but others, such as the tenotomy, are also used. This muscle-lengthening technique is often applied to several muscles crossing the joint. By performing this procedure, the muscles heal with noncontractile elements that cannot contribute to the tension-generating capacity of the surgically incised muscle. Because the muscles are now weaker, the joint resultant force will be decreased, allowing time for healing in the joint to occur.

Another mechanical alternative in management of the degenerated hip joint is a femoral osteotomy. Two choices exist: the varus or the valgus procedure. A varus osteotomy may indeed increase the load-bearing surface of the joint (Fig. 9.12) and the moment arm for the abductor muscles. For reasons previously discussed, these increases are highly desirable by-products of the technique. Also note that this method will cause the operated leg to be shorter than the contralateral limb. A short leg causes the pelvis to drop on the involved side and results in greater contact area of the articular surfaces (31). Although a valgus osteotomy may also increase the total joint contact area, its decrease of the abductor moment arm may necessitate a tenotomy to offset this disadvantage (Fig. 9.13) (17).

Total Joint Replacement

Degenerative and rheumatoid arthritis of the hip has led to the development and refinement of procedures for joint surface and total joint replacement. Extensive analyses of both anatomical and mechanical factors have been completed that provide data that improve clinical outcomes. Total joint replacement is, in fact, an excellent example of mechanics applied to the biological specimen. As a result of the procedure, anatomy cannot be totally compromised. Freeman pointed out the importance of adequate blood supply to the head of the femur (10). Elaborations earlier in this chapter explained the need for caution against indiscriminant sectioning of muscles or translocation of bony prominences to which muscles attach. Some surgeons use techniques that remove and reattach the greater trochanter of the femur. The reattachment site is usually more distal

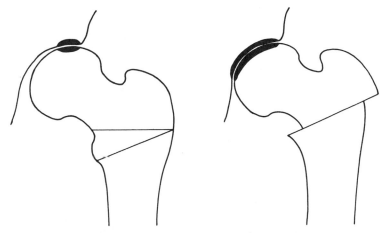

Figure 9.12. A varus osteotomy of the hip removes the wedge of bone shown in the left portion of the figure. Note the change in load-bearing surface and the moment arm for the abductor muscles. (From Radin EL, Simon SR, Rose RM, Paul IL: *Practical Biomechanics for the Orthopedic Surgeon*. New York, John Wiley & Sons, 1979).

and lateral than the original, therefore providing a larger abductor moment arm (Fig. 9.14).

A further matter of import is prosthesis design. Certain alloys of lesser strength may have the advantage of being lighter in weight when compared to other

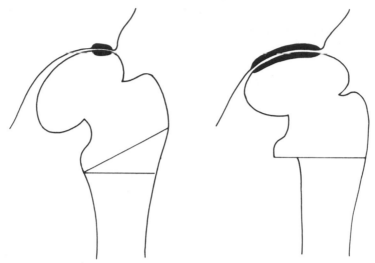

Figure 9.13. A valgus osteotomy, due to difference in the shape of the joint surface as for Figure 9.12, has been performed by means of removal of the wedge-shaped piece of bone. Note that the moment arm of the abductor muscles has been shortened. (From Radin EL, Simon SR, Rose RM, Paul IL: *Practical Biomechanics for the Orthopedic Surgeon.* New York, John Wiley & Sons, 1979.)

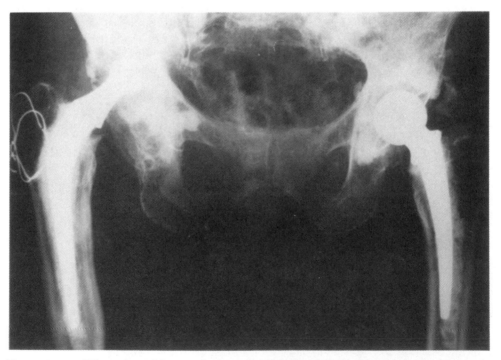

Figure 9.14. Bilateral total hip replacement. Note the differing angles in the hips as a result of the two procedures. The thread-like appearance in the location of the greater trochanter is a result of reattaching the greater trochanter with wire.

materials. In view of the incidence of fracture in the components used in total hip arthroplasty, strength of the materials used is of great importance to the patient. For example, the femoral neck may have a small range of tolerance for a bending moment. In general, the success or failure of total joint replacement is dependent upon the stresses imposed by loading. Stresses exist not only in the prosthetic components themselves but also at the interfaces among the components' cement and bone. Stress caused by bending of the femoral component could be alleviated by increasing the valgus in the femoral component or by decreasing the length of the neck of the prosthesis. Strength could also be increased by increasing the cross section of the prosthetic component, but the weight also will be commensurately increased (32). Debate continues as to the mechanisms responsible for prosthesis loosening. Extensive experimental work is being conducted in an attempt to determine the nature and magnitude of the forces responsible.

Shear forces probably are responsible for the stress occurring at the interfaces. One mechanism used to offset this problem is to decrease the size of the femoral head, serving to commensurately reduce shear forces in the joint. Clarke also speculates that other reasons include socket impingement by the femoral neck at extremes of motion and contact forces generated by joint forces (5).

Stauffer, in a 10-yr follow-up study of total hip replacements, states that the most common type of loosening resulted from prosthesis-cement interface failure due to splitting of the cement mantle (Fig. 9.15). Circumferential stresses are generated due to the axial loading of the tapered and wedge-shaped component inserted into the femur. The incidence of loosening at 10 yr was 11.3% for the acetabular component and 29.9% for the femoral component (37). Johnston and Crowninshield also reported a 10-yr follow-up of total hip arthroplasty patients and stated that component loosening is the major long-term problem of the procedure. Their assessment of bone resorption and radiolucency as related to prosthesis loosening showed that 9% of the patients had femoral component loosening at 10 yr postreplacement, but they observed no correlation between femoral loosening and calcar resorption. Although the incidence of acetabular loosening was only 7.9%, the data indicated that the association of calcar resorption and acetabular loosening was important (17). Each of these studies points out that both the loading of the hip and the components used in the replacement procedures are significant. The actual mechanisms causing the changes and the resulting loosening are not yet precisely clear. Radin has indicated that components not adequately supported or fixed on the femur also may loosen. As further understanding of the conditions that produce component loosening is made possible through clinical, experimental, and theoretical testing, higher success rates will be achieved.

Alternative forms of reconstruction are being offered as means of overcoming the biomechanical faults of the earlier techniques (4). Cementless total hip arthroplasty involves different designs and fixation by threads, pegs, screws, self-locking mechanisms, or a pore-coated prosthesis-bone interface. These models essentially use the principle of increased surface area for facilitating fixation by bony ingrowth. There is also a trend for using less rigid, elastic implants that overcome stress propagation of more rigid implants. Others prefer to use cementless arthroplasty for the patient 40 yr old or less who requires an arthroplasty, as newer materials undergo less wear, and the absence of cement allows bony ingrowth directly into the prosthesis, resulting in less loosening (24). Principles associated with the treatment of the joint all remain fundamentally similar,

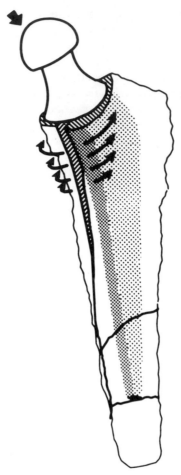

Figure 9.15. Schematic drawing of loosening at the cement-prosthesis interface. See text for further description. (From Stauffer RN: Ten-year follow-up study of total hip replacement. *J Bone Joint Surg* [*Am*] 64:983–990, 1982.)

focusing on minimizing the likelihood of component loosening. However, a cementless prosthesis requires a much longer nonweight-bearing period, to allow component fixation to occur. This presents a considerable problem for the physical therapist to gain or maintain motion without disturbing alignment, while concurrently avoiding extreme losses of muscle strength due to disuse.

Finally, comment about wear needs to be included. Numerous laboratory and clinical retrieval studies demonstrate the import of this consideration in the performance of total joint arthroplasties. Principles of friction must also be applied because the mechanical systems implanted cannot match the low friction of natural human joints. Wear, craters, and the role of debris all have been associated with changes in articular surfaces and lead to potentially undesirable results. In addressing some of the aspects associated with polyethylene wear, Rose and Radin remark that relatively high wear may occur even in the absence of acrylic debris (34). Materials are being refined with an aim to significantly reduce friction and resultant wear.

For the present, knowledge of the role of these factors in disrupting normal joint kinematics is essential for effective function of the therapist in the clinical environment. Further, little is known as to how these factors influence the treatment that the therapist provides. One can only speculate that the extremes of the range of motion, particularly those with forceful movements, should be avoided. The same may be said for impact loading. That is, the extremities which contain the prostheses should not have high loads placed on it in short periods of time. Virtually no data exist as to whether range of motion is best gained with active exercise or passive stretch. Neither do we know whether the patient's ability to generate torque should be accomplished with isometric or dynamic exercise. Only after sufficient data have been generated and communicated will the therapist have a sufficient pool of knowledge on which to judge the clinical selections necessary for the most effective patient care.

Fractures

Biomechanics and material properties also play a role in the treatment of fractures. Extensive analyses of materials, insertion site, failure, and other biomechanical features have been aggressively evaluated by surgeons as well as by manufacturers. In failures of adequate treatment of the intertrochanteric fracture, the clinician is often reminded of the large magnitude of force that must be transmitted across the fracture site. Many of these fractures have been treated by closed techniques that require prolonged inactivity before healing allows weight bearing through the fracture site. Thus, treatment by internal fixation (open reduction) is often the treatment of choice, because improved mobility avoids unsatisfactory results. The fixation device and method must be able to

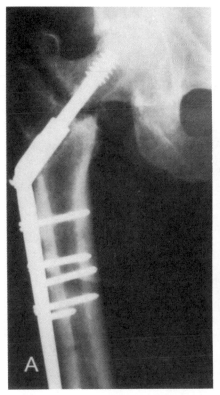
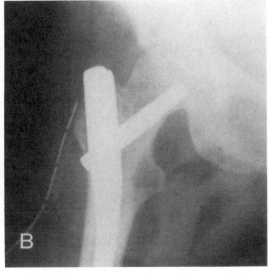

Figure 9.16. Compression screw-plate for fractured femur (A) and a Zickel nail in a patient with metastasis in the femur secondary to breast cancer (B). The nailing was performed to prevent fracture and prolong function.

tolerate loading by body weight and that created by frequent and high muscle forces. In discussing the treatment of hip fractures, Kaufer states that of five possible variables, only bony quality and fragment geometry cannot be modified. The other factors, reduction, the implant, and implant placement, all are controllable. In all cases the ideal is to achieve a stable reduction. Usually this requires sufficient medial and posterior cortical contact between the proximal and distal segments to oppose the tendency toward varus and posterior displacement that occurs in intertrochanteric fractures (19).

Figure 9.16 presents two of the most commonly used implant devices: the compression plate and intramedullary devices. Note that both are inserted into the trabecular bone of the proximal segment. The distal fragment is reattached to the external femoral cortex by the angulated nail plate, and the intramedullary device contacts the internal cortical surface. These devices offer either a fixed or adjustable angle of inclination between 130 and 150°. Provision of an option that would allow greater varus in the hip would only invite complications caused by large bending moments during lower limb loading. So, the choice of device that provides the fracture patient with a stable hip is determined by the consideration given to material properties and their ability to tolerate loading. Upon thorough evaluation of all aspects of mechanics, treatment will more likely yield a positive result.

SUMMARY

The hip joint, by virtue of its location in the body, has the unenviable task of providing both large ranges of motion and large torques in attempting to meet the requirements imposed by human motion. Loads that must be tolerated by the joint create special degenerative pathologies that provide applications of biomechanics. As further information becomes available on load-bearing joints and their clinical management, the application of biomechanical principles will become even more important in assuring that patients are left with minimal dysfunction.

References

1. Backman S: The proximal end of the femur. *Acta Radiol [Suppl]* 146:1–166, 1957.
2. Brand RA, Crowninshield RD, Johnston RC, Pedersen DR: Forces on the femoral head during activities of daily living. *Iowa Orthop J* 2:43–49, 1982.
3. Cabaud HE, Westin GW, Connelly S: Tendon transfers in the paralytic hip. *J Bone Joint Surg [Am]* 61:1035–1041, 1979.
4. Capello WN: Surface replacement. *Iowa Orthop J* 3:50–54, 1983.
5. Clarke IC: Biomechanics. *Orthop Clin North Am* 13:681–707, 1982.
6. Dostal WF: The Prediction of Coordinates of Bony Landmark and Hip Muscle Attachment Points. Ph.D. thesis, Graduate College, University of Iowa, Iowa City, Iowa, 1979.
7. Dostal WF, Andrews JG: A three dimensional biomechanical model of hip musculature. *J Biomech* 14:803–812, 1981.
8. Favill J: *Outline of the Spinal Nerves*. Springfield, IL, Charles C Thomas, 1946.
9. Fischer FJ, Houtz SJ: Evaluation and function of the gluteus maximus muscle. *Am J Phys Med* 47:182–191, 1968.
10. Freeman MAR: Some anatomical and mechanical considerations relevant to the surface replacement of the femoral head. *Clin Orthop* 134:19–24, 1978.
11. Haley ET: Range of hip rotation and torque of hip rotator muscle groups. *Am J Phys Med* 32:261–270, 1953.
12. Hjelmstedt A, Asplund S: Congenital dislocation of the hip: a biomechanical study in autopsy specimens. *J Pediatr Orthop* 3:491–497, 1983.

13. Hoaglund FT, Low WD: Anatomy of the femoral neck and head, with comparative data from caucasians and Hong Kong Chinese. *Clin Orthop* 152:10–16, 1980.
14. Inman VT: Functional aspects of the abductor muscles of the hip. *J Bone Joint Surg [Am]* 29:607–619, 1947.
15. Jarvis DK: Relative strength of the hip rotator muscle groups. *J Am Phys Ther Assoc* 32:500–503, 1952.
16. Johnston RC: Mechanical considerations of the hip joint. *Arch Surg* 107:411–417, 1973.
17. Johnston RC, Crowninshield RD: Roentgenologic results of total hip arthroplasty. *Clin Orthop* 181:92–98, 1983.
18. Kapandji IA: *The Physiology of the Joint: Lower Limb*, vol 2. Baltimore, Williams & Wilkins, 1971.
19. Kaufer H: Mechanics of the treatment of hip injuries. *Clin Orthop* 146:53–61, 1980.
20. Kessler R, Hertling D: *Management of Common Musculoskeletal Disorders*. New York, Harper & Row, 1983.
21. Lehmkuhl LD, Smith L: *Brunnstrom's Clinical Kinesiology*. Philadelphia, FA Davis, 1983.
22. Markhede G, Stener B: Function after removal of various hip and thigh muscles for extirpation of tumors. *Acta Orthop Scand* 52:373–395, 1981.
23. Merchant AC: Hip abductor muscle force. *J Bone Joint Surg [Am]* 47:462–476, 1965.
24. Moreland DW: Cement in total hip arthroplasty. *Clin Orthop* 141:70–41, 1983.
25. Murray MP, Sepic SB: Maximum isometric torque of hip abductor and adductor muscles. *Phys Ther* 48:1327–1335, 1968.
26. Nemeth G, Ekholm J, Arborelius UP, et al: Influence of knee flexion on isometric hip extensor strength. *Scand J Rehabil Med* 15:97–101, 1983.
27. Olson VL, Smidt GL, Johnston RC: The maximum torque generated by the eccentric, isometric, and concentric contractions of the hip abductor muscles. *Phys Ther* 52:149–157, 1972.
28. Pare EB, Stern JT, Schwartz JM: Functional differentiation within the tensor fasciae latae. *J Bone Joint Surg [Am]* 63:1457–1471, 1981.
29. Pauwels F: *Biomechanics of the Normal and Diseased Hip*. Berlin, Springer-Verlag, 1976.
30. Radin EL: Biomechanics of the human hip. *Clin Orthop* 152:28–34, 1980.
31. Radin EL, Paul IL: The biomechanics of congenital dislocated hips and their treatment. *Clin Orthop* 98:32–38, 1974.
32. Radin EL, Simon SR, Rose RM, Paul IL: *Practical Biomechanics for the Orthopedic Surgeon*. New York, Wiley, 1979.
33. Rodnan GP, Schumacher HR (eds): *Primer on the Rheumatic Diseases*. Atlanta, Arthritis Foundation, 1983.
34. Rose RM, Radin EL: Wear of polyethylene in the total hip prosthesis. *Clin Orthop* 170:107–115, 1982.
35. Rydell N: Biomechanics of the hip joint. *Clin Orthop* 92:6–15, 1973.
36. Soderberg GL, Dostal WF: Electromyographic study of three parts of the gluteus medius muscle during functional activities. *Phys Ther* 58:691–696, 1978.
37. Stauffer RN: Ten-year follow-up study of total hip replacement. *J Bone Joint Surg [Am]* 64:983–990, 1982.
38. Williams PL, Warwick R (eds): *Gray's Anatomy*, ed 36. Philadelphia, WB Saunders, 1980.

10

Knee

Compared to any other joint the knee has been subjected to the greatest amount of attention, both clinical and investigative. The joint, by virtue of bony and soft tissue structure, epitomizes arthrokinematics that demand motion beyond the typical 1° of freedom. In addition, the inclusion of cartilageneous pads between the joint surfaces makes for an interesting study of load transmission and injuries. Finally, the fact that the joint is located between the body's longest bony segments predisposes the joint to traumatic injury and other pathologies. This chapter will discuss these and other aspects of the kinesiology and pathokinesiology of the knee.

MUSCULAR ACTIONS

There has been considerable attention given to the quadriceps because of the importance of these muscles in controlling the joint. Little information is available on the flexor musculature because of a comparatively less significant role in knee control. Considered as a whole, the extensors are composed of a cross sectional area approximately 148 cm^2, approximately three times that of the hamstring musculature (46). The flexor group is supported functionally by the sartorius, gracilis, popliteus, and gastrocnemius muscles. Each of these has at least one additional function and therefore cannot be considered as a primary knee flexor.

Special note should be taken of the musculature responsible for controlling knee motion, because most of the key components also serve at either the hip or the ankle. Of all the flexor musculature only the popliteus can claim a single joint action. Conversely, on the extensor side, the rectus femoris can play an important role in hip motion. Thus, in any considerations of knee motion the therapist must be aware of both the proximal and distal joint positions in order to accurately test or interpret patient performance. Considering the possible combinations used by patients in generating joint torques will assist the therapist with understanding how the interactions produce effective function in the lower limb.

Most frequently used are the knee extension-hip extension and hip flexion-knee flexion combinations. The extension "synergy" is commonly found in activities such as rising from a chair or in ascending stairs. Gait is also a useful example, because if appropriate moments were not simultaneously generated during stance phase at the hip and knee, flexor moments would result in the tendency for the upper body to rotate around the most distally fixed segment. Control of the extended position at each of these joints is by the hamstrings at the hip and the quadriceps at the knee. However, note that these muscles also have antagonistic actions, i.e., knee flexion and hip flexion for the hamstrings and the rectus femoris, respectively. So, if both muscle groups generate tension, motion tends to be prevented and isometric contractions result. From this situation, an important lesson in mechanics can be learned. The explanation for our ability to complete the simultaneous knee and hip extension movement appears to rest in the finding of Elftman, who in 1939 published the lengths of moment arms for the muscle groups for a representative individual. He stated that the 4.4-cm rectus femoris moment arm at the knee exceeds the moment arm of 3.9 cm at the hip. Conversely, the 6.7-cm moment arm of the hamstrings at the hip exceeded the moment arm of 3.4 cm at the knee. Because the moment arms favor knee extension for the rectus femoris and hip extension for the hamstrings, simultaneous motions can be achieved (22). Achieving both motions concurrently has another beneficial effect. As the knee is extended, the hamstring musculature is actually being lengthened at the knee. Thus, because the muscle is lengthened at the knee while tension is needed at the hip, the motions maintain the muscle at an appropriate length for tension generation. A similar explanation can be given for the function of the rectus femoris, with the exception being that the muscle is being lengthened at the hip.

One further extension of the multiple joint phenomenon is apparent if consideration is given to the effects on the gastrocnemius muscle. The preceding information shows that hip extension in essence facilitates knee extension. Thus, it should also be clear that knee extension puts the gastrocnemius muscle in a lengthened position. The overall result is that the gastrocnemius is then able to effectively exert tension for the purpose of plantar flexion of the ankle, commonly done with the hip and knee in extension. The result is an interdependency among the joints which are responsible for propulsion and maintaining the upright posture. These relationships also hold true during eccentric phases of muscle activity and are demonstrated easily by assuming a sitting position from upright standing.

The combined motions of hip flexion and knee flexion occur in ascending stairs, the latter being accomplished passively. Active control of both motions is frequently achieved by eccentric contractions of the hip and knee extensors. With this combination the rectus femoris is shortening at the hip while simultaneously elongating at the knee.

The knee extension-hip flexion motion can be completed by the quadriceps. This straight leg-raising maneuver is limited, however, for two reasons. First, the musculature comprising the quadriceps is shortening at both the hip and the knee, therefore limiting the muscle's tension-generating ability. This limitation has been referred to as active insufficiency (54). Secondly, the antagonistic hamstrings are being stretched to the point of limiting the range of motion. Thus, passive insufficiency is involved. Similar comments can be made for the reciprocal situations as they apply to the hamstrings during the motions of knee flexion and hip extension. In fact, active insufficiency can be easily demonstrated by noting, while single limb standing, one's inability to touch the heel to the buttock by actively contracting the knee flexors of the free lower limb.

Many analyses of the function of the components of the quadriceps have been completed. Most have used electromyographic techniques to make determinations of level and duration of muscle activity. Brunnstrom, however, used descriptive anatomy and palpation to conclude that the rectus femoris is activated after the early part of the knee extension range of motion and particularly when considerable resistance had to be overcome (54). Other more extensive works have since been completed that provide more objective data. Of some interest has been the influence of hip position upon the performance of the rectus femoris. Close, in a 1964 study, evaluated the EMG activity of the rectus femoris during knee extension performed in the supine and sitting positions. Rectus femoris and vasti activity occurred simultaneously during supine knee extension, but sitting knee extension produced rectus femoris activity only at terminal extension (16). The trend would likely be confirmed by visual analysis of supine and sitting position data presented by Okamoto, at least for the trials completed from the supine position. The sitting trials do not corroborate the Close data (74). However, a 1980 study showed that the rectus femoris contracted only near the limit of knee extension. In analyzing the quadriceps during other activities these investigators also found high levels of activity in the rectus femoris during the initial range of the straight leg raise and throughout hip flexion with the knee flexed (27).

Because the function of the quadriceps is regarded with great import as a measure of rehabilitation, some work has been done to assess the actions of the quadriceps muscle during exercises. The primary purpose of these works has been to determine whether there is a differential role of the musculature in various portions of the range of motion. Pocock investigated the temporal phase of action of the three superficial quadriceps femoris muscle components during various clinically useful quadriceps exercises. EMG activity was measured during active knee extension under several resistive loading conditions. The most important conclusion was that there was little variation in temporal sequence among the three quadriceps components and that the EMG patterns were similar throughout the entire range of knee extension (80). These findings have since been verified by other investigators who have evaluated the potential specificity of activity of the vastus medialis muscle in the terminal portion of knee extension (8, 21, 41).

Other studies have evaluated levels of muscle activity during exercises used for purposes of rehabilitation. The straight leg raise and the isometric quadriceps setting exercise frequently have been compared. Gough and Ladley demonstrated that quadriceps activity was greater during isometric contraction in 25 subjects as opposed to only 6 subjects for the straight leg raise maneuver (35). Knight et al concluded that none of the three superficial quadriceps muscles are as active during straight leg raising as during knee extension at the same relative workload (50). Most recently Soderberg and Cook reported the results of a study comparing the two exercises while EMG was recorded from the vastus medialis and the rectus femoris muscles. As a result of the maximal effort trials completed by the 40 normal subjects, highly significant differences were demonstrated between the activity levels of the two muscles. In the straight leg raise, the mean normalized level of rectus activity was 93% of the maximum, while that of the vastus medialis was only 63% of its maximum. Conversely, for the quadriceps-setting exercise the rectus activity was only 52% as compared to 103% for the vastus medialis. Because of differences demonstrated in the quadriceps and in the biceps femoris and gluteus medius muscles the exercise selected should be based on therapeutic purposes (92).

The distal, and most oblique, portion of the vastus medialis has also been of interest because of potential functions resulting from the alignment of the muscle fibers. Due to the position of the fibers this portion of the muscle is better located to provide a medial force on the patella rather than assist the quadriceps muscle with knee extension. Some speculation as to the importance of this function in resisting lateral displacements, or even dislocations, of the patella has been offered.

Because of the undefined role of the oblique fibers of the vastus medialis, Lieb and Perry derived EMG data simultaneously from the three other components of the quadriceps and from the long and oblique portions of the vastus medialis. Results showed that the EMG signal amplitude derived from the oblique was twice that of the other components. There were, however, no other differences in respect to the other components tested. These authors also commented that there was no consistent variation in EMG pattern to suggest that any one of the muscles studied had a "predominant" responsibility for knee extension in any part of the range of motion (58). Offering an opposite view, Reynolds et al confirmed the lack of a specific role of the oblique in their study of muscle function during terminal knee extension. Comparison of the EMG derived from the medialis oblique and the lateralis showed low and insignificant differences between the activity of the two muscles (83).

Other muscles that affect the knee have also been studied. Because the flexors are attached either medially or laterally to the tibia, they have some tendency to rotate the knee. Lateral rotators include the biceps femoris and the tensor fascia latae. Kapandji states that the tensor muscle loses the ability to flex and rotate when the knee is extended, in effect becoming only a knee extensor (46). Of all the muscles posterior to the knee that may have a role in rotation, only the short head of the biceps femoris (lateral rotation) and the popliteus (medial rotation) are monarticular muscles.

Specifically, the popliteus is potentially important because of the role that the muscle may serve in "unlocking" the knee. Other functions of this muscle have been purported to be posterior displacement of the lateral meniscus and the control of forward motion of the femur on the tibia. To more thoroughly investigate the function of the popliteus Basmajian and Lovejoy used EMG while a number of different activities were performed. Results showed the muscle to be most active on medial rotation of the shank segment. Flexion action appeared to be minimal. Prevention of forward displacement of the femur and posterior motion of the meniscus, although not unequivocally established, were supported by the findings of this study (5). More recently Mann and Hagy studied the popliteus during planned exercises and gait. Their work confirmed the medial rotation function of the muscle, partly via the phasic activity associated with internal tibial rotation required during the gait cycle. The internally rotated position of the tibia on the femur throughout most of the stance phase was also apparently maintained by the popliteus (63).

Little information is available as to the function of the gastrocnemius at the knee. Because of the bilateral composition of the muscular insertion into the femur little rotary component could be mustered. The ability of the muscle to create knee flexion is well recognized, however, and may be demonstrated in the control of knee hyperextension.

ARTHROLOGY AND ARTHROKINEMATICS

The knee joint has major responsibility for carrying out the functional activities required for normal daily function. Joint surfaces and structures must, of necessity, successfully tolerate loads of magnitudes similar to those cited for the hip joint. However, inherent stability such as exists at the hip is not present at the knee joint. Further, the joint is located between the two longest levers in the body, therefore subjecting the joint to or requiring great torques. Because the joint has a large range of motion in only one plane the bony and soft tissue structures must be capable of withstanding considerable loads and/or externally applied torques. A thorough understanding of the arthrology and arthrokinematics is required, therefore, to comprehend the import of the structure on the normal and abnormal function.

Arthrology

Osteology

The bony makeup of the tibiofemoral joint appears, from the superficial standpoint, to be rather simple. However, the femoral condyles should be considered as individual convex surfaces. This is necessitated by the marked differences in the shape of the condyles, both femoral and tibial. Gross examination of the femur shows that the medial condyle projects extensively, both longitudinally and medially. This is required to offset the lateral to medial migration of the femur as the shaft of the bone progresses distally. The femoral condyles differ in anterior-posterior dimension and configuration, a factor that is important when joint movement takes place. For example, the medial and lateral condyles both decrease their radii from anterior to posterior. That is, the distance from the center of rotation in the condyles is greatest towards the anterior bony surface, progressively decreasing as one moves along the distal edge of the bone to the posterior surface. Other differences exist, however, in that the medial condyle is longer anteroposteriorly while the lateral condyle is flatter (46). The lateral condyle is more prominent anteriorly, probably to control the tendency for lateral displacement of the patella via the pull of the quadriceps.

The medial and lateral compartments of the tibial plateau also have demonstrable bony differences. Some texts state that the tibial plateaus are convex in both the mediolateral and the anteroposterior directions, although the latter direction is not uniform (103). Kapandji states that anteroposteriorly the medial tibial condyle is concave superiorly, while the lateral condyle is convex superiorly. Further, because the radii of curvature of these bony segments are not equal, the articular surfaces are not congruent. That the medial tibial surface is longer than the lateral anteroposteriorly, and slightly concave to the lateral side, may have implication for knee kinematics (103). Neither can the intercondylar eminence be ignored because of the mechanical resistance that may be offered to the femoral condyles during rotatory motions of the knee.

The patella must also be considered because of the significant role that the bone plays in knee mechanics and pathologies. Imbedded in the patellar tendon, the posterior aspect of the bone is well endowed with articular cartilage. Agreement exists that respective facets articulate with the femoral condyles, while some indicate special locations during specific points in the range of motion of flexion and extension (7, 103).

Finally, osteologic considerations at the knee would be incomplete without a brief discussion of the proximal tibiofibular joint. Although not a part of the knee joint proper, this joint has distinct soft tissue connections that have bearing on the arthrokinematics of the knee. Little information is available on the specific impact of the anatomy and kinematics of this joint. One study, however, supplied both radiographic and anatomic data that classified the joint geometry into either horizontal or oblique configurations. The horizontal was associated with increased surface area and greater rotary mobility while the oblique type had less of each of these characteristics. Based on the results of this study the author concluded that the primary functions of the proximal tibiofibular joint are to dissipate lateral tibial bending moments and torsional stresses applied at the ankle. The role of the joint in tensile versus compressive loading is probably not clear or of any particular significance (73).

Ligaments

Anatomic locations of soft tissue structures are relevant because of the effects that they have on the resulting joint motion. Ligaments of primary interest are the tibial and fibular collateral and the anterior and posterior cruciate ligaments. The tibial or medial collateral ligament extends from a posterosuperior position on the femur to the medial aspect of the medial tibial plateau. There is general agreement that the tibial collateral and its posterior oblique fibers blend with the capsule of the joint. Consensus also exists that the ligament is attached to the medial meniscus (46, 103). The lateral collateral ligament is much smaller than the medial as it traverses the joint from the posterior and superior lateral femoral condyle to the fibular head. In general, the shape of this ligament is much rounder and thinner than the medial collateral ligament (103).

The anterior and posterior cruciate ligaments, believed to control anterior and posterior translatory movement of the two bony segments on each other, also need to be considered. As implied by name, the anterior cruciate runs from the anterior middle portion of the tibia in a superior and posterior direction to an attachment on the medial aspect of the lateral femoral condyle. Conversely, the posterior cruciate has attachments between the middle of the posterior tibial plateau and the anterolateral aspect of the medial femoral condyle. The import of these attachment sites will become clear when the kinematics of the joint are presented.

One additional ligament deserving mention is the ligamentum patellae. Forming the central portion of the common tendon of the quadriceps, this ligament is approximately 8 cm in length from the patella to the tibial tuberosity (103). Tensile strength is considered to be very high.

Specific mention must also be made of the meniscofemoral ligaments. Both anterior and posterior portions emanate from the lateral meniscus, ultimately running in close association with the posterior cruciate ligament. Their effects will also be explained in later sections of this chapter.

Capsule

The complicated and very large capsule of the knee receives extensive reinforcement, particularly from the collateral and patellar ligaments. One area of interest is the posterolateral aspect, since this segment is frequently damaged in traumatic injuries. Reinforcement of the capsule is provided by the arcuate or fabellofibular ligaments alone or collectively. In over two-thirds of the knees studied the fabellofibular ligaments were responsible for the reinforcement (87). Few detailed studies of this region have been undertaken. One such study, including 35 dissections, has shown that the lateral structures of the knee can be divided into three layers. The deepest part of the lateral aspect of the capsule divides into two laminae just posterior to the overlying iliotibial tract. These laminae encompass the arcuate, fabellofibular, and lateral collateral ligaments.

Also recall that the posterior capsule is specifically reinforced by the deep and posterior oblique portions of the medial collateral ligament (48). Further reinforcement posteriorly is provided by the oblique popliteal ligament, derived from the semimembranosus muscle (103). Further strength is gained via muscular tendons, for example the patellar and quadriceps tendons anteriorly, the iliotibial band laterally, and the tendons of the pes anserine medially. The most important additional posterior support is derived from the tendons of the biceps femoris, the gastrocnemius, and the popliteus muscles. For further descriptions of the intricacies of the knee joint the reader should resort to an anatomy text.

Menisci

When considering the knee joint the menisci must also be included. Both the medial and lateral menisci are semilunar in shape, although the lateral forms a greater part of a circle than does the medial. These wedge-shaped structures have been credited with serving as a protector for the capsule while at the same time deepening the articulation and providing a buffer for pressure (94). The peripheral tibial and ligamentous attachments, and lack of central attachments are critical to the understanding of the joint arthrokinematics. That is, the unattached internal edge of a meniscus allows for considerable freedom of movement. On the other hand, because of the attachment of the medial meniscus to the semimembranosus and the medial collateral ligament, mobility of the peripheral portion is limited, thus potentially affecting the type of internal derangement that frequently results from traumatic injury of the knee. Generally, the lateral meniscus is considered to be the more mobile of the two, in spite of the attachment to the popliteus muscle.

Arthrokinematics

Rotation

Movement of the knee, whether active or passive, demands interaction among a variety of the structures detailed in earlier sections of this chapter. Although the largest magnitude of movement is in the sagittal plane, i.e., flexion-extension, rotational movements are crucial to normal function. Consensus exists that during extension of the nonweight-bearing knee, external rotation of the tibia occurs during the last 30° of extension. Circumstances are different in the case of weight bearing, however, because the tibia is now the fixed segment. As a result, the 5 to 7° of rotation that occur under the later condition most probably result from combined tibial external rotation and femoral internal rotation. The overall resultant effect of this motion is the achievement of the close-packed position of the knee joint, indicative of maximum congruity of the surfaces. Many explanations have been offered as to the reasons why this rotational movement occurs. The unequal curvature of the femoral condyles has been suggested, because different degrees of rotation would be required by the different bony geometry. Similar rationale can be applied to the different anteroposterior femoral condyle dimensions as a reason for the rotation. Soft tissue influences have also been cited. Included in this category are tightening of either or both the anterior and posterior cruciate ligaments. Perhaps the ligaments wind on themselves during the terminal phases of knee extension. Even a tightening of the collateral ligaments has been postulated. Perhaps the most likely explanation is that change in position or length of these and other structures combine to produce the close-packed position.

Menisci and their motion also are a factor in knee arthrokinematics. Because they are deformable and mobile, reconfiguration of the joint produces relocation of the horns of the menisci. Also recall that various muscles send slips to the menisci, producing a direct effect on the motion that occurs. Steindler has stated that in knee extension the menisci are forced forward and stretched, increasing the pressure on these cartilagenous discs (94). Although essentially in agreement, Kapandji specifies that during active knee extension the menisci are pulled forward by the meniscopatellar fibers. Even the posterior horn of the lateral meniscus is pulled anteriorly, during extension, by tension developed in the meniscofemoral ligament as the posterior cruciate ligament becomes taut. Active knee flexion also causes posterior menisci movement, the medial via tension in the semimembranosus and the lateral by tension in the popliteus expansion. In rotational movements and during passive knee motion the menisci are considered to follow the femoral condyles (46).

Surface Motions

The femoral, or convex surface, in articulation with the tibial or concave surface, provides an excellent example to study joint movements. As has been discussed in Chapter 3, "Articular Mechanics and Function," the surfaces act in a prescribed manner. Considering specifically the knee, as the tibia is extended on the femur, note that rolling and sliding occur in the same direction (Fig. 10.1). Now consider the movement in which the femoral condyles move. Note that unless the femur slides anteriorly on the tibia during the joint flexion the femur would literally roll off the posterior margin of the tibia (Fig. 10.2). Accomplishing this sliding motion allows the femur to use the total surface of the femoral condyle. Thus, in the case of the convex moving on the concave, the roll and

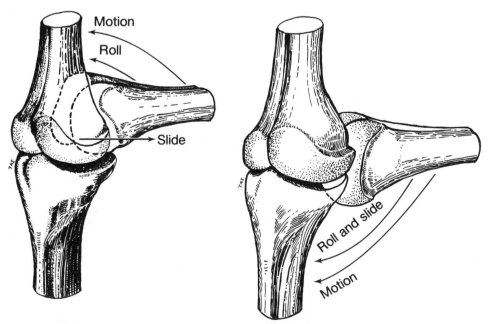

Figure 10.1.   A schematic drawing of the motions between the tibia and femur. During movement of the concave on the convex surface, as for the tibia on the femur, the rolling and sliding are in the same direction. If the femur moves on the tibia the roll and slide are in opposite directions for normal movement to occur.

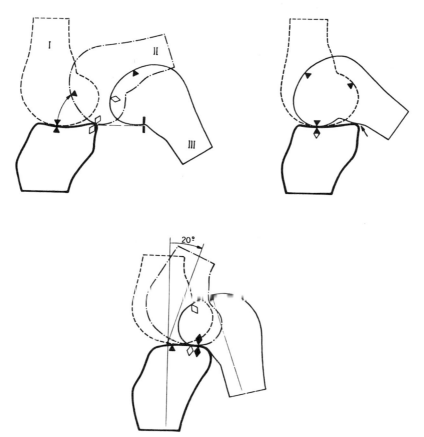

Figure 10.2. A graphic depiction of the results of lack of the normal mechanism shown in Figure 10.1. The *upper left* shows that the femur would fall off the posterior aspect of the tibia if slide did not occur in the opposite direction. The *upper right* shows the effect of too much slide, while the *bottom figure* shows the normal condition. The diamonds are contact points for the respective portions of the range of motion. (From Kapandji IA: *The Physiology of the Joints.* New York, Churchill Livingstone, 1970, vol 2.)

slide occur in opposite directions. In moving these surfaces on each other congruity has been maintained. Without the existence of such a mechanism joint integrity would be sacrificed so much so that little or no stability would remain.

The patellofemoral joint cannot be ignored, primarily because of the mechanical effect in both normal and pathological motion. During flexion and extension of the knee the patella moves vertically as much as 8 cm in the intercondylar groove. While flexion is accomplished the patella and patellar tendon are also displaced posteriorly. This occurs because as viewed from a lateral projection the angle of attachment of the tendon to the tibial tuberosity is progressively diminished (Fig. 10.3). Finally, during rotation of the knee the patella is displaced laterally during internal rotation of the tibia and medially during lateral rotation of the tibia (46). Without these motions, considered accessory by some, the normal arthrokinematics cannot be demonstrated in the knee.

BIOMECHANICS

The pertinent anatomical considerations have been described in the previous section. An understanding of these features leads to the mechanical events that

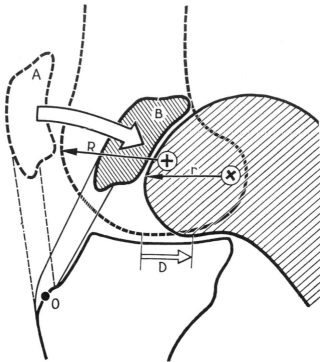

Figure 10.3.   Two superimposed lateral views of the knee. The position of the patella in extension (*A*) and in flexion (*B*) is shown. The decreased distance (*R* and *r*) of the patella from the axes of rotation (+ and ×) is also shown. *D* is the displacement of the contact point between the two bones, and *0* signifies the attachment of the patellar ligament. (From Kapandji IA: *The Physiology of the Joints.* New York, Churchill Livingstone, 1970, vol 2.)

occur at the knee joint. Discussed in this section of the chapter are the instant center of rotation and the influence of the length of various knee ligaments on the resultant motion. Information on the biomechanical effect of the patella and the patellar ligament will also be presented.

Kinematics

The kinematics of the knee have been well described by many clinicians and investigators. The sagittal plane range of motion consists of approximately 10° of hyperextension to 145° of flexion. The fully extended or close-packed position negates rotation and adduction and abduction (valgus and varus). However, up to 45° each of internal and external rotation are available when the knee is at 90° of flexion. Laubenthal et al, using electrogoniometry, quantified the knee motion necessary to perform activities of daily living. Eighty-three degrees was the mean value recorded for stair climbing, 93° for sitting, and 106 for shoe tying (53). Observation indicates that 65 to 70° of knee flexion is required during normal gait.

Instant Center of Rotation

Several attempts have been made to identify the location of the instant center of rotation for the sagittal plane motion of the knee. The technique and the results are thoroughly described in the volume by Frankel and Burstein (28).

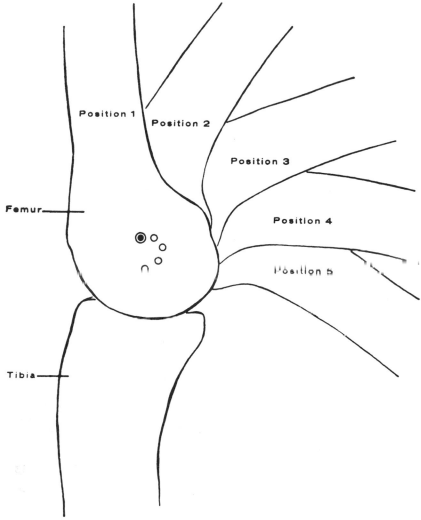

Figure 10.4. The instant center of rotation is plotted with respect to both the femur and tibia. The *encircled solid circle* represents the location for position 1. (From Frankel VH, Burstein AH: *Orthopaedic Biomechanics*. Philadelphia, Lea & Febiger, 1970.)

Their method established the semicircular pathway shown in Figure 10.4. Smidt also completed an instant center analysis for the knee and determined a slightly different locus (Fig. 10.5). He noted that the centers fell within a circle with a diameter of 2.3 cm. All points were located on axes that penetrated the lateral femoral condyle (91). Little information is available as to the axis for transverse plane knee rotation. According to Steindler the vertical axis of the knee passes through the medial condyle (94). Work by Wang and Walker, accomplished while assessing changes in ligament lengths, confirmed this in several specimens for several joint angles (102). More recently, with the knee being used as an example, the difficulties associated with instant center analysis have been addressed (93). Regardless of the precise location for the instant center, the knee cannot be considered to be a true hinge joint. Further, and perhaps more importantly, bony and soft tissues produce changes in the arthrokinematics during a range of motion because the location of the center of rotation moves.

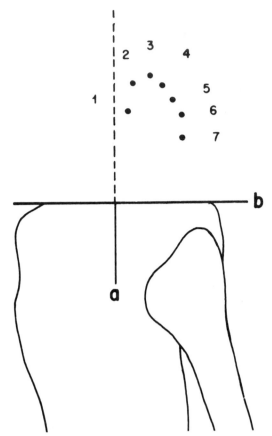

Figure 10.5. Pathway of the instant centers with respect to the tibia and femur for full extension to 90° of flexion in increments of 15°. (From Smidt GL: Biomechanical analysis of knee flexion and extension. *J Biomech* 6:79–92, 1973.)

Effects of Motion on Ligaments

Consider the position of the medial collateral ligament as shown in knee extension in Figure 10.6. Then, study the ligament configuration with the knee in the flexed position and note that several events have occurred. First, the contact point of the femur on the tibia has moved posteriorly. In addition, the menisci have also been required to assume a new position. The mechanisms available for these movements were discussed in a previous section of this chapter. As mentioned previously, the patellar ligament can be seen to have decreased the angle of insertion in relationship to the tibia. Finally, the joint motion has necessitated changes in the length of the anterior and posterior segments of the long fibers of the medial collateral ligament. These changes, even though relatively small, create stretching of the anterior portion of the ligament and concurrent slack in the posterior segment. Realize also that length changes concurrently take place in the lateral collateral and cruciate ligaments of the knee. Changes also occur in the capsule, the most important of which is the slack produced in the posterior portion.

Because of the stress in the ligaments and the capsule a large amount of work has been undertaken to evaluate the role of ligaments in restraining motion in the knee. In vitro and in vivo studies have been performed during anteroposte-

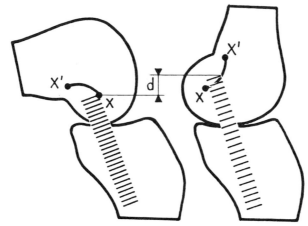

Figure 10.6.   Lateral view of the knee in flexion and extension, showing the effects on the medial collateral ligament. Due to the location of the center of rotation the anterior portion of the ligament may become taut during flexion, while the posterior is placed on a slack. The length of the ligament is shown as d, the centers of curvature of the condyles as X and X'. (From Kapandji IA: *The Physiology of the Joints.* New York, Churchill Livingstone, 1970, vol 2.)

rior, valgus, and varus motion and during induced torques. Results from some of these studies improve our understanding of knee function and have implications for treatment indications and contraindications. Table 10.1 summarizes the results of some of the studies that have been reported.

In regard to the cruciate ligaments, Cabaud has provided a summary of the function of the anterior ligament. There is strong documentation that this ligament resists anterior displacement of the tibia on the femur. Probably less recognized is the anterior cruciate's primary role in resisting internal rotation (12). This function has been reinforced by the findings of Lipke and associates who determined that in 7 of 17 cadaver knees significant increases in rotation occurred with sectioning of this ligament (60). Cabaud further summarizes, while ignoring any twist within the ligament, that the posterior fibers of this ligament are longest in the position of knee extension while the anterior fibers are most tense in flexion (12). Conversely, the posterior cruciate is given primary credit for resisting posterior displacement of the tibia on the femur. Less appears to be known about the rotation function of this ligament, although Fukubayashi et al have shown a marked loss of rotation with insufficiency of the cruciate ligaments. That is, intact ligaments produced concurrent rotation. As a result, they concluded that the cruciates also constitute a primary mechanism in the production and control of rotation during anterior and posterior knee motion (32). An example of their results is shown in Figure 10.7.

Because sometimes the cruciate ligaments are deficient, there is also some interest in determining which structures provide secondary restraint to motion. Butler and coworkers specifically addressed this issue in performing the antero-posterior drawer sign in human knees. With the loss of the anterior cruciate and the iliotibial tract and band, the mid one-third of the medial and lateral capsules and the medial and lateral collateral ligaments all serve to restrain this motion. Secondary restraints for posterior motion were provided by the posterior lateral capsule and popliteus complex combined and also by the medial collateral ligament. The authors noted, however, that if the cruciates are torn, only minimal

Table 10.1.   Ligaments

	Medial collateral	Lateral collateral	Ant. cruciate	Post. cruciate
Steindler 1955	Checks both rotations	Tight in ext. Checks rot. and ext. in ext. Checks in rot. late. No checking effect in flexion.	Tight in extension, loose in flexion 30–90°. >90° wound with post. and tight.	Tight in flexion after 30°
Brantigan and Voshell 1941	Tight in ext. and flex. Limits rot. motion in ext.	Tight in ext. only. Limits rot. motion in ext.	Prevents lat. motion (i.e., tight?). Limits rot. motion in ext.	Prevents lat. motion (i.e., tight?) Limits rot. motion in ext.
Kapandji 1970	Taut during ext., slack during flex. Med. rot. relaxes, lat. rot. tightens (when extended)	Taut during ext. Slack during flex. Med. rot. relaxes, lat. rot. tightens (when extended)	Slackened in full flex. Stretched in hyperext. Lat. rot. relaxes, med. rot. tightens (when extended) Says have constant length ratio 3:5 with posterior shorter	Stretched during ext. and hyperext. Lat. rot. relaxes, med. rot. tightens (when extended)
Wang and Walker 1974	Collaterals 2× as effective in controlling rotation laxity		Note: Cite Roud who says is some tension in all positions	
Girgis et al 1975			Cruciates wound in flex., unwound in ext. Becomes loose once flexed. In 25 cases, 14 had ant. longer, 11 had post. longer.	Bulk of loose in ext. Bulk becomes tight once 30° of flexion.
Markolf et al 1976	Section creates greatest torsional laxity and increase in int. rot. Main contributor to valgus stiffness. Section with posterior capsule produced large ↑ in AP laxity.	Section with posterior capsule decreased ext. rot. stiffness. No effect on varus stiffness.	Isolated section produced greatest ↑ in AP laxity at full ext.	Isolated section produced greatest ↑ at 90° flexion

Table 10.1.—*Continued*

	Medial collateral	Lateral collateral	Ant. cruciate	Post. cruciate
Grood et al 1977	Tensile strength 590 N		Tensile strength 830 N	
Kennedy et al 1977	Most lax in full flex. Stretches with ext., valgus and ext. rot.		Most lax at 35° flex. Stretch with flexion and ext. Int. rot. and varus also stretch	Most lax at 35° flex. Stretch with flex. and ext.
Butler et al 1980			Provides 86% of ant. restraining force.	Provides 95% of restraint
Piziali et al 1980	Resists lateral tibial displacement	Resists medial tibial displacement	Resists medial tibial displacement until apply up to 200 N force on femur	Resists lateral tibial displacement
Fukubayashi and Kurosawa 1980			Maximum laxity at 30° of knee flexion.	
			Section produced more than double the amount of anterior displaced.	Section tripled amount of posterior displacement
Summary of above plus others	Tight in ext. and ext. rot. Perhaps some responsibility in AP motion	Tight in ext. and probably ext. rot.	Tight in ext. Controls ant. glide of tibia on femur	Tight in flexion. Limits post. glide of tibia

support exists from these secondary structures (11). Finally, Kapandji describes the mechanical role of the cruciates and makes a case that during flexion the anterior cruciate is responsible for the anterior sliding movement of the femur as the condyles roll posteriorly. This is achieved via induced ligamentous tension as the femoral attachment of the ligament attempts to move further away from the tibial attachment. Because the ligament will not significantly elongate, the resulting motion is the anterior movement of the femur. Similar mechanics can be applied for the explanation of the posterior cruciate ligament producing posterior slide of the femur during knee extension (46).

Additional work has been completed on the effects of rotary testing of the knee, partly for discovering the role of the capsule in restraining motion. Lipke and coworkers included sectionings of the posterolateral complex and found increased internal rotation in specimens with concurrently destroyed anterior cruciate ligaments. Their work also revealed that section of the anterolateral capsule produced no increase in either internal or external rotation. However,

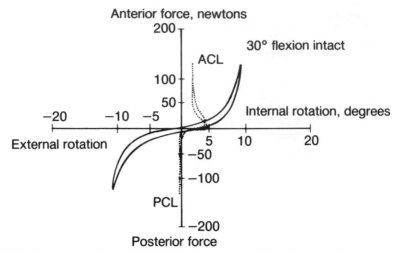

Figure 10.7. Representation of the tibial rotation resulting from application of antero-posterior force with the knee at 30° of flexion. The *dotted line* shows the result after either isolated section of the anterior or posterior cruciate ligament (*ACL, PCL*). (From Fukubayashi T, Torzilli PA, Sherman MF, Warren RF: An in vitro biomechanical evaluation of anterior-posterior motion of the knee. *J Bone Joint Surg [Am]* 64:258–264, 1981.)

when the posterolateral capsule was divided, external rotation was significantly increased (60). This latter result confirmed earlier work by the Markolf group that also demonstrated large increases in anteroposterior laxity when the medial collateral ligament and posterior capsule were sectioned in combination (66). Similar results, i.e., large increases in anterior posterior motion, have also been found when the medial meniscus is sacrificed after the isolated section of the anterior cruciate ligament (55). The position of the knee has also been varied for the different tests. As expected, the posterior capsule is less prone to injury when the knee is in the flexed position because the structure is relatively slack (36). As may also be anticipated, axial load and intact menisci reduce rotary laxity (101).

Three-dimensional laxity of the anterior cruciate deficient knee has been evaluated by a group of investigators collaborating with Noyes. Their study used commonly employed clinical tests to study anterolateral and anterior laxity in cadaver knees before and after cutting the anterior cruciate ligament. Results from the translatory tests demonstrated more than twice as much movement when the anterior cruciate ligament was sectioned alone. Relatively minor effects were seen when the iliotibial band and lateral capsule were sectioned. Rotation tests showed similar results. In general, their data suggest that the primary laxity, whether in translatory or rotary motion, results from an approximately 100% increase in anteroposterior translatory and only a 15% increase in rotation laxity. An example of the results for the pivot shift maneuver is shown in Figure 10.8 (70).

Patellofemoral Joint

Two key biomechanical features of the patellofemoral joint should be understood. The first is that the patella increases the moment arm of the quadriceps tendon so that adequate extensor torques can be generated. That the moment arm varies over the range of motion has been shown by Smidt. From 90 to 45°

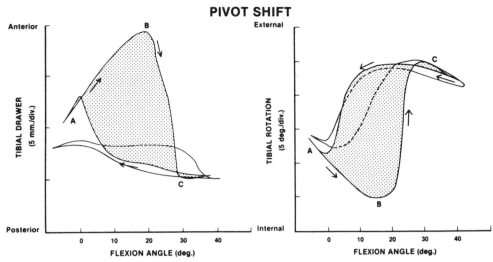

PIVOT SHIFT

Figure 10.8. Knee motion for anteroposterior motion (drawer) and rotation plotted versus knee flexion prior to (open circle) and after (dotted circle) hip joint reaching. Starting position is A, maximum subluxated, B; and C, the reduced position. (From Noyes FR, Grood ES, Suntay WJ, Butler DL: The three dimensional laxity of the anterior cruciate deficient knee as determined by clinical laxity tests. *Iowa Orthop J* 3:32–44, 1983.)

of flexion, the moment arm increases from 3.8 to 4.9 cm and then decreases to 4.4 cm at full extension (91). This factor may be the reason why greatest quadriceps torques can be generated at about 45° of flexion. A decreased moment arm and shortened muscle length would account for the smaller torques that can be generated at the end of the range of movement.

A second feature is the generation of patellofemoral joint forces. Because the patella is not pulled strictly vertical in the patellar groove on the femur, there is a resultant contact force between these two bones. Therefore, assuming the same quadriceps tension, patellofemoral contact force decreases as the knee is extended (Fig. 10.9). Conversely, with greater knee flexion, such as during stair climbing and the squat exercise, patellofemoral contact forces will rise markedly due to both the mechanics and increased quadriceps tension (29). Apparently, however, the tension in the quadriceps tendon and patellar ligament cannot be considered as being of the same magnitude. Ellis and coworkers have found that a ratio of the tensions in the two structures changes little in the first 15° of flexion but that patellar ligament tension was reduced to 50% of that in the quadriceps tendon when the knee was flexed from 80 to 100° (23). These results have implications for analyses that calculate patellofemoral joint reaction force.

Although subjected to degenerative and other disease processes, the patellofemoral joint is capable of withstanding high loads while assuring that friction is minimal as the tendon and inferior surface of the patella move over the femur. A discussion of the effect of pathologies on the patellofemoral joint will be included in a later section of this chapter.

Rotation

Now that the arthrology and joint mechanics have been discussed let us return to the topic of conjunct rotation in the knee. As discussed in previous sections of this chapter completion of the last few degrees of knee extension includes a rotation of 5 to 7°. Numerous explanations are now available because there are

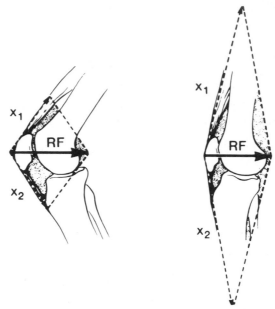

Figure 10.9.   Lateral view of the knee, depicting the alteration in the patellofemoral joint reaction force (*RF*) with knee angle. Quadriceps tendon and patellar ligament tensions are indicated with x_1 and x_2, respectively. (From Paulos L, Rusche K, Johnson C, Noyes FR: Patellar malalignment: a treatment rationale. *Phys Ther* 60:1624–1632, 1980.)

legitimate mechanical reasons for the end result. Whether the rotation is caused by bony structures, soft tissue, muscular forces, or a combination of all of these factors, the debate will probably continue, because no precise experimental techniques exist to allow accurate answers to the problem.

Frequently cited as a classic study of knee mechanics is the study of Lieb and Perry. They undertook an analysis of the knee in order to clarify the role of muscular forces in creating knee extension. Among the parameters assessed were the fascial coverings and fiber alignments of the quadriceps muscles. The vastus medialis was divided into a longus section and an oblique section, because the angle of pull of the longus was 15 to 18° from the long axis of the femur as compared to 50 to 55° for the oblique segment. To study mechanical effects cables were inserted into the tendons of each of the five muscular components. Results demonstrated that almost twice as much quadriceps force was required to produce full extension than to extend the knee 15° short of the full range of motion. To assess the capability of the vastus medialis oblique in performing the terminal phase of extension, isolated loads were applied to this muscle. Because this isolated loading did not produce extension and other testing demonstrated medial alignment effects, the authors concluded that the only selective function of the vastus medialis is patellar alignment. Even though there is early and clinically recognizable atrophy of the vastus medialis, the prominence of the muscle and the thinness of the fascial covering mislead the therapist into believing that there is specific rather than general quadriceps atrophy (57).

KINETICS

The tibiofemoral and patellofemoral joints are both capable of tolerating considerable load. Weight bearing requires the tibiofemoral joint to bear considerable load during activities of daily living. Shear forces are also a factor, both at the patellofemoral joint and between the tibial and femoral surfaces during joint movement. Presented in this section of the chapter will be information on joint torque, forces incurred during compression and shear, and the role of the joint structures in distributing pressure.

Torque

Numerous studies have evaluated torque of the knee extensors and flexors. Recorded values have varied due to differences in techniques used to record data. With the advent of sophisticated dynamometers, more data are being gathered by means of isokinetic testing. Because the testing of both normal and pathological subjects has been done under isometric, concentric, and eccentric conditions, torque differences resulting from the different contractions can be studied. Application of data resulting from these contractions is relevant, however, because all contraction forms are used in completion of activities required for effective human function.

Comparison of isometric torques are complicated by the variance caused by altering the angle of the knee joint. For knee extensors the highest maximum values have usually been recorded at a position of 45° of flexion. With normal subjects in the sidelying position, Smidt recorded values close to 1200 kg cm (120 Nm) (91). Lindahl and coworkers calculated the maximal extending moment to be 226 Nm, a value not usually attained in experimental studies (59). The Wahrenberg group assessed the moment during the vigorous knee extension required during kicking and determined the highest torque achieved by any subject to be 260 Nm. The mean value for all the kicks was 151 Nm (99). Considering that the kicking movement is a dynamic activity that requires concentric contraction, the determination of a value that exceeds the isometric value could be considered unusual.

The recently published data of Scudder show a maximum value of 398 Nm generated while at 60° short of knee extension when the subject was in the seated position. Mean maximal values were 291 Nm, obtained at the same joint position (86). Comparisons completed across sexes for 70 yr olds have also been done. Results for contractions performed in positions similar to those of Scudder showed 191 Nm for men and 108 Nm for women tested at 60° short of complete extension. At 90° the values fell to 161 and 89 Nm, respectively (3). The differences shown with age and between the sexes are not surprising because they have been well documented previously. Compared to the normal population little data are available for the description of the pathological subject. Lankhorst and collaborators included isometric torque as one of the variables in a study of 24 osteoarthritics. These patients, while seated, averaged between 70 and 92 Nm of extension torque (52). Thus, therapists need to continue to establish normative data for all groups, the primary determinants being pathology, age, and sex.

Maximal torque has also been reported for the knee flexors. Maximal torque recorded by Smidt at 0° was 63 Nm, a value that does not closely agree with the 39-Nm value reported by Lunnen et al (62, 91). Values from the Scudder data decrease from a high of about 157 Nm at 30° short of full extension to 142 Nm at 60° short of full extension (86). Part of the large discrepancy in torque is due to the fact that male versus predominantly female subjects were used. Walmsley and Yang also used female subjects in determining knee flexion torque, reporting an isometric maximum of 93 Nm for a position of 30° of flexion. Testing was also completed with the subjects supine, i.e., in 0° of hip flexion, and the resultant torque was always markedly less for comparable points in the range of motion (100). Lunnen et al varied the hip position while the subject remained seated and recorded 39 Nm at 0° of hip flexion, 49 Nm at 45°, 57 Nm at 90°, and 65 Nm at 135° (62). Thus, there is clear demonstration that hip angle influences knee flexion torque. Sitting upright distinctly stretches the hamstrings across the posterior aspect of the hip, allowing for greater torque generation. The implication is that therapists must be consistent in their procedures, since not only knee position, but also hip position exert a powerful influence on the recorded torque.

Torque measured during isokinetic movement has more recently become available with the advent of devices to assess unidirectional and bidirectional concentric and eccentric contractions. Smidt, using a specially made dynamometer, recorded a mean maximal eccentric knee flexor torque of about 54 Nm at 30° of flexion. Conversely the eccentric torque for the quadriceps reached a maximum of 120 Nm at the range of 60 to 75° of flexion. Concentric contractions for the hamstrings registered torque of 42 Nm in a range from 20 to 35° while the quadriceps' maximal value of about 90 Nm was reached in the 35 to 60° range of motion. All data were collected at a constant angular velocity of 13°/sec (91). Scudder tested a number of velocities and found that torque progressively decreased as the velocity of movement increased. Figure 10.10 shows the torque curves produced throughout the range of motion over the velocities tested (86). Several features of the curves deserve attention. First, the data should reinforce knowledge of the force-velocity relationship, because for any location in the range of motion, the torque decreased as the velocity of contraction increased. Also observe that the peak torque for any given velocity occurs at or very near 120°. Although the quadriceps muscles are not as long at this position as at the 90° angle, the torque is markedly higher. The supposition is that the mechanical advantage produced by the patella and patellar ligament is optimal at the 120° location, sufficiently so as to offset the decreased muscle length that occurs at this range of motion.

If comparisons across contraction types are completed from torque data presented, other features are demonstrable. For example, the flexor and extensor data of Smidt show a rather specific pattern in that the eccentric torque exceeds the isometric torque, which both exceed concentric torque (91). Further evidence has been provided by the work of van Eijden et al in their efforts to develop a dynamometer to measure knee extension torque during static and dynamic contractions. Figure 10.11, selected from their results, definitively shows the relationship according to contraction type (98). One may question the graph, however, since it shows no angular displacement. This can be explained by the fact that the dynamometer moved at a constant slow velocity during the course of the contraction. If contractions were completed at higher velocities the separation of the values would be greater than those shown. Reasons for increased tension have been explained in Chapter 2, "Muscle Mechanics and Neurology."

Torque measurements have also been used for purposes of evaluating the quadriceps to hamstrings ratio. This parameter is of some interest because reconditioning of athletes and others is occasionally based on returning torques to a normal ratio. Although data are more commonly available for males, studies have now begun to surface for female athletes (40). Goslin and Charteris have attempted to use isokinetic dynamometry of the knee to establish normative

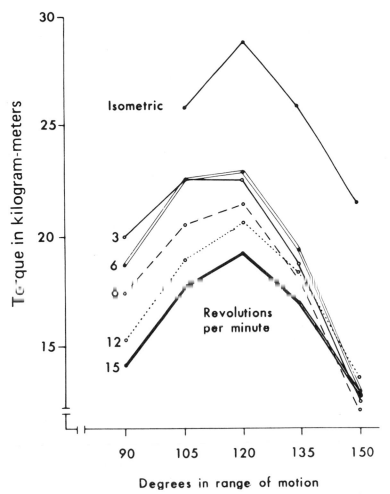

Figure 10.10. Average maximal knee extension torques for isometric and several velocities of isokinetic trials. See text for discussion. (From Scudder GN: Torque curves produced at the knee during isometric and isokinetic exercise. *Arch Phys Med Rehabil* 61:68–72, 1980.)

data for use in the clinical setting. Maximal extension to flexion torque ratios were 2.19:1 for males and 2.32:1 for females. These authors also use their data to develop norms so that at 30°/sec the ratio of 2.25:1 is normal, 3.25:1 is abnormally high, and 1.25:1 is abnormally low. Further, they (arbitrarily) contend that rehabilitation is not complete unless the extensor to flexor ratio is approximately 2:1, with the weaker extensors not less than 60% as strong as the extensors of the opposite limb (34). Use of a higher percentage may clinically be more justifiable. Wyatt and Edwards have also assessed this ratio, reporting values for both males and females. Ratios, reported in percentages, were virtually the same in each of the two samples of 50 men and 50 women. For all testing, the hamstring values were less. Hamstring to quadriceps ratios at tests of 60°/sec were 71 to 72% at 60°/sec, increasing to 83 to 85% at the highest test speed of 300°/sec. Wyatt and Edwards comment that their results show higher values than the ratio of 63% at 60°/sec as reported by Scudder. As the test velocity was increased, the differences in torque values decreased (105). As evidenced by

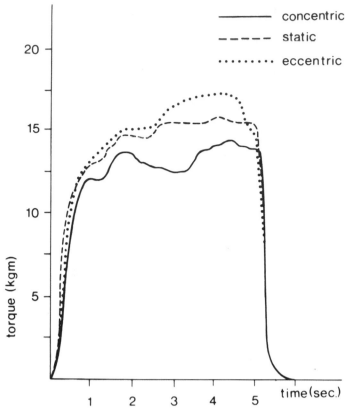

Figure 10.11.   Torque curves for maximal voluntary contractions of one subject. See text for further description. (From van Eijden TMGJ, de Boer W, Verburg J: A dynamometer for the measurement of the extension torque of the lower leg during static and dynamic contractions of the quadriceps femoris muscle. *J Biomech* 16:1019–1024, 1983.)

the data, the population from which the information is collected is obviously a primary factor in determining the appropriate ratio to use clinically.

Because rotation of the knee is often involved in the production of pathology, rotary torque data may assist the therapist in making a determination of the criterion level to be used in treatment of the unstable knee. To establish such norms Osternig et al tested 28 young adult subjects for purposes of determining both internal and external rotation torques. Testing was completed at both 45 and 90° of knee flexion. Mean torques, greater at the 90° position, ranged from 121 to 151 Nm, with little difference between knees or between direction of rotation (75). Shoemaker and Markolf measured rotary torques at 20 and 90° of flexion. At the neutral position of rotation values ranged from 25 to 31 Nm, again with little difference between direction of rotation (88). The large differences between the results of the two studies may be partly accounted for by differing methodologies. This discrepancy makes it extremely difficult for therapists to apply these data to their own clinical situations, probably necessitating that normative data be developed in accordance with individual testing protocols.

Joint Loading

As has been implied above, load transmission by the knee is important because of the repetitive loading cycles that are required during locomotion. The work of Morrison is the most frequently cited when loading of the knee during gait is considered. He has reported mean peak compression force of just over three times body weight for the early and late phases of stance. When ramps or stairs were ascended, the peak values increased to 4 to 4.25 times body weight (68). The values reported for the knee are somewhat less than those for the hip, probably because of the decreased need for muscular forces. The resultant effect of the need for minimal muscle force is to decrease the compressive effect at the joint.

It is well known, however, that muscular contraction of the extensors and flexors do affect compression and shear at the knee. Magnitudes of these forces are dependent on loading conditions, such as weight bearing or nonweight bearing, point of load application, and intensity of muscular contraction. For example, Smidt determined that in extension the quadriceps was responsible for 132 kg of compression. The hamstrings produced 268 kg compression at the position of knee extension but less than 10 kg compression when the knee was positioned at 90° of flexion. In a flexed position the quadriceps contributed 274 kg of compression effect. Taking into account muscle length change and angle of insertion, the relative changes in magnitude could have been predicted. Shear production, of ultimate importance in rehabilitation exercises, was at a maximum of 34.7 kg for the quadriceps with a distally applied load when the nonweight bearing knee was 15° short of full extension. The ability of the hamstrings to exert a maximum posterior shear of 151 kg at 90° of flexion is of considerably less importance, unless the posterior cruciate ligament is injured or unless this force is considered to be a potential restraint to the anterior motion of the tibia on the femur as a result of quadriceps contraction (91).

How loads are transmitted through the joint is another factor to consider. Because the contact area determines the pressure per unit area, the fully extended position that offers maximal contact area would appear to be the position of choice. Further, Kettelkamp has noted that the area of the medial plateau is about 60% larger than that of the lateral plateau (49). Considering that the cartilage of the medial plateau is approximately three times thicker than the lateral the combined effect is that the medial aspect can more easily tolerate higher imposed forces (29).

Although debated before more sophisticated analytical techniques became available, evidence now exists that the menisci participate in load bearing. There is indication that distribution of the load is more effective and that pressure is of less magnitude when the menisci are intact. Fukubayashi and Kurosawa have provided specific data on this problem, noting that the peak pressures were 3 MPa with the menisci and 6 MPa without them at compressing loads of 1000 N. Their work also demonstrated that the contact area decreased to less than one-half of that of the intact knee. Figure 10.12 shows an example from their data. Note both the shape and magnitude of the pressure patterns (31). The tibial fixation, meniscal structure, and femoral condyle geometry all would seem to indicate that the menisci bear load throughout the knee range of motion, perhaps as much as 45% of the total in the human knee joint (89).

Stability of the knee when the joint is in a condition of loading is of practical concern because the joint is almost always loaded to some extent in situations that create pathologies. In fact, in clinical circles, the effect of loading has been well accepted. In examination of the knee, for example, apparent ligamentous laxity created by the destruction of the articular cartilage requires that traction (distraction) loads be exerted in order to rule out the possibility of pseudolaxity. Conversely, the knee loaded in compression assumes a more close-packed

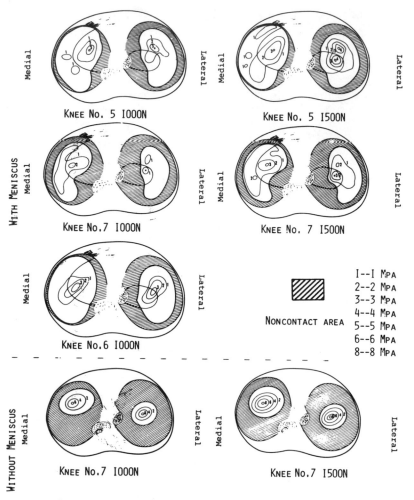

Figure 10.12. Schematic views of pressure distribution patterns with and without the meniscus. Note changes, particularly on the lateral side. (From Fukubayashi T, Kurosawa H: The contact area and pressure distribution pattern of the knee. *Acta Orthop Scand* 51:871–879, 1980.)

position and thus a greater degree of stability is noted upon examination. Markolf and coworkers have been among those that have established the effect of joint load on stability. They found that while a tibiofemoral compressive force was applied, stiffness was increased. Laxities decreased in anteroposterior, mediolateral, torsional, and varus-valgus testing. Apparently no matter whether the joint load is produced by gravitational, dynamic, or muscular force, the effect is to protect the ligaments from strain. As a result of meniscal removal the authors also noted that the knee is looser in the unloaded, but not in the loaded knee (65).

Patellofemoral Joint

The kinetics of the patellofemoral joint are also a factor in consideration of knee motion because often the levels of the forces exceed tolerable limits and/ or produce pathology. A frequently cited work relative to the patellofemoral joint is that of Reilly and Martens, who in 1972 studied the joint reaction forces and the quadriceps forces during straight leg raising and other activities. The lowest value for patellofemoral joint reaction force (PFJR) was during walking, amounting to 0.5 times body weight. Stair climbing required PFJR of 3.3 times body weight, while the largest force of 7.6 times body weight was produced during the squat activity (82). These values appear to have been confirmed via radiographic and mathematical analysis of 15 normal knees (67). Figure 10.9 showed the mechanical effects of differing joint positions on the patellofemoral joint reaction force.

Other consideration needs to be given to conditions of weight bearing versus knee extension of the free distal portion of the extremity. Specifically note that in standing with full knee extension the quadriceps force is minimal, but increases with greater knee flexion (i.e., the squat). If extending against resistance while in the sitting position with the knee at 90° of flexion the quadriceps force requirement is zero, increasing as extension ensues (39). These factors, coupled with changes in contact area of the patella on the femur, offer potential explanation for understanding that some exercises can produce significant forces at this joint. Further discussion of these features are contained in the section on pathokine-siology

Because these magnitudes of forces are distributed over a potentially limited area, i.e., the inferior surface of the patella, the contact stresses per unit area can be very large. Investigators have determined that between 13 and 38% of the patellar surface bears joint load, and have calculated patellofemoral contact stresses to vary between 1.3 and 12.6 N/mm^2 (67). Methods of reducing these forces resort to altering the mechanical conditions producing the high loads. One technique utilized is to reduce the load supported, for example by decreasing the weight of the patient or avoiding maneuvers such as the squat. Another technique that has been used is the advancement of the tibial tuberosity. This surgical procedure has been shown to reduce the PFJR force by about 50%, thereby potentially resulting in diminished pain in patients suffering from osteoarthritis of this joint (64).

PATHOKINESIOLOGY

Due to a wide range of injuries to the knee many conditions that demonstrate pathological motion are available for discussion. This section of the chapter will be primarily devoted to the effects induced by damage or repair of soft tissue. Joint replacement procedures will also be discussed, as will the mechanical implications resulting from changes in the patellofemoral joint.

Pes Anserine Transfer

One surgical procedure, although now used less commonly, is the proximal transfer of the pes anserine insertion at the tibia. The pes is made up of tendinous insertions of the sartorius, gracilis, and semitendinosus muscles, and its location on the proximal tibia makes for assessibility for surgical relocation. Noyes and Sonstegard have depicted the mechanical effects, shown in Figure 10.13. The basic premise of the transfer is to provide additional stability during terminal knee extension (screw-home mechanism). As predicted by the result shown in Figure 10.13, proximal transposition of the pes causes an increased moment arm for rotation. Assuming that the muscle lengths have not been significantly shortened, causing reduced tension generation, the effective moment for rotation should be increased. To test such an hypothesis both flexion and rotation forces

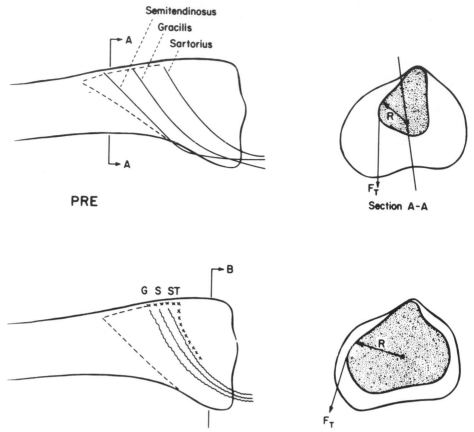

Figure 10.13. Effect of the transplantation of the pes anserine to a more proximal location on the tibia. Cross sections are shown for two locations. Note the change in the moment arm R. Force (F_T) is also represented. (From Noyes FR, Sonstegard DA: Biomechanical function of the pes anserinus at the knee and the effect of its transplantation. *J Bone Joint Surg [Am]* 55:1225–1241, 1973.)

were measured in cadaver specimens. As was anticipated when all test positions were considered, the flexion force was decreased by as much as 36%. This loss of flexion force is due to the fact that the moment arm for flexion is decreased as a result of the proximal relocation of the pes insertion. However, rotation forces were significantly increased at 90, 60, and 30° of flexion, but not in the fully extended position. This "wind up" effect was considered to be advantageous in the control of rotation in the knee (71).

A number of laboratory and clinically based studies have evaluated the effectiveness of the procedure. DiStefano and coworkers evaluated 15 postsurgical subjects for changes in torque generated in internal rotation. Although the 60° knee angle produced the greatest torque of 28.5 Nm in the postsurgical knee, the only test position that produced an increased torque pre- to postoperatively was the 30° test position (+9.2%) (20). Osternig et al also evaluated 15 postsurgical subjects and found no significant differences between postsurgical and nonsurgical contralateral limbs for any of the positions tested. Internal rotation torque for nonsurgical limbs tested at 90° of flexion, while in 5° of tibial rotation, were about 37 Nm (76). Others have performed clinical evaluations of the results of the transfer. Retrospective analyses have provided mixed results.

D'Arcy found improvement of stability during activity in 42 of 51 knees, while Chick et al stated that 89% of patients followed after 6.1 yr had a combined rotary instability of the knee (14, 18). More positive results are reported by the Freeman group, in that symptomatic improvements occurred in many patients. However, the results were not felt to be adequate for the patients used in the population in which the procedure was completed (30). In spite of these results function of the pes in providing stability has been demonstrated. Electromyographic comparison of normals with those in which the pes had been transferred demonstrated that increased levels of activity occurred in those with transfers. Thus, the conclusion was that these muscles were being used to control any potential instability in the knee (78).

In summary, attempts have been made to control anteromedial knee instability with transfers of the pes anserine. Although the procedure is based on known mechanical effects the results have generally been discouraging. Because elongation of transposed muscle tendon can occur with time the long-term effect of this procedure is perhaps not optimal.

Anterolateral Instability

Although anterolateral instability has been recognized since 1972, only recently has more attention been given to this relatively common problem. The instability, also known as the pivot shift, is considered to be either the subluxation or reduction, or both in rapid succession, of the loaded joint. The pathology is manifested (as subluxation) as the femur twists externally or the tibia rotates internally. Occurring mainly in the lateral compartment of the knee, the anterior cruciate ligament and the lateral and posterolateral segments of the capsule are considered to be deficient. Because the joint is in the close-packed position in full extension and because the iliotibial band may control the subluxation after 40 or 50° of flexion has been attained, the shift should be evaluated within this range of motion (61). Noyes et al indicate that the mechanics are significantly influenced via the position of the iliotibial band. They point out that this band, as an extension of the tensor fascia lata muscle, is an extensor until 30° of flexion and a flexor beyond 40° (70). Anterior drawer movement of the lateral tibial component followed by sudden reduction of the tibiofemoral joint at about 30 to 40° produces the abnormal rotation seen (69). Although there is some suggestion that under low stress translational motion dominates angular motion (1), there is also evidence available that changes can be seen during the pivot shift in the movement pattern of the instant axis of rotation within the sagittal condylar silhouette. The findings indicate that in the late stages of extension rolling predominated, followed by a marked change to a gliding motion. Data reduced from the radiographs also indicated that excessive friction and compressive forces existed in patients with anterolateral instability (97).

Ligamentous function and passive restraints that may produce certain joint motion can be related to the pivot shift by way of analyzing which structures are deficient in the knee demonstrating abnormal motion. As could be anticipated from the earlier section in this chapter, the anterior cruciate ligament is the most commonly disrupted structure in the knee. There is also evidence that the posterolateral capsule is stretched in order to allow room for the lateral femoral condyle during subluxation. Changes may occur in the fabellofibular and arcuate ligaments, but consistent findings in this area have not been shown (61), except in the series of 12 cases surgically repaired by DeLee et al (19).

As a result of pathological motion, various procedures have been attempted for purposes of controlling abnormal rotation. Among the surgical procedures that have been attempted are surgical advancement of the biceps femoris insertion toward Gerdy's tubercle and the Ellison and Losee methods, both of which involve transferring the iliotibial band. The latter procedure involves transposition of the tendon of the iliotibial band by passing the attachment and bone fragment under the fibular collateral ligament to an insertion on the anterolateral aspect of the tibia (24).

The effectiveness of these transfers has differed depending upon the patient population and the precise procedure used. For example, Odenstein and co-workers reported on a group of 60 patients in which the distal iliotibial band was transferred to the fibular collateral ligaments. Although early scores that rated such factors as instability and pain were improved, the results at the end of a 40-month period indicated that the transfer did not function satisfactorily (72). Contrary to the Odenstein work Benum used a segment of the patellar ligament and adjoining patella on six patients, five of which had increased stability and good function (6). Perhaps if Benum had followed patients for more than 17 months the results for his patient group would have demonstrated similar deterioration. As with many transfers the primary deterrent to a continuing good result is elongation of the tissue due to stretch, whether such is applied incidentally or intentionally. Knowing the surgical procedure and the motion required, indications and contraindications may assist with yielding better long-term results from transfer procedures.

Control of the pivot shift is normally by passive restraint, but in the abnormal case functional control may be achieved by dynamic, muscular control of rotation. Training programs, particularly for the athletic population have included some elements that address this feature by way of incorporating hamstring exercises in the rehabilitation or treatment of knees with demonstrated shifts. EMG data now being collected is expected to elucidate the role of the leg musculature in the control of the pivot shift.

Ligamentous Reconstructions

Due to any number of injuries to the knee ligaments, reconstructions may be advised. Generally, these techniques are designed to increase stability and improve joint function. Ligamentous, capsular, and musculotendinous units have all been used in procedures designed to achieve these end results. In all cases, surgical repairs should be designed such that joint kinematics and the resulting kinetics will not be altered, particularly in structures that are used in the repair procedure. Mechanics, either those required by functional activities or invoked by well-meaning therapeutic exercises, can produce abnormal forces that will lead to potential failure of the procedure. Translocation may also lead to abnormal shear forces at locations where ligaments or structures are required to pass through or over bone or over new soft tissue structures (42). Knowing the procedure is thus important in attempting to thoroughly understand knee function requiring therapeutic procedures.

Although simple ligament relocations are done, such as the anterior and distal advancement of the medial collateral ligament for instances of medial instability, the majority of this section will deal with reconstructions associated with anterior cruciate ligament insufficiencies. The type of reconstruction can be direct or by extraarticular substitution and intraarticular augmentation. Fascia latae allografts and temporary supportive prostheses are also available but less frequently used (85). In any case, Butler has developed criteria for replacement of the anterior cruciate ligament, such that the tissue has (a) adequate mechanical properties (strength and stiffness); (b) vascular viability; (c) availability; and (d) access to bone at both ends of the graft (Butler DL, personal communication, University of Iowa, Iowa City, Iowa, 1983). In addition, the procedure should be (e) technically feasible and (f) have a low morbidity (74). Whether the procedures have developed the criteria or vice versa, the patellar ligament, iliotibial band, and semitendinosus tendon have all been used in the surgical procedures (15, 106, 107). Judging function on the basis of functional activities, and in some cases on the return to competitive sports, results could be considered to be encouraging at the least. One example is the follow-up by Johnson et al who used the patellar tendon for the reconstruction. Sixty-nine percent of the patients had good to excellent results. Arthrosis and parapatellar pain were the most frequent factors that contributed to failure (45). Unsuccessful reconstructions are due to lack of attention to the classic criteria or to reasons cited in the section on anterolateral instabilities.

Regardless of the debilitating nature of the injury and the subsequent surgical procedure, rehabilitative techniques should be instituted. However, consideration must be given to both the extraarticular and intraarticular mechanics associated with any therapeutic procedure. Consider, as has been discussed earlier, the ability of the quadriceps to generate tension of sufficient magnitude that will cause anterior shear of the tibia upon the femur. An analysis by Johnson, for example, has indicated that for knee extension performed with a long leg cast or knee brace as much as 12.3 kgf would be applied in the direction of anterior shear (44). If in fact the anterior cruciate had been injured or if surgical reconstructions had been completed, there is a clear danger that muscle contraction can induce unwanted or too great a stress in the tissues (4). This is apparently true for the last 30° of knee extension (38). Thus, for these reasons there is serious question about the efficacy of quadriceps exercises during the rehabilitative phases. Because ligamentous strength may take more than a year to return to reasonable levels, the time for use of quadriceps exercises must at least be cautiously approached.

In recognition of this problem many therapists will limit the range of motion to only 60° of flexion or use exercise programs that require cocontraction of the hamstrings. These exercises are thought to resist or restrain the tendency for anterior shear of the tibia. One such exercise suggested for use is the step-up exercise. A purported advantage of this exercise is that contractions of both the quadriceps and hamstrings are required, reducing the tendency for joint shear. Because little evidence existed as to the level of tension required in these muscles to perform the step-up and down, Brask et al performed an electromyographic study on these muscles during the exercise. Their results revealed that the average values for muscular activity, depending on the height and the direction of the step, ranged from 24 to 60% of maximum EMG for the vastus medialis and 8 to 23% for the rectus femoris. Activity in the biceps femoris was only 3 to 9% and in the semimembranosus/semitendinosus muscles of the order of 4 to 9%. Thus, in spite of the attempt to control for shear, the hamstrings may not be generating sufficient tension to be able to do so (10). Rather, the fact that the patient is weight bearing may be the critical factor in controlling shear, since the joint is more congruous under these conditions.

Other mechanisms have also become available for control of anterior shear during resistive exercises, allowing the therapist to limit the amount of forward movement of the tibia (43). This and other methodologies must continually be developed for purposes of allowing therapeutic procedures to specifically address the needs of the patient. Understanding potential and real mechanical effects must be the responsibility of therapists to assure that outcomes are consistent with the therapeutic intent.

Patellar Mechanics

As discussed earlier in this chapter the patella is responsible for mechanical effects that are facilitative to knee extension. Losses, such as in patellectomy (Fig. 10.14), thus have an influence on the ability of the patient to perform knee

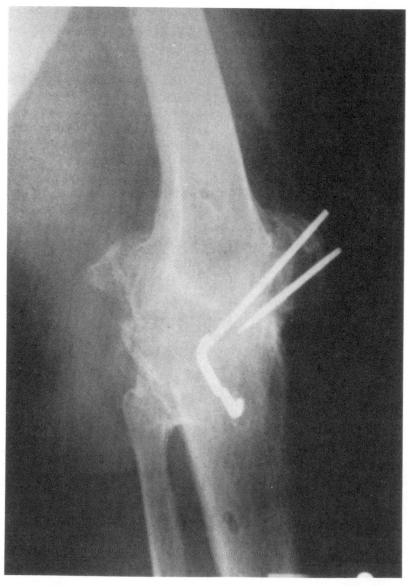

Figure 10.14. AP radiograph of a fused knee, necessary after a poor functional result from a patellectomy. Due to excessive bone formation absence of the patella is difficult to discern.

extension, resulting in the common condition known as extensor lag (Fig. 10.15). Although Peeples and Margo contend that such a lag should not be seen if proper surgical technique, postoperative immobilization in extension, and rehabilitation procedures are observed, the losses are difficult to overcome. Both theoretical and clinical studies have revealed that extension capability is reduced from 15 to 49% (77, 96). The primary reason for this loss appears to be due to the decreased moment arm through which the quadriceps mechanism can now act. Thus, a significant loss in moment arm means that higher tensions must be generated in the extensors to offset the loss. Because these patients are likely to suffer from quadriceps weakness due to factors that precipitated the patellectomy, the therapist is forced to deal with a doubly difficult problem: loss of tension and loss of the adequate moment arm.

Contrasted to the patellectomy is the procedure of elevation or displacement of the tibial tubercle. This technique is done for purposes of relieving abnormally high patellofemoral joint forces and pain that may result. Figure 10.16 shows a free body diagram of the pre- and postoperative conditions. With the tibial tubercle elevated and maintained by the assistance of a bone block, two significant mechanical changes have occurred. First, note that the distance (d) from F(p) to the instant center of rotation has increased, resulting in the improved ability for the generation of an extension moment. Secondly, note that the angle between F(p) and F(q) has increased, the result of which is a decreased magnitude of patellofemoral contact force as demonstrated by a reduction in the magnitude of vector F(c). Thus, the procedure achieves two changes that should facilitate extension moments in the knee (Fig. 10.17). Although there is some disadvantage associated with slow return to full function and poor cosmesis, the results seem to justify the continued use of the procedure. That ½ inch of elevation appears

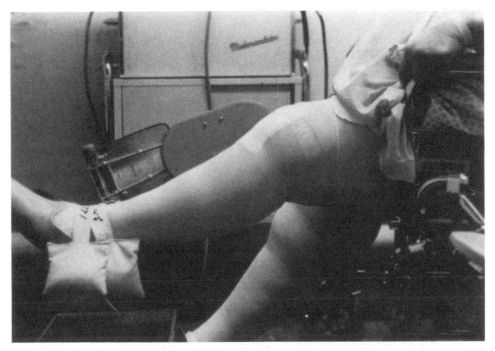

Figure 10.15. Postpatellectomy patient attempting to extend the knee with 3 lbs suspended at the distal shank. Although the center of the hip is difficult to locate, significant extensor lag exists due to insufficient extensor moment.

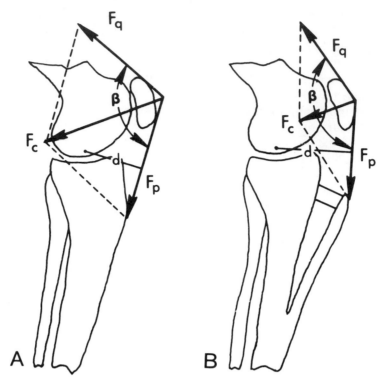

Figure 10.16.   Lateral view of the knee, pre (*A*) and post (*B*) elevation of the tibial tubercle. Compared to preoperatively the contact force F_c is decreased due to change in angle of β and the increase in the patellar moment arm *d*. Force in the quadriceps and patellar ligament are shown with F_q and F_P, respectively. (From Maquet P: Mechanics and osteoarthritis of the patellofemoral joint. *Clin Orthop* 133:70–73, 1979.)

to be the optimum amount of elevation is at least of some help in controlling the unsightly tibial prominence (25, 26).

Patellofemoral joint reaction forces are a factor to be considered in exercise techniques, not only because some patients' pathologies are associated with the patella. On many occasions patients cannot tolerate a dynamic knee extension movement due to pain/discomfort from the reaction forces. Because the area of the patella in contact with the femur increases with knee flexion, the area over which forces are distributed also increases. The effect is to distribute the load over a broader area. Conversely, during extension the opposite occurs. The result is that at some point in the range the compression will exceed the physiological loading occurring during weight bearing. This has been demonstrated to be at 52° short of complete knee extension. A practical example can be produced from a plot of the patellofemoral joint reaction forces during knee extension with a resistance of a 9-kg weight boot added to the foot of the subject (Fig. 10.18). Note that the peak force would occur approximately 40° from complete knee extension, a point in the range of motion that may be difficult for a patient with patellofemoral joint pathology. Also note that after this point in the range of motion the force decreases rapidly because at this joint position tension in the quadriceps and patellar tendon produce mostly shear in the joint rather than compressive force (39). Thus, therapists need to consider pressure rather than force in order to make a conclusion. Even though contact force decreases with extension, if contact area decreases at a faster rate there is a

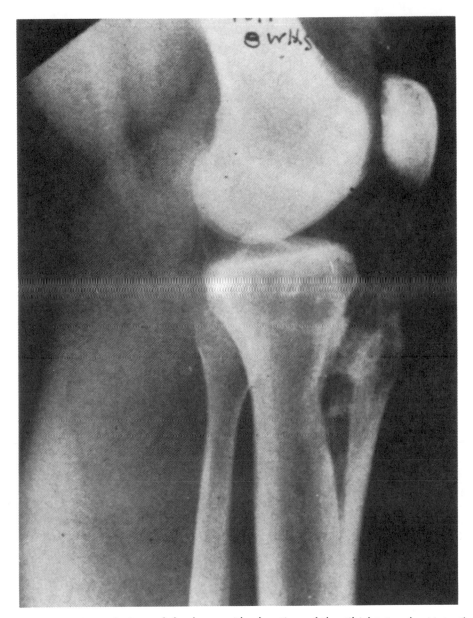

Figure 10.17.   Lateral view of the knee with elevation of the tibial tubercle. Note the bone block used to maintain the position of the tubercle.

resultant increase in pressure. These mechanics offer the reason why many patellofemoral patients have no symptoms at 52° or greater, and severe pain at angles of less than 52°.

Other pathologies of the extensor mechanism also occur with regularity. Patellar malalignment problems can be of such severity that the patella can dislocate laterally. In these cases, transposition tightening or "reefing" of medial structures may best solve a problem that tends to be recurring. In malalignments of lesser magnitudes, functional training of the quadriceps with setting and straight leg raising exercises may arrest the persistent symptoms. Another useful

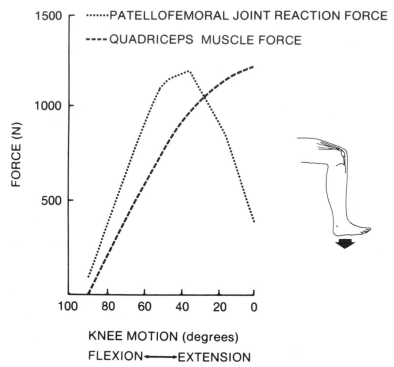

Figure 10.18. Force in the patellofemoral joint and the quadriceps for knee extension completed with a 9-kg weight boot with the subject seated and the lower leg free. See text for further discussion. (From Frankel VH, Nordin M: *Basic Biomechanics of the Skeletal System*. Philadelphia, Lea & Febiger, 1980.)

exercise is the manual displacement of the patella slightly laterally, having the patient return it to neutral via quadriceps muscle contraction.

Ruptures of the extensor mechanisms, both in the quadriceps tendon and in the patellar ligament, have been reported. In either case the therapist will face a difficult task of rehabilitating to the point of normal extensor torque because of temporal delays required to allow sufficient healing before resistive exercise can be started. Caution would certainly have to be exhibited to minimize the opportunity for dynamic loading that increases the tension in the tendon or ligament to a point where the high tensile stress would lead to rupture (Fig. 10.19).

Therapists should also be aware that evidence is now surfacing that joint position and state of effusion apparently influence the level of contraction that can be produced (104). This is of significance because many knee patients demonstrate effusions as a result of either trauma or surgery or both. In one study, decreased EMG activity was demonstrated at the fully extended position when compared to the position of 30° of flexion (95). Another, completed by Krebs and coworkers, established that when operated and nonoperated limbs were compared, types of exercise and joint position caused differences in the resulting EMG values (51).

Note should be taken though that the fully extended position, being close-packed, provides a decreased area of volume available for joint fluid. Therefore, the effused knee often adopts a degree of flexion and is inhibited from full extension by increased fluid pressure that distends the capsule. These results

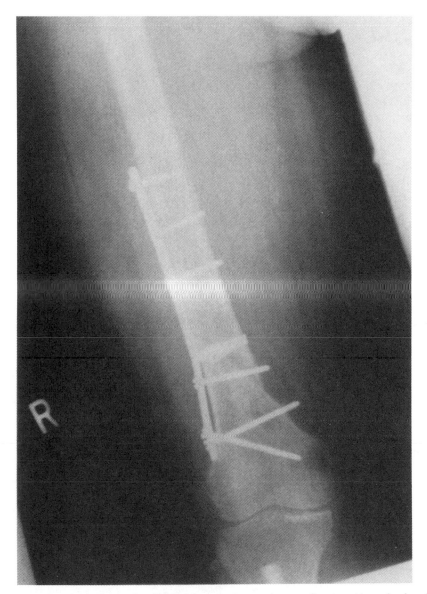

Figure 10.19. AP radiograph of distal femur, 7 months postfixation. Knee had only 30° of flexion, and caution with active and passive movement had to be taken because of the fracture. Soft tissue limitations in the extensor appratus limited range of motion.

point to the importance of taking into account information relative to neural control mechanisms when applying therapeutic interventions.

Total Joint Replacements

Since the advent of joint replacements, the knee has been a popular joint for this procedure because of the high incidence of degenerative disease and problems of malalignment. These arthroplasties are completed primarily for purposes of reducing pain and improving range of motion. Stability, however, must be maintained. Multiple prosthetic designs are available to the surgeon. One classification system of these replacements includes three major types (81).

The unconstrained type of implants are intended for those patients with ligamentous integrity because these passive structures will, of necessity, be responsible for maintaining the stability of the joint. At the other extreme is the constrained device which is not dependent upon ligaments for alignment. These components, however, may be more likely to loosen due to the inability of other joint structures to manage the forces. A compromise of these two designs is the semiconstrained (Fig. 10.20). These devices can attempt to select the positive features associated with each of the other two devices. Regardless of the procedure, failure rates, for a variety of reasons, have continued to be a concern. Cameron and Hunter summarize some of these mechanisms and discuss tibial loosenings as related to tilt and sink, compression, torsion, and other mechanical groupings. Further confounding problems of these procedures include infection, loss of bone, patellar subluxation, and other factors (13). In general, therapists can expect that additional designs will be marketed, tested, and implanted in the patients that they treat. Clinical results to date have certainly had sufficient desirability to establish effectiveness of the total knee replacement, thereby indicating that continued and even more widespread use can be anticipated.

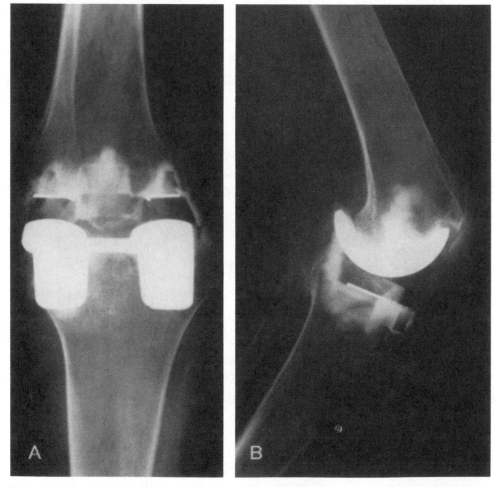

Figure 10.20.   AP (A) and lateral (B) views of total knee replacement. Note shape of new femoral condyles that allow for some rotation and varus and valgus. Tibial plateaus can be discerned by using wire inserts in the components.

The effects of the arthroplasty on the kinematics and kinetics of the joint are of interest to therapists. Generally, patients and therapists will concede that pain is diminished and functional performance improved. In fact, specific studies evaluating patient performance have been completed. Range of knee motion has been improved, unchanged, or diminished, depending on the source cited. The same can be said for the ability of the patient to achieve complete extension, resulting in many cases in the functional difficulties associated with loss of terminal extension (17). According to Ritter and Stringer the total knee arthroplasty can be expected to correct 5 to 7° of valgus deformity and return the knee to full extension within 1 yr. Further, because less improvement is seen in patients whose preoperative flexion was less than 75°, less ultimate flexion can be anticipated in patients with less initial flexion (84).

An example of the difficulties encountered with patients whose knees have undergone arthroplasty as a result of arthritis will point out the difficulties of therapeutic treatment. Osteoarthritic patients generated from 56 to 103 Nm of extension torque before surgery and from 21 to 102 Nm after surgery. Rheumatoids had an increased range of values, 4 to 76 Nm preoperatively and 23 to 109 Nm 1 yr after surgery (17). Not only is the range very large, but the values are quite below the values of 191 and 108 Nm for 70-yr-old asymptomatic men and women, respectively (2). Since the age range for the operative group is generally comparable with the normative data, significant problems may exist for the therapist in restoring normal torque values to the surgical group.

Other measures postarthroplasty have also been evaluated. In monarticular degenerative arthritis, the measurements of gait had returned to normal levels within 2 yr of the surgery. Specifically noted were the normality of velocity, stride lengths, and kinematics of the hip, knee, and ankle. The data did determine, however, that the patients spent about 30% longer for double stance and had increased cycle times (90). Shorter than normal stride lengths, reduced midstance knee flexion, and uncharacteristic flexion-extension moments at the knee have also been demonstrated (2). That the type of prosthesis can influence the results is also established. Five types of prostheses have been used to analyze the effect of the design on walking and stair climbing. Differences could be discerned on the basis of the design. For example, a normal range of motion during stair ascent and descent was achieved with only the least constrained, cruciate-retaining prosthesis. Even though all the implants were considered to be clinically successful, all patients had abnormalities of gait (2). At least a part of this result may be due to the geometry of the prosthetic components. It is interesting that the mechanics of the cruciate ligaments are altered to varying degrees, depending on the prosthetic design involved. Apparently, components with single radius of curvature geometry cause constraint forces to exist in the posterior cruciate ligament. Such a problem is nonexistent if multicurvature designs simulating the actual configuration of the femoral condyles are used (56). These findings further establish the nature of the interaction between the bony and soft tissue structures. Cognizance of these features must be included if effective planning and treatment is to be realized from the therapeutic intervention necessary to redeem normal joint kinetics and kinematics.

SUMMARY

The knee is an interesting joint to study because the anatomical conditions produce a great variety of kinetic and kinematic events. These events are often altered by pathology, producing abnormal motion that is often difficult to restore to normal. Factors that alter the normal mechanics of the joint and the surrounding structures will continue to be modified by surgical and other therapeutic interventions. As patients are likely to continue to be subjected to trauma and degenerative conditions, the understanding of normal and abnormal mechanics of the knee will likely remain of considerable import to practicing therapists.

References

1. Allum R, Jones D, Mowbray MAS, Galway HR: Triaxial electrogoniometric examination of the pivot shift sign for rotatory instability of the knee. *Clin Orthop* 183:144–146, 1984.
2. Andriacchi TP, Galante JO, Fermier RW: The influence of total knee-replacement design on walking and stair-climbing. *J Bone Joint Surg [Am]* 64:1328–1335, 1982.
3. Aniansson A, Grimby G, Rundgren A: Isometric and isokinetic quadriceps muscle strength in 70 year old men and women. *Scand J Rehabil Med* 12:161–168, 1980.
4. Arms SW, Pope MH, Johnson RJ, Fischer RA, Arvidsson I, Eriksson E: The biomechanics of anterior cruciate ligament rehabilitation and reconstruction. *Am J Sports Med* 12:8–18, 1984.
5. Basmajian JV, Lovejoy JF: Functions of the popliteus muscle in man. *J Bone Joint Surg [Am]* 53:557–562, 1971.
6. Benum P: Anterolateral rotary instability of the knee joint. *Acta Orthop Scand* 53:613–617, 1982.
7. Blackburn TA, Craig E: Knee anatomy—a brief review. *Phys Ther* 60:1556–1560, 1980.
8. Bos RR, Blosser TG: An electromyographic study of vastus medialis and vastus lateralis during selected isometric exercises. *Med Sci Sports* 2:218–223, 1970.
9. Brantigan OC, Voshell AF: The mechanics of the ligaments and menisci of the knee joint. *J Bone Joint Surg* 23:44–66, 1941.
10. Brask B, Lueke RH, Soderberg GL: Electromyographic analysis of selected muscles during the lateral step-up exercise. *Phys Ther* 64:324–329, 1984.
11. Butler DL, Noyes FR, Grood ES: Ligamentous restraints to anterior-posterior drawer in the human knee. *J Bone Joint Surg [Am]* 62:259–270, 1980.
12. Cabaud HE: Biomechanics of the anterior cruciate ligament. *Clin Orthop* 172:26–31, 1983.
13. Cameron HU, Hunter GA: Failure in total knee arthroplasty. *Clin Orthop* 170:141–146, 1982.
14. Chick RP, Collins HR, Rubin BD, et al: The pes anserinus transfer. *J Bone Joint Surg [Am]* 63:1449–1452, 1981.
15. Clancy WG, Nelson DA, Reider B, Narechania RG: Anterior cruciate ligament reconstruction using one-third of the patellar ligament, augmented by extra-articular tendon transfers. *J Bone Joint Surg [Am]* 64:352–359, 1982.
16. Close JR: *Motor Function in the Lower Extremity: Analyses by Electronic Instrumentation.* Springfield, IL, Charles C Thomas, 1964.
17. Collopy MC, Murray MP, Gardner GM, et al: Kinesiologic measurements of functional performance before and after geometric total knee replacement: one year follow up of twenty cases. *Clin Orthop* 126:196–202, 1977.
18. D'Arcy J: Pes anserinus transposition for chronic anteromedial rotational instability of the knee. *J Bone Joint Surg [Br]* 60:66–70, 1978.
19. DeLee JC, Riley MB, Rockwood CA: Acute posterolateral rotatory instability of the knee. *Am J Sports Med* 11:199–207, 1983.
20. DiStefano V, Nixon JE, O'Neil R, Davis O: Pes anserinus transfer: an in vivo biomechanical analysis. *Am J Sports Med* 5:204–208, 1977.
21. Duarte-Cintra AI, Furlani J: Electromyographic study of quadriceps femoris in man. *Electromyogr Clin Neurophysiol* 21:539–554, 1981.
22. Elftman H: The function of the muscles in locomotion. *Am J Physiol* 125:357–366, 1939.
23. Ellis MI, Seedhom BB, Wright V, Dowson D: An evaluation of the ratio between the tensions along the quadriceps tendon and the patellar ligament. *Eng Med* 9:189–194, 1980.
24. Ellison AE: Distal iliotibial band transfer for anterolateral rotatory instability of the knee. *J Bone Joint Surg [Am]* 61:330–337, 1979.

25. Ferguson AB: Elevation of the insertion of the patellar ligament for patellofemoral pain. *J Bone Joint Surg [Am]* 64:766–771, 1982.
26. Ferguson A, Brown TD, Fu FH, Rutkowski R: Relief of patellofemoral contact stress by anterior displacement of the tibial tubercle. *J Bone Joint Surg [Am]* 61:159–166, 1979.
27. Fisk R, Wells J: The quadriceps complex in bipedal man. *J Am Osteopath Assoc* 80:291–294, 1980.
28. Frankel VH, Burstein AH: *Orthopaedic Biomechanics.* Philadelphia, Lea & Febiger, 1970.
29. Frankel VH, Nordin M: *Basic Biomechanics of the Skeletal System.* Philadelphia, Lea & Febiger, 1980.
30. Freeman BL, Beaty JH, Haynes DB: The pes anserinus transfer. *J Bone Joint Surg [Am]* 64:202–207, 1982.
31. Fukubayashi T, Kurosawa H: The contact area and pressure distribution pattern of the knee. *Acta Orthop Scand* 51:871–879, 1980.
32. Fukubayashi T, Torzilli PA, Sherman MF, Warren RF: An in vitro biomechanical evaluation of anterior-posterior motion of the knee. *J Bone Joint Surg [Am]* 64:258–264, 1982.
33. Girgis FG, Marshall JL, Al Monajem ARS: The cruciate ligaments of the knee joint, anatomical, functional and experimental analysis. *Clin Orthop* 106:216–231, 1975
34. Goslin BR, Charteris J: Isokinetic dynamometry: normative data for clinical use in lower extremity (knee) cases. *Scand J Rehabil Med* 11:105–109, 1979.
35. Gough JV, Ladley G: An investigation into the effectiveness of various forms of quadriceps exercises. *Physiotherapy* 57:356–361, 1971.
36. Grood ES, Noyes FR, Butler DL, Suntay WJ: Ligamentous and capsular restraints preventing straight medial and lateral laxity in intact human cadaver knees. *J Bone Joint Surg [Am]* 63:1257–1269, 1981.
37. Grood ES, Noyes FR, Miller EH: Comparative Mechanical Properties of the Medial Collateral and Capsular Structures of the Knee. 23rd Annual Orthopaedic Research Society, Las Vegas, 1977. Dependable Printing Co., Chicago, 1977.
38. Grood ES, Suntay WJ, Noyes FR, Butler DL: Biomechanics of the knee-extension exercise. *J Bone Joint Surg [Am]* 66:725–734, 1984.
39. Hungerford DS, Barry M: Biomechanics of the patellofemoral joint. *Clin Orthop* 144:9–15, 1979.
40. Imwold CH, Rider RA, Haymes EM, Green KD: Isokinetic torque differences between college female varsity basketball and track athletes. *J Sports Med Phys Fitness* 23:67–73, 1983.
41. Jackson RT, Merrifield HH: Electromyographic assessment of quadriceps muscle group during knee extension with weighted boot. *Med Sci Sports* 4:116–119, 1972.
42. James SL: Biomechanics of knee ligament reconstruction. *Clin Orthop* 146:90–101, 1980.
43. Johnson D: Controlling anterior shear during isokinetic knee extension exercise. *J Orthop Sports Phys Ther* 4:23–31, 1982.
44. Johnson RJ: The effect of immobilization on ligaments and ligamentous healing. *Contemp Orthop* 2:237–241, 1980.
45. Johnson RJ, Eriksson E, Haggmark T, Pope MH: Five- to ten-year follow-up evaluation after reconstruction of the anterior cruciate ligament. *Clin Orthop* 183:122–140, 1984.
46. Kapandji IA: *The Physiology of the Joints.* New York, Churchill Livingstone, 1970, vol 2.
47. Kennedy JC, Hawkins RJ, Willis RB: Strain gauge analysis of knee ligaments. *Clin Orthop* 129:225–229, 1977.
48. Kessler R, Hertling D: *Management of Common Musculoskeletal Disorders.* New York, Harper & Row, 1983.
49. Kettelkamp DB, Jacobs AW: Tibiofemoral contact area determination and implications. *J Bone Joint Surg [Am]* 54:349–356, 1972.
50. Knight KL, Martin JA, Londeree BR: EMG comparison of quadriceps femoris activity during knee extension and straight leg raises. *Am J Phys Med* 58:57–69, 1979.
51. Krebs DE, Staples WH, Cuttita D, Zickel RE: Knee joint angle: its relationship to quadriceps femoris activity in normal and postarthrotomy limbs. *Arch Phys Med Rehabil* 64:441–447, 1983.

52. Lankhorst GJ, van de Stadt RJ, van der Korst JK, et al: Relationship of isometric knee extension torque and functional variable in osteoarthrosis of the knee. Scand J Rehabil Med 14:7–10, 1982.
53. Laubenthal KN, Smidt GL, Kettelkamp DB: A quantitative analysis of knee motion during activities of daily living. Phys Ther 52:34–42, 1972.
54. Lehmkuhl LD, Smith LK: Brunnstrom's Clinical Kinesiology. Philadelphia, FA Davis, 1983.
55. Levy IM, Torzilli PA, Warren RF: The effect of medial meniscectomy on anterior-posterior motion of the knee. J Bone Joint Surg [Am] 64:883–888, 1982.
56. Lew WD, Lewis JL: The effect of knee prosthesis geometry on ligament mechanics during flexion. J Bone Joint Surg [Am] 64:734–739, 1982.
57. Lieb FJ, Perry J: Quadriceps function—an anatomical and mechanical study using amputated limbs. J Bone Joint Surg [Am] 50:1535–1548, 1968.
58. Lieb FJ, Perry J: Quadriceps function—an electromyographic study under isometric conditions. J Bone Joint Surg [Am] 53:749–758, 1971.
59. Lindahl O, Movin A, Ringqvist I: Knee extension: measurement of the isometric force in different positions of the knee joint. Acta Orthop Scand 40:79–85, 1969.
60. Lipke JM, Janecke CJ, Nelson CL, et al: The role of incompetence of the anterior cruciate and lateral ligaments in anterolateral and anteromedial instability. J Bone Joint Surg [Am] 63:954–960, 1981.
61. Losee RE: Concepts of the pivot shift. Clin Orthop 172:45–51, 1983.
62. Lunnen JD, Yack J, LeVeau BF: Relationship between muscle length, muscle activity, and torque of the hamstring muscles. Phys Ther 61:190–195, 1981.
63. Mann RA, Hagy JL: The popliteus muscle. J Bone Joint Surg [Am] 59:924–927, 1977.
64. Maquet P: Mechanics and osteoarthritis of the patellofemoral joint. Clin Orthop 144:70–73, 1979.
65. Markolf KL, Bargar WL, Shoemaker SC, Amstutz HC: The role of joint load in knee stability. J Bone Joint Surg [Am] 63:570–585, 1981.
66. Markolf KL, Mensch JS, Amstutz HC: Stiffness and laxity of the knee—the contributions of the supporting structures. J Bone Joint Surg [Am] 58:583–594, 1976.
67. Matthews LS, Sonstegard DA, Henke JA: Load bearing characteristics of the patellofemoral joint. Acta Orthop Scand 48:511–516, 1977.
68. Morrison JB: The mechanics of the knee joint in relation to normal walking. J Biomech 3:51–61, 1970.
69. Müller W: The Knee:Form, Function and Ligament Reconstruction. Berlin, Springer-Verlag, 1983.
70. Noyes FR, Grood ES, Suntay WJ, Butler DL: The three dimensional laxity of the anterior cruciate deficient knee as determined by clinical laxity tests. Iowa Orthop J 3:32–44, 1983.
71. Noyes FR, Sonstegard DA: Biomechanical function of the pes anserinus at the knee and the effect of its transplantation. J Bone Joint Surg [Am] 55:1225–1241, 1973.
72. Odenstein M, Lysholm J, Gillquist J: Long-term follow up study of a distal iliotibial band transfer (DIT) for anterolateral knee instability. Clin Orthop 176:129–135, 1983.
73. Ogden JA: The anatomy and function of the proximal tibiofibular joint. Clin Orthop 101:186–191, 1974.
74. Okamoto T: Electromyographic study of the function of muscle rectus femoris. Res J Phys Educ 12:175–182, 1968.
75. Osternig LR, Bates BT, James SL: Patterns of tibial rotary torque in knees of healthy subjects. Med Sci Sports Exerc 12:195–199, 1980.
76. Osternig LR, Bates BT, Tseng YL, James SL: Relationship between tibial rotary torque and knee flexion/extension after tendon transplant surgery. Arch Phys Med Rehabil 62:381–385, 1981.
77. Peeples RE, Margo MK: Function after patellectomy. Clin Orthop 132:180–186, 1978.
78. Perry J, Fox JM, Boitano MA, et al: Functional evaluation of the pes anserinus transfer by electromyography and gait analysis. J Bone Joint Surg [Am] 62:973–980, 1980.
79. Piziali RL, Seering WP, Nagel DA, Schurman DJ: The function of the primary ligaments of the knee in anterior-posterior and medial-lateral motions. J Biomech 13:777–784, 1980.
80. Pocock GS: Electromyographic study of the quadriceps during resistive exercise. J Am Phys Ther Assoc 43:427–434, 1963.

81. Radin EL, Simon SR, Rose RM, Paul IL: *Practical Biomechanics for the Orthopedic Surgeon.* New York, Wiley, 1979.
82. Reilly DT, Martens M: Experimental analysis of the quadriceps muscle force and patello-femoral joint reaction force for various activities. *Acta Orthop Scand* 43:126–137, 1972.
83. Reynolds L, Levin TA, Medeiros JM, et al: EMG activity of the vastus medialis oblique and the vastus lateralis in their role in patellar alignment. *Am J Phys Med* 62:61–70, 1983.
84. Ritter MA, Stringer EA: Predictive range of motion after total knee replacement. *Clin Orthop* 143:115–119, 1979.
85. Rovere GD, Adair DM: Anterior cruciate-deficient knees: a review of the literature. *Am J Sports Med* 11:412–419, 1983.
86. Scudder GN: Torque curves produced at the knee during isometric and isokinetic exercise. *Arch Phys Med Rehabil* 61:68–72, 1980.
87. Seebacher JR, Inglis AE, Marshall JL, Warren RF: The structure of the posterolateral aspect of the knee. *J Bone Joint Surg [Am]* 64:536–541, 1982.
88. Shoemaker SC, Markolf KL: In vivo rotatory knee stability. *J Bone Joint Surg [Am]* 64:208–216, 1982.
89. Shrive NG, O'Connor JJ, Goodfellow JW: Load-bearing in the knee joint. *Clin Orthop* 131:279–287, 1978.
90. Simon SR, Trieshmann HW, Burdett RG, et al: Quantitative gait analysis after total knee arthroplasty for monarticular degenerative arthritis. *J Bone Joint Surg [Am]* 65:605–613, 1983.
91. Smidt GL: Biomechanical analysis of knee flexion and extension. *J Biomech* 6:79–92, 1973.
92. Soderberg GL, Cook TM: An electromyographic analysis of quadriceps femoris muscle setting and straight leg raising. *Phys Ther* 63:1434–1438, 1983.
93. Soudan K, Van Audekercke R: Methods, difficulties and inaccuracies in the study of human joint kinematics and pathokinematics by the instant axis concept. Example: the knee joint. *J Biomech* 12:27–33, 1979.
94. Steindler A: *Kinesiology of the Human Body under Normal and Pathological Conditions.* Springfield, IL, Charles C Thomas, 1955.
95. Stratford P: Electromyography of the quadriceps femoris muscles in subjects with normal knees and acutely effused knees. *Phys Ther* 62:279–283, 1982.
96. Sutton FS, Thompson CH, Lipke J, Kettelkamp DB: The effect of patellectomy on knee function. *J Bone Joint Surg [Am]* 58:537–540, 1976.
97. Tamea CD, Henning CE: Pathomechanics of the pivot shift maneuver—an instant center analysis. *Am J Sports Med* 9:31–37, 1981.
98. van Eijden TMGJ, de Boer W, Verburg J: A dynamometer for the measurement of the extension torque of the lower leg during static and dynamic contractions of the quadriceps femoris muscle. *J Biomech* 16:1019–1024, 1983.
99. Wahrenberg H, Lindbeck L, Ekholm J: Knee muscular moment, tendon tension force and EMG during a vigorous movement in man. *Scand J Rehabil Med* 10:99–106, 1978.
100. Walmsley RP, Yang JF: Measurement of maximum isometric knee flexor moment. *Physiother Can* 32:83–86, 1980.
101. Wang CJ, Walker PS: Rotatory laxity of the human knee joint. *J Bone Joint Surg [Am]* 56:161–170, 1974.
102. Wang CJ, Walker PS, Wolf B: The effects of flexion and rotation on the length patterns of the ligaments of the knee. *J Biomech* 6:587–596, 1973.
103. Warwick H, Williams PL (eds): *Gray's Anatomy,* ed 35. Philadelphia, WB Saunders, 1973.
104. Wild JJ, Franklin TD, Woods GW: Patellar pain and quadriceps rehabilitation: an emg study. *Am J Sports Med* 10:12–15, 1982.
105. Wyatt MP, Edwards AM: Comparison of quadriceps and hamstring torque values during isokinetic exercise. *J Orthop Sports Phys Ther* 3:48–56, 1981.
106. Yost JG, Chekofsky K, Schoscheim P, et al: Intraarticular iliotibial band reconstruction for anterior cruciate ligament insufficiency. *Am J Sports Med* 9:220–224, 1981.
107. Zaricznyj B: Reconstruction of the anterior cruciate ligament using free tendon graft. *Am J Sports Med* 11:164–176, 1983.

11

Ankle and Foot

The ankle and foot are a complex series of joints whose integrity is maintained primarily by an expansive ligamentous network. Yet, these joints and their interactions are responsible for ambulation and the rapid elevation of the body into space in activities such as jumping. Compared to the knee, little is known about the ankle and foot. In fact, much of what is known about the ankle and foot has resulted from studies associated with gait. However, in the all too frequent pathological circumstance, the effect is incapacitating. This chapter will focus on normal function before describing the biomechanics of the ankle and foot. The final section will deal with pathokinesiology.

Because of the multiplicity of joints and varied terminologies that are used to describe the ankle and foot, there is necessity to define the commonly used descriptors of ankle and foot motion. The ankle is considered to be the joint formed by the tibia, fibula, and talus. The foot includes all the joints distal to the ankle, and in general the five metatarsals and the phalanges constitute the forefoot. The midfoot consists of the cuneiform, navicular, and cuboid bones, while the hindfood (rearfoot) includes the talus and calcaneus (32). Plantar flexion and dorsiflexion will be considered to be the motion about a horizontal axis through the ankle that lies in the frontal plane. Subtalar joint motion occurs about an axis oblique to the three axes around which the usual flexion-extension, abduction-adduction, and rotation occur. Special terminology has been adopted in that pronation consists of dorsiflexion, eversion, and abduction. Eversion occurs about an axis running in the anteroposterior direction of the foot. Abduction, in the special case of the foot, occurs around a vertical axis. Supination, in contrast, is the result of combined inversion, adduction, and plantar flexion. Note that eversion and inversion are components of pronation and supination, respectively. Reference is also commonly made to forefoot adduction and abduction, but realize that these movements take place about a vertical axis. Similarly, hindfoot "valgus" and "eversion" are synonymous. Many attempts have been made to standardize the descriptors; yet there is currently no one system that is universally accepted. Although the most common systems will be presented in this volume, the reader is advised to be prepared to interpret and make applications to other systems that may appear in the literature.

MUSCULAR ACTIONS

The actions of the muscles affecting the ankle and foot complex are difficult to interpret in any simple fashion for several reasons. First, the muscles originate from an area ranging from the posterior, distal aspect of the femur to the small bones of the distal foot. In addition, most muscles cross numerous joints, therefore giving the potential actions a great diversity. The multiple joint crossings also have implications for length-tension considerations. Finally, whether the foot is fixed (closed kinetic chain) or free (open chain) will determine if the leg will move about the foot, such as in gait, or the foot about the leg. Although some of the early work on muscle function was hampered by little information on the position of the axes of the joints of the ankle and foot, some determinations have been made as to muscle function.

Ankle

Any muscle attached to the femur or to any structures in the lower leg and projecting to the foot will have some effect on the ankle. Often considered to be of primary interest are the gastrocnemius and the soleus muscles, collectively labeled as the triceps surae. Due to the femoral attachment of the gastrocnemius, this muscle can have a more profound effect on plantar flexion of the ankle when the knee is in an extended (muscle lengthened) position. In essence, then, quadriceps contraction facilitates an increased plantar flexion moment by virtue of stretch applied to the gastrocnemius muscle. Many manual muscle tests and clinical tests used for assessing the level of force exerted by the gastrocnemius and soleus muscles offer knee flexion as a means to differentiate the abilities of the two muscles. Whether the 44-mm shortening of the soleus versus the 39-mm shortening of the gastrocnemius has an effect on the tension generated is unclear (22). The importance of the triceps surae can be realized from presentation of the 1911 Fick data. That work identified cross sections of 23 and 20 cm^2 for the gastrocnemius and soleus, respectively. These values compare to the total value of 21 cm^2 for the flexors hallucis and digitorum longus, the tibialis posterior, and the peroneus longus and brevis (26). Because these muscles all pass relatively close to the axis for plantar flexion, clearly the most important musculature for propulsive activities is the triceps surae. Some significance may also exist in the finding that the triceps surae concurrently supinates the foot during plantar flexion (22). Even this is in dispute since Campbell et al have reported that the medial soleus is active during foot eversion. The fact that this muscle was more active during eversion than inversion was perhaps due to the muscle acting as a restraint to hypereversion by the peroneals (5). This eversion may be due to the fact that the axis for subtalar motion lies lateral to the insertion of the Achilles tendon on the posterior aspect of the calcaneus. Electromyographic evidence that the gastrocnemius muscle is active in inversion also exists (14).

Note should also be made of the differential role of the gastrocnemius and soleus during standing posture. Although both muscles would be in an anatomically advantageous position to generate tension, there is considerable EMG and histochemical information available that would indicate that the soleus muscle is primarily responsible for producing the plantar flexion moment at the ankle. Some attention should also be given to the fact that during support of the body by the foot, the leg is moving over the fixed distal segments that are usually considered as the muscle insertion. Whether this reversal has any specific meaning in terms of muscle function is not clear, but Sutherland has performed work that shows that the plantar flexors play a role in maintaining the knee in extension during the stance phase of gait (54). Simon and coworkers have also done complex analyses, suggesting that calf muscle activity is used to restrain forward momentum rather than to propel the body further. More specific attention will be given to this matter in Chapter 13, Posture and Gait (45).

The roles of the other muscles in plantar flexion and their additional motions also raise some interesting points. In considering plantar flexion the minimal contribution of the muscles other than the triceps surae has already been pointed out. However, of the five remaining muscles, the peroneals contribute about one-half of the remaining torque (22). Further evidence for the necessity of effective plantar flexion is the stiffness of the sagittal plane motion of the subtalar joint, allowing for transfer of torque to the ankle (12).

The peronei are given credit for primary production of forefoot eversion. Yet, the longus reaches all the way to the inner aspect of the foot, demonstrating the capability to pull the medial aspect of the foot down into the supporting surface. Other explanations for muscle function in arch control can be offered. The peroneus longus tendon passed under the "keystone" or apex of the lateral longitudinal arch and thereby provides a supportive function. The peroneus longus also bowstrings across the transverse arch as the tendon projects to the medial border of the foot. By pulling the medial border toward the lateral border it supports the transverse arch that bridges between the two longitudinal arches. Further, the tibialis posterior inserts at the apex of the medial longitudinal arch, also serving a supportive role. Considered together the peroneus longus and posterior tibialis make a sling arrangement.

Note that in the functional closed kinetic chain situation, though, body weight passively produces pronation, rather than requiring muscle activity to pull the bones down. This action, combined with the motions of the triceps surae, provides a beautiful example of the synergistic action of muscles in producing more effective plantar flexion. This is probably true in spite of the fact that plantar flexion was found to be a secondary function of the peroneus longus and the posterior tibialis muscles (1).

Supinator muscles include the group on the medial aspect of the ankle mortise. The posterior tibialis is clearly an important muscle in completing this function. Although the anterior tibialis is still regarded as being responsible for inversion, its line of action lies almost precisely along the subtalar axis, thereby negating motion around this axis. The anterior tibialis, and the extensors digitorum and hallucis longus, together provide an excellent balance for dorsiflexion of the foot. Generally, small cross sections are observed in these muscles because of the low torques required in this direction of motion. Returning to the medial aspect of the ankle, the role of these muscles in supporting the longitudinal arch has been long debated. EMG data show that the muscles potentially responsible are active only at low levels and over very short time intervals (3). The attachment of the posterior tibialis, by means of a sling-type arrangement spanning several tarsal bones, is in an anatomically advantageous position to support the longitudinal arch. Evidence that loss of this muscle leads to a collapse of the arch provides support for the role of this muscle (12). Perhaps the muscle, tendon, and other soft tissues are also elongated if direct and/or aperiodic muscle support is lost. Other muscular actions of these extrinsic muscles are specific to the locus of attachment. For example, a long toe extensor serves to extend the toes, whether the muscle is attached to the hallux or the remaining digits.

The other muscles affecting the function of the foot are the intrinsic muscles. Found predominantly on the plantar aspect of the foot, these muscles assist in propulsion and potentially have an impact on the position of the arch. Although there are differences in the structure of the interossei and lumbricals in comparison to those of the hand, their positions and functions are very similar. Imbalance of forces among these muscles can lead to decreased function and abnormal joint position as seen in the hand; yet the import is much less because of the relatively course function of the foot. Some attention should, however, be given to the influence of the plantar fascia and ligaments, because attachments spanning the tarsals allow the structures to act much like a truss (Fig. 11.1). The extremely high tensile strength of the fascia, coupled with its tensile stiffness, makes the fascia an ideal structure for the receipt of repetitive loads such as occur during walking. In such dynamic cases the toes are brought, by either an active or passive process, into dorsiflexion. Because the fascia inserts distally at the metatarsophalangeal joints, the fascia becomes tighter as the toes are dorsiflexed. Thus, as body weight passes forward over the foot the fascia tightens and raises the longitudinal arch (12).

Others, such as Elftman, consider supination to occur simultaneously with this windlass effect of the plantar fascia. Supination is responsible for the close-packed position of the tarsals and produces a "rigid lever" for propulsion (10). By this mechanism the foot provides a stable segment about which the rest of the body may move. Without such a rigid system in the most distal segment, motion in the more proximal segments could not be carried out as effectively. Static conditions produce a similar effect in that tarsal bones have relatively tight interfaces that assist in constraining motion. Although there is a large number of joints in which motion can occur, the ligaments of the foot also are partly responsible for limiting motion, thus providing a rigid structure under static as well as dynamic conditions (12).

ARTHROLOGY AND ARTHROKINEMATICS

The ankle and foot form a complex series of joints that has anatomy, and subsequent arthrokinematics, peculiar to the joint under consideration. For convenience and for reasons of functional importance the ankle, subtalar, and transverse joints will be specifically discussed.

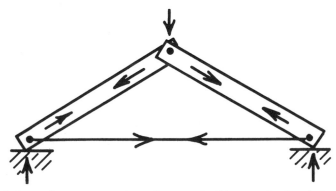

Figure 11.1.   Schematic representation of a truss. In this case the two bony segments are pinned together and at each end. The tie across the bottom depicts the plantar fascia. (From Hicks JH: The three weight-bearing mechanisms of the foot. In Evans FG (ed): *Biomechanical Studies of the Musculoskeletal System.* Springfield, IL, Charles C Thomas, 1961.)

Ankle

The ankle mortise, also known as the talocrural joint, is composed of three bones: the tibia, fibula, and talus. The distal end of the tibia is expanded in both anteroposterior and mediolateral directions. Matching the inferior aspect of the tibia is the convex surface of the talus. Often referred to as the dome of the talus or as the trochlear region, the articular surface is wider anteriorly than posteriorly. Perhaps most important is that the radius of curvature of the medial segment is smaller anteriorly than posteriorly, as compared to the lateral trochlea whose radius appears to be constant from anterior to posterior (19). This mediolateral difference in radius is responsible for the ankle kinematics described below. Mention should also be made of the articulations of the talus with the medial and lateral malleoli and of the inferior tibiofibular joint, perhaps relatively unimportant except when stability is considered. Also of import in pathological situations is the fact that the lateral malleolus is smaller and projects more distally than does the medial.

Stability of the joint, primarily in medial and lateral directions, is maintained by the expansive medial and the smaller, more specific lateral ligaments. By connecting specific bony structures, each set of ligaments normalizes joint kinematics and prevents abnormal ranges of movement. Detailed presentation of these ligaments is outside the scope of this text, although references to several structures are included in the section on pathokinesiology.

Understanding the kinematics of the ankle is dependent upon a knowledge of the bony shapes as presented in the previous paragraphs. The tapering of the trochlea from anterior to posterior and the different radii of curvature of the medial and lateral aspects account for asymmetry and thus the conjunct rotation that is seen with dorsi- and plantar flexion of the ankle. The greater length of the trochlear surface in the posterior direction also determines that plantar flexion has a greater range of motion than does dorsiflexion. Extremes of motion in either direction are limited either by bony impingement, capsular or ligamentous constraints, or available length of muscles and tendons antagonistic to the attempted motion (22).

Other principles of joint motion such as the movement of convex on concave surfaces (or vice versa) also apply to the ankle and do not need reiteration. The close-packed position of the ankle is considered to be at the position of extreme dorsiflexion. According to Kapandji, the slight spreading of the malleoli and rotation of the fibula, occurring upon extreme dorsiflexion become important only if such spreading is severely restricted (22). Conversely, excess spread can lead to a widened mortise and an unstable ankle.

Subtalar

The subtalar joint is complicated by virtue of the fact that two or three talar facets, depending upon how they are considered, articulate with the calcaneus. In essence, both the posterior and anterior facets (perhaps further divided into anterior and medial) are complex, slightly curved surfaces. The posterior articulation of the calcaneus on the talus is convex on concave, respectively. The anteromedial facet surfaces also are convex on concave (24). The latter surface, or surfaces, are supported by the bony shelf of the calcaneus, the sustentaculum tali. Kapandji maintains that the most essential ligament of this joint is the interosseus talocalcaneal ligament consisting of anterior and posterior segments. This structure passes from the sulcus tali to the sulcus calcanei and becomes tight during the motion of eversion (56). It also has been identified as playing a role in stabilizing this joint during both static and dynamic activities (22).

Motions of the subtalar joint are produced by the combined action of the posterior and anterior surfaces. Recall from the opening paragraphs of this chapter that the orientation of the axis of subtalar motion (Fig. 11.2) requires a three-plane description of the resulting movement. Therefore, during supination the calcaneus moves distally (plantar flexion) medially (adduction), and rotates around the longitudinal axis of the foot to lie on the lateral surface (inversion).

Transverse Tarsal

This joint, also referred to as the midtarsal joint, is composed of the articulation of the talus with the navicular and the calcaneus with the cuboid bone. In most cases the two joints are considered together because they are functionally similar. The talonavicular joint is unremarkable as the rounded head of the talus matches the concavity of the posterior surface of the navicular bone. The calcaneocuboid joint is relatively complex, and like the talonavicular joint is tightly bound with multiple ligaments.

Motion at the midtarsal joint is constrained by means of ligaments and the matching of articular surfaces. Although the talonavicular joint is considered to have 3° of freedom, the adjacent calcaneocuboid joint (with only 2° of freedom) and the tightness of the joint between the calcaneus and navicular restrict midtarsal movement. Note also that the axis for motion is similar in location and orientation to the axis of the subtalar joint. Because of the interaction of these two joints, the motions of most relevance are inversion and eversion (24).

Summary of Ankle and Foot Arthrokinematics

The motions of many bones of the ankle and foot are difficult to describe because of the multiple articular surfaces of most bones, the various locations of the axes of rotation, and interactions that occur among the joints when movements are undertaken. To understand that gliding and rotation occur between all surfaces is fundamental. If, for example, one attempts to elevate the medial

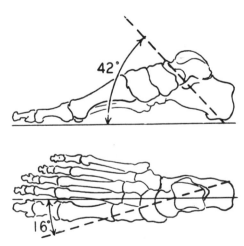

Figure 11.2.   The position of the axis of the subtalar joint is shown by the *dashed line* in each of two projections. (From Manter JT: Movements of the subtalar and transverse tarsal joints. *Anat Rec* 80:397–410, 1941.)

border of the foot so that the sole faces medially, these gliding and rotary motions take place. The greater part of supination is in the mechanism of the subtalar joint. However, the motion of the calcaneus around the talus facilitates movement at the transverse tarsal joint, the net effect of which is to increase the overall range of inversion. The latter is accomplished by rotation in the talonavicular joint and the downward gliding of the cuboid on the calcaneus. Finally, recall that in plantar flexion the dome of the talus is narrower, allowing for additional inversion range through talar tilt within the ankle mortise (56). Thus, motions of the ankle and foot are composites, meaning that isolated movements of individual segments cannot occur without interacting with other joints and causing changes in the amount of surface congruity. A more complete description of foot arthrokinematics may also include the other joints not addressed in this volume. However, most motion in the tarsal and metatarsal joints and the phalanges is planar and probably of much less total import than the motions in the three joints described. More detailed accounts can be located in Kapandji and in such compendia as those authored by Sgarlato (22, 43). At any rate, effective management of the patient with involvement of the distal aspects of the lower limb will surely depend on the knowledge of the normal arthrokinematics of the ankle and foot.

BIOMECHANICS
Kinematics

Angular displacements of the ankle and foot have been extensively described. Sagittal plane motion in the ankle appears to total about 80°, 50 of which is available in plantar flexion (22). Lesser values have been reported, particularly if the limb is bearing weight. Less range is also required in the ankle during such functional activities as gait. Functionally, a greater range is available due to the contribution of the forefoot, as in the ability of an adept ballerina. Motion at the subtalar joint is more difficult to isolate and quantify. Total range of values are generally reported to be from 17 to 24°, but Kapandji states that supination range is 52°, while pronation is limited to 25 to 30° (22). Subotnick, however, indicates that a minimum of 18° of supination is necessary for subtalar joint function (52). Transverse tarsal joint motion has also been determined. Hicks specified that midtarsal range was 8° about the longitudinal foot axis and 22° about an oblique axis (described in the instant center section of this chapter) (17).

Arches of the Foot

Most descriptions of the foot include a discussion of three arches, a transverse and both a medial and lateral longitudinal. The medial is seemingly the most important because of the ramifications for alterations in total foot mechanics should the medial longitudinal arch undergo significant change. MacConaill and Basmajian describe the foot as a twisted plate that generates what most refer to as the longitudinal arches. For the lateral arch the posterior support is the calcaneus, the keystone is the cuboid, and the fourth and fifth metatarsal head the anterior support. Further twisting or untwisting of the arches can be accomplished by muscular actions and/or by combined motions of the ankle and foot. These mechanisms will be discussed in subsequent paragraphs (27).

The longitudinal arches of the foot have been extensively discussed in relation to the ability to bear weight. Three potential mechanisms exist in the foot for this purpose. First, note that the bony configuration of the metatarsals is such that together they form a transverse bow that is convex superiorly. This arrangement allows the bones to act as beams for the purpose of effectively supporting body weight. Although bone size of the middle three metatarsals may appear to be too small to effectively resist loading, the collective ability of these bones shows them capable of supporting at least three or four times body weight. A second mechanism capable of load bearing appears to be the truss-like configuration of the foot. In this situation the longitudinal bony configuration is supported by ligaments and the planar aponeurosis. If in fact the bones were not constrained by these soft tissues the bones would be able to spread apart, leading to the demise of the longitudinal arches. Recall also that the configuration of the longitudinal arches can be altered by means of changes in tension in the plantar aponeurosis as detailed in previous sections of this chapter. The third possible mechanism for arch control, muscular tension, has been discussed previously. In any event, if muscles such as the peroneus longus and tibialis posterior were active, about 15 to 20% of the body weight could be supported (21). Summarizing, a number of mechanisms are available for purposes of managing the load created by body weight. In all probability, no single factor accounts for the ability of the foot to manage the repetitive and relatively high loads that must be tolerated. Hicks has even suggested that management may be in combination, for example, 25% by beam, and 50 to 75% by arch (18).

Axes and Instant Centers of Rotation

The analyses of the ankle, subtalar, and midtarsal joints all have included study of the axes of rotation of the respective joints. Relative to the ankle Mann has specified the location of the axes in the transverse and frontal planes. The respective ranges of the axis location are shown in Figure 11.3. And, although the ankle axis is 20 to 30° displaced relative to the axis of the knee, this fact bears little apparent implication for the arthrokinematics of the ankle or foot

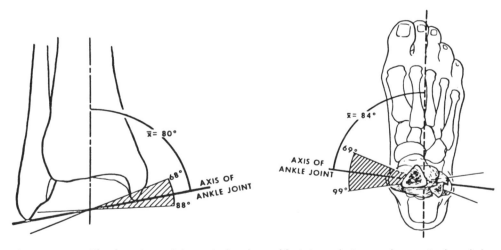

Figure 11.3.   The location of the axis for the ankle joint relative to the vertical and the anteroposterior directions. Both the means and the extreme locations of the axis are shown for both planes. (From Mann RA: Biomechanics of the foot. In *Atlas of Orthotics: Biomechanical Principles and Application*. American Academy of Orthopedic Surgeons. St. Louis, CV Mosby, 1975, pp 257–266.)

(28). Some years ago rather extensive work was completed by a team of investigators on the location of the instant center of rotation of the ankle. For the 22 ankles studied from positions of plantar flexion through dorsiflexion, in only 12 ankles did the ICR remain in the talus throughout the range of motion. Sample determinations for weight- and nonweight-bearing ankles are shown in Figures 11.4 and 11.5. Note that in the weight-bearing ankle an ICR lies outside of the body of the talus. The investigators also remarked that the normal ankle showed distraction tendencies in the early range of plantar flexion, followed by sliding in the midportion, and compression as the close-packed position was reached toward the limit of dorsiflexion (40).

The position of the subtalar axis has been defined since 1941, at which time Manter studied 16 cadavers. He used both a vertical and a horizontal reference frame to define the axis position relative to the foot. The axis was inclined anteriorly by 42° with respect to the plantar surface of the foot. In the other plane it was medially deviated an average of 16° from the plane that bisected the calcaneus and the first web space (Fig. 11.2). Manter further observed that the plane of rotation of the subtalar joint was not at a right angle to the joint axis. Because sideways slipping could not occur the conclusion was reached that subtalar motion was rotational with an average helix of 12°. Thus, the screw-like action of the subtalar joint is created by the osteokinematics shown in Figure 11.6 (31). Numerous studies have been completed since the original work of Manter, among those being Inman's work. In this case only 20 of 58 specimens showed constant increments of linear displacement that would be consistent with a true screw. Although the helix angle was determined to be only 7.9°, the deviation of these data from the original work is considered to be small (19). One other concept is important to describe. Because the interaction of the tibia and foot is important for control of the body on the foot, i.e., in posture and

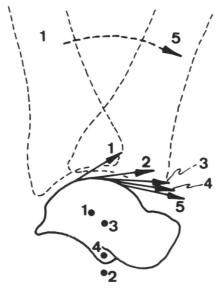

Figure 11.4. Points *1* through *4* show the location of the instant center of rotation for the ankle joint during dorsiflexion in the weight-bearing ankle. The vectors represent surface velocities, indicating that primarily shear is taking place. See text for further detail. (From Sammarco GJ, Burstein AH, Frankel VH: Biomechanics of the ankle: a kinematic study. *Orthop Clin North Am* 4:75–96, 1973.)

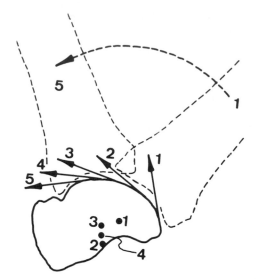

Figure 11.5. Same as for Figure 11.4 except in the nonweight-bearing ankle. (From Sammarco GJ, Burstein AH, Frankel VH: Biomechanics of the ankle: a kinematic study. *Orthop Clin North Am* 4:75–96, 1973.)

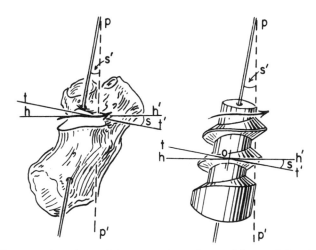

Figure 11.6. Comparative view of the posterior calcaneal facet of the right subtalar joint with a right-hand screw. The horizontal plane in which the motion is occurring is indicated with *hh'*, and *tt'* is a plane perpendicular to the screw axis. The angle *s'* is equal to *s*, the helix angle of the screw. Note that *s'* is determined by dropping a vertical line from point *p* to *p'*. The *arrow* depicts the path of the body following the screw. (From Manter JT: Movements of the subtalar and transverse tarsal joints. *Anat Rec* 80:397–410, 1941.)

gait, an understanding of the movements involved may prove helpful. In order to emphasize that the subtalar joint provides rotation between the foot and tibia, the joint can be described as an oblique hinge. In essence, what happens is that as the tibia is externally rotated the foot assumes a more supinated position. This phenomenon can be easily demonstrated by placing the foot lightly on the floor and rotating the tibia. Conversely, internal rotation of the tibia will produce pronation and a subsequent flattening of the medial longitudinal arch (27).

Axes at the transverse tarsal joint have also been defined. This work led to the

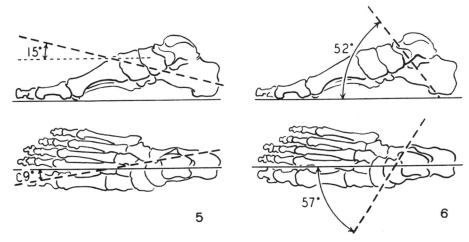

Figure 11.7. Depiction of the two axes of the transverse tarsal joints for two views of the foot. The portion to the *left* shows a more longitudinal axis when compared to the more oblique axis shown in the two *right-hand* figures. (From Manter IT: Movements of the subtalar and transverse tarsal joints. Anat Rec 80:397–410, 1941.)

identification of two composite axes, a longitudinal and an oblique (Fig. 11.7). Forefoot inversion and eversion would be the movements about the former axis, while plantar flexion combined with adduction and dorsiflexion combined with abduction would occur about the oblique axis. More extensive work was done by Elftman, who was able to identify two axes each for the calcaneocuboid and the talonavicular joints. He was able to demonstrate that, because of the orientation of the axes, pronation of the subtalar joint forced the axes into a parallel position and subsequently allowed free movement of the forefoot. Supination caused a limitation of motion in the forefoot because the movements at the calcaneocuboid and talonavicular joints opposed each other (10). The interactions of tibial rotation, subtalar, and midtarsal motion are summarized in Figure 11.8.

Torque

The measurement of torque at the ankle must be interpreted with some caution due to the fact that multiple joints are included in the determinations. If testing conditions are not similar across trials, clinics, or studies, comparisons are difficult or impossible to make. Partly for these reasons Nistor et al completed a methodological study of ankle torque, finding that errors varied between 5 and 10%. They noted that changes in ankle position caused great differences in the recorded torque values, leading to larger errors when measurements were made of peak torque values (36).

Several data sets are available in the literature that allow for some assessment of ankle plantar flexion torque. The study by Nistor and coworkers on ten adult subjects determined that with the ankle in the neutral position, 113 Nm of isometric torque were produced in an open kinetic chain arrangement. Plantar flexion of 15 and 30° decreased the values to 83 and 65 Nm, respectively. However, 15° of dorsiflexion caused the torque to increase to 134 Nm (36). Fugl-Meyer and assistants also provided information on the plantar flexors, showing torque to be greater by 15% when the knee was extended as compared

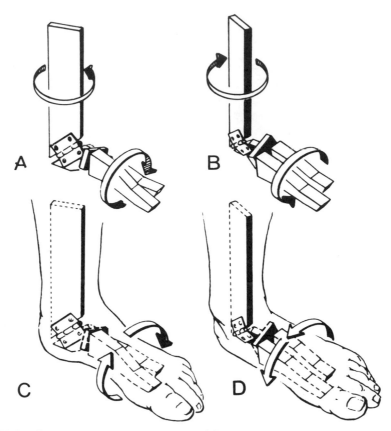

Figure 11.8. Diagrammatic representation of the effects of internal and external rotation on the subtalar and transverse tarsal joints. Consider *A* and *C* together, in which case the tibia is externally rotated. Concurrently, the subtalar joint supinates. The transverse tarsal joint is made more rigid because the two axes of this joint, shown in Figure 11.7, become less parallel to each other. In *B* + *D* the opposite occur, including laxity in the transverse tarsal joint because the axes are now more parallel to each other. (From Mann RA: Biomechanics of the foot. In *Atlas of Orthotics: Biomechanical Principles and Application.* American Academy of Orthopedic Surgeons. St. Louis, CV Mosby, 1975, pp 257–266.)

to 90° of knee flexion. Isometric plantar flexion values ranged from 110 to 140 Nm for their group of 30 young men (13). Another study, using various age groups of both sexes, has shown torque values for young men and women to range from 30 to 122 Nm when isometric testing was performed in the neutral position. These investigators concluded that significant torque differences were due to weight and age and not to sex or height of the subjects (11).

Isokinetic dynamometers have also been used to study ankle plantar flexion torque. Nistor et al tested at 30, 90, and 180°/sec and found values of 101, 54, and 27 Nm, respectively (36). Fugl-Meyer and coworkers provided similar results in that torque was about 100 Nm at 30°/sec and diminished to 40 Nm at 180°/sec. The Falkel work tested only at 30°/sec and determined values that ranged from 29 to 106 Nm for young adult men and women (11).

Less objective data are available for dorsiflexion, perhaps because of the relatively small torque needed for effective function. Representative findings for dorsiflexion performed isometrically by normal young adult subjects range from

29 to 31 Nm in the neutral position of the ankle. As could be anticipated, data from 60 and 180°/sec isokinetic trials were less: 24 and 13 Nm, respectively (4).

KINETICS
Ankle

Information about the kinetics of the ankle and foot is sparse when compared with that available for the knee and hip. The primary reason is that the ankle is less prone to osteoarthritic (osteoarthrotic) changes, therefore creating less joint pathology than encountered in other joints of the lower limb. Considerable attention has been paid, however, to the transmission of loads and the mechanics of the foot during gait. Thus, in most circumstances the kinetics of the ankle and foot have been considered under dynamic conditions.

Under static conditions, such as in the assumption of the symmetrical standing posture, the joint reaction forces are rather easy to determine. The magnitudes of these forces would be one-half body weight plus the force resulting from contraction of musculature that crosses the joint. Because there is minimal muscle contraction required during normal standing posture the joint reaction forces are of a relatively low magnitude. Rising to tiptoe on one leg will increase the force to over two times body weight for two reasons: the entire body weight is supported by one limb and the plantar flexors are now required to sustain a strong contraction (12). One would expect forces during gait and other dynamic activities to increase the compressive force in the ankle joint. Stauffer and coworkers have indeed shown this to occur in their analytic work on the ankle. Their data showed a compressive force of about three times body weight from heel-strike to foot-flat and a further rise to a peak value of 4.5 to 5.5 times body weight during heel-off when the plantar flexors were undergoing strong contraction (Fig. 11.9) (48). These data agree well with the maximal ankle joint reaction forces of 5.2 times body weight derived from the mathematical model of Seireg and Arvikar, but differ slightly from the 3.9 times body weight peak found by

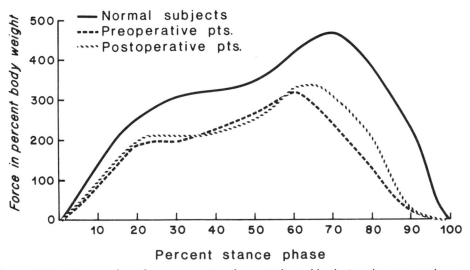

Figure 11.9. Mean values for compressive force at the ankle during the stance phase of gait. Note the similar pattern but smaller forces in the patient groups. (From Stauffer RN, Chao EYS, Brewster RC: Force and motion analysis of the normal, diseased, and prosthetic ankle joint. *Clin Orthop* 127:189–196, 1977.)

Procter and Paul (39, 42). Consideration of the ankle cannot ignore the presence of tangential or shear force. This force was found to be in the posterior direction, i.e., the talus tending toward posterior movement on the mortise, during the majority of the stance phase of gait. Magnitude was just over 0.6 times body weight. After 80% of stance phase had passed, talocrural shear was anterior and less than 50% of the magnitude produced in the early weight bearing phases (48).

Also of relevance is the amount of contact area available in the ankle. The unpublished data of Greenwald, cited in the Stauffer et al work, show that the load-bearing surface of the ankle is from 11 to 13 cm^2 (48). This relatively large area can be responsible for the low loads per unit area, potentially offering a sound reason for the low incidence of osteoarthrosis. Of further interest is the demonstration that under small loads achieved during the early stance phase of gait, the contact areas on the talus are two distinct oblong areas located on its medial and lateral aspects. As the load is increased the distribution of the pressure changes so that the load is distributed over the entire superior surface of the talus. Thus, the maximal area for load transfer is used, minimizing the force per unit area (59).

Subtalar

Little information is available on the kinetics of the subtalar or other joints of the foot, probably because of the complexities associated with the joint mechanics. Little truly objective data are available, and the analyses usually result from either clinical evaluations or mathematical models. The former category includes the analysis discussed by Perry. To describe the events functionally, the mechanisms can be discussed in terms of the gait cycle. Eversion in the subtalar joint is precipitated at heel-strike by means of two mechanisms. The first is caused by off-center (eccentric) loading of the foot, that is, when body weight is considered relative to the center of rotation in the subtalar joint (Fig. 11.10). Thus, in such circumstances the calcaneus is forced somewhat anteriorly and also laterally into a valgus position. Simultaneously, the talus is shifting medially and downward. Further, this internal rotation of the talus is responsible for inducing internal rotation of the tibia and thus perpetuating eversion in the subtalar joints (37). Apparently these 10° of motion occur within the first 8% of the stance phase of the average walking cycle (58). Only during the terminal stance phase does supination reverse the cycle (37).

The only objective data that exist on the subtalar joint have been provided by means of mathematical modeling. In this case the peak resultant force in the anterior facet of the talocalcaneonavicular joint was 2.4 times body weight. The average peak force for the posterior facet was 2.8 times body weight and also occurred in the late stance phase of the gait cycle (39).

Soft Tissues

A discussion of the forces in the ankle and foot would be incomplete without the inclusion of tendinous and ligamentous forces. Little information is available in regard to the forces of such structures. The Stauffer group thought the tibialis anterior tendon force to be of negligible import in their study of the ankle joint, since the magnitude of tensile loading is probably 20% of body weight or less. Further, electromyographic data show that the muscle contracts for a very short duration, primarily at the end of the swing phase of the gait cycle. Force in the

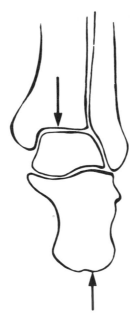

Figure 11.10.   Representation of the loading effect on the ankle. Calcaneal floor contact is lateral to the force due to body weight, causing potential eversion in the subtalar joint. (From Perry J: Anatomy and biomechanics of the hindfoot. *Clin Orthop* 177:9–15, 1983.)

Achilles tendon is considerably greater and accounts for a good portion of the compressive force across the ankle (48).

Analyses of restraining effects and failure in the ligaments of the foot and ankle have also been performed. One of these ligaments, the anterior talofibular ligament, is considered to be of particular significance because of the control this ligament may have on talar motion. The literature disagrees somewhat as to the role of the ligament, primarily in the amount of allowed talar tilt. Johnson and Markolf have studied 30 cadaver ankles in an attempt to more definitively determine the effects of section of the anterior talofibular ligament. In general, they found that ankle laxity was dependent upon position. Least motion was found in the dorsiflexed position, confirming that this is the close-packed position of the joint. Section of the ligament significantly increased anterior-posterior laxity, but greatest increases in motion in inversion-eversion (5.2°) and in internal-external rotation (10.8°) were seen in the position of plantar flexion. Because of the importance of the anterior talofibular ligament in controlling these motions the ligament is felt to be one of the prime stabilizers of the ankle and an indirect stabilizer of the subtalar joint (20).

An understanding of the ligaments has also been aided by evaluation of their tensile strength, in that cadaver tests have shown a wide variation in the tensile strength of the anterior talofibular ligament. The mean value of 206 N was derived from a range of 58 to 556 N, identifying almost a ten-fold increase in the difference found among ankles. Midsubstance failures and bony attachment site failures were about equally divided, creating greater difficulty in the ability to account for the variability seen across specimens (51). That a low tensile failure level of 3 N was established after anterior talofibular ligament section in some specimens has some potential impact for cases of ankle sprains, many of which will injure the anterior tibiofibular ligaments (20).

PATHOKINESIOLOGY

Many pathologies produce abnormalities in the foot that lead to disruptions of normal mechanics. Such conditions lead to potentially disabling circumstances, because motion of the proximal segments of the body are dependent upon the most distal segment of the lower limb being adequately related to the supporting surface. Discussed in this section will be common mechanical problems, the influence of muscular function, and the effect of overuse syndromes. Results of arthroplasties and the changes produced by various pathologies on the forces measured under the foot will also be presented.

Mechanical Behavior

Because the foot and ankle are located most distally in the limb, the joints comprising these segments are responsible for allowing effective weight reception and for generating the torque required for propulsion. Thus, as in most other joints, there must be allowance for flexibility and yet a mechanism for adequate control. Various pathologies, whether in the forefoot or hindfoot, are known to affect a large percentage of the population. Although hindfoot varus has been identified, a far more pervasive problem is forefoot varus. This condition contributes to abnormal compensatory pronation in the subtalar joint so that a more equal weight distribution may occur on the metatarsal heads during stance. Such pronation, coupled with midtarsal joint unlocking, causes instability of the forefoot and renders this segment of the propulsive device ineffective. Sgarlato states that pronation beyond 50% of stance phase in gait causes foot unlocking and instability at heel lift, as well as shearing and subluxation at the subtalar joint (43).

A significant ramification of pronation is the effect on the arches of the foot and the implications for changes in these arches on the mechanics of the foot and ankle. Long-term stress on the soft tissues most likely elongates them and alters the positions of the bony segments relative to each other. Subsequently, pronation can lead to poor positioning, manifested most often as loss of height of the medial longitudinal arch of the foot. Since there is a reasonable amount of evidence that musculature provides little support of the arch, the maintenance of joint integrity and control would appear to be of fundamental importance. This flatfoot condition can occur in children as a result of alterations in connective tissue composition, bony structure, or inadequate development of muscular mechanisms (2). In adults the most common etiologies of acquired flatfoot have been identified as arthritis, rupture of the posterior tibial tendon, or profound peripheral neuritis conditions that affect the foot (30). According to McPoil and Brocato, five foot types cause subtalar joint compensation as manifested by abnormal pronation: forefoot varus, forefoot valgus, rearfoot varus, tibia vara, and equinus deformity (32).

Management of the pronated foot consists of numerous methods, including surgery, exercise, and the use of a foot orthosis. In many surgical cases, joint mechanics is significantly altered, and in some cases bones are fused. Exercise has been generally conceded to be ineffective because of the apparent inability of the musculature to adequately support the arch, particularly over extended periods of time. The most recently developed treatment mode, that of the balanced foot orthosis, achieves forefoot equilibrium by placing a wedge or post under the medial forefoot (43). This technique thus can eliminate the necessity for abnormal compensatory pronation during the stance phase of gait. There is, however, some controversy as to the effectiveness of this method. Sims has shown that use of an orthosis significantly decreased mean foot pronation during standing immediately after and 4 weeks after application of the orthosis. Other results showed an orthosis to be ineffective in decreasing mean foot pronation during walking when testing was done immediately after application. However, significant decreases were noted in the midstance and late stance phases of gait after 4 weeks of use (46). Whether additional changes or long-term effects are manifested as a result of this treatment is awaiting further research.

Gait

The motion patterns of the subtalar joint were described in the previous section on subtalar kinetics. A more functional view, as summarized in Figure 11.11, has been provided by Mann. During the first 15% of the cycle the foot rapidly adapts to the supporting surface. Note that many of the changes in motions or levels of muscular activity occur at 15% of the cycle, the point at which foot flat is achieved. Inversion, indicated earlier as part of supination of the subtalar joint, is accompanied by increased stability in the transverse tarsal

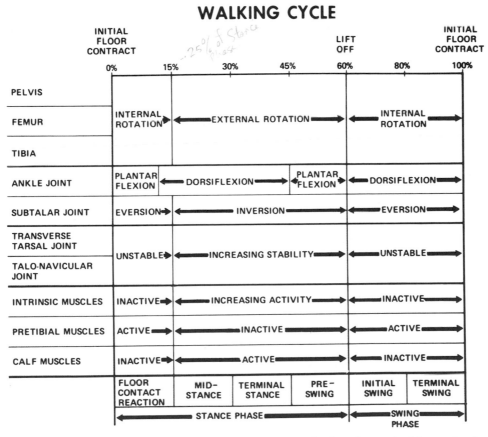

Figure 11.11. Summary diagram for the entire gait cycle that shows the kinematics for the subtalar joint as well as for other segments. General descriptions of levels of muscle activity are also provided. (From Mann RA: Biomechanics of the foot. In *Atlas of Orthotics: Biomechanical Principles and Application.* American Academy of Orthopedic Surgeons, St. Louis, CV Mosby, 1975, pp 257–266.)

and the talonavicular joints. Although not shown on the chart, recall that extension of the toes occurs as a result of the natural progression of the body over the foot, leading to elongation of the tension in the plantar fascia. Thus, additional stability is given to the foot. The net effect of the events of late stance is stabilization of the longitudinal arches of the foot at the time of toe-off. The remaining events of the cycle are accomplished in the nonweight-bearing position and proceed in order to position the foot for the next contact with the supporting surface (28). The course of the interactive events that take place in the foot and ankle must be understood, because the proper event and the order of occurrence will be the determinant of normal or pathological motion. Realizing the complexity of the events and the fact that the entire cycle is completed in about 1 sec emphasizes the import of both proper arthrokinematics and muscular control required for normal function of the ankle and foot.

One of the manifestations of nearly all pathologies is altered gait. Such changes are usually demonstrated in a number of ways, including but not limited to kinematic and kinetic effects. For example, Katoh and coworkers showed that patients with painful heel pads and plantar fasciitis had altered temporal and distance parameters during gait. These same patients also had altered kinetics, manifested in decreased vertical loading components at heel-strike and at toe-off, as well as decreased anterior shear at the shoe-force plate interface during early stance. These same investigators evaluated patients with isolated talonavicular fusion and determined there to be decreased pronation, especially during side-slope walking with the involved foot on the upper side. Their data support the clinical observation that subtalar motion is coupled with motion occurring at the transverse tarsal joint (23).

Alterations in gait are also commonly associated with the rheumatoid patient. Hindfoot instability may be a contributing factor in other difficulties and therefore may require specific evaluation. Other difficulties that are frequently encountered by these patients include the pronated foot, valgus of the great toe, painful heel, and toe deformities. The pathomechanics associated with pronation have been discussed in earlier sections. Hallux valgus influences gait because of the import of the great toe during push-off. As a result of discomfort the patient is likely to attempt to push off with greater loading through the lateral aspect of the foot than is usually required or desired. Another possibility is that these patients just do not achieve much heel-off but instead propel themselves with the foot flat. Changes in the toes can lead to multiple problems, such as diminished propulsive force during terminal stance (9). That these conditions with an etiology of muscular imbalances are the major initiating factor in foot deformities has also been identified by D'Amico (8).

How loads are transmitted through the foot has received considerable attention. Some of the debate centers on whether all the metatarsals are loaded during stance. In static postures the load is apparently distributed throughout the foot. Approximately 50% of the load is borne by the heel. The remaining 50% is distributed across the metatarsal heads, with twice as much load being taken on the first metatarsal head as on the others.

Transmission of loads during gait has also been evaluated in subjects with normal and pathological feet. In general, the pattern for progression of the center of pressure through the foot is as follows. Upon receipt of the pressure just slightly lateral to the midline of the heel, the path moves forward in virtually a straight line towards the head of the third metatarsal. Toward the end of stance the pressure is directed medially, and at toe-off it leaves the foot at the first web space (23). Collis and Jayson provided more specific data relative to the metatarsal heads, showing the highest pressures under the heads of the second and third metatarsals of normal subjects. Patterns for the three rheumatoid patients studied showed a wide variance, probably indicative of the differences produced by the total disease process (6). Presumably a number of the patients that Stokes et al studied before and after surgery for hallux valgus also suffered from rheumatoid arthritis. Their predictable results showed significantly reduced loads imposed on the toes and the medial side of the forefoot when compared to healthy feet. An additional factor found to be of importance was metatarsal length, there being a direct relationship between length and receipt of load (50).

Muscle Function and Overuse

As noted in the section of this chapter on muscle function, the foot is kinetically balanced by muscle tensions and their respective moment arms in relationship to the joints that the muscles cross. As long as there is no disruption of this balance, the foot and ankle can function effectively. Under any circumstances creating changes in this balance, the therapist must be prepared to deal with pathological motion. Some of these potential changes have been discussed in terms of imbalances resulting from rheumatoid arthritis. The remainder of this section will discuss other muscular dysfunctions and losses.

In general the loss of any given muscle or group of muscles tends to create ankle and foot deformity or dysfunction consistent with the loss. For example, loss of the musculature of the anterior tibial compartment resulting from injury to the peroneal nerve will leave no dorsiflexion capability. The foot drifts into a plantar-flexed and supinated position due to the unopposed pull of the tibialis posterior muscle. Conversely, tibial nerve injury paralyzes calf musculature and leads to extreme and usually continuous positioning of the foot in dorsiflexion, termed the calcaneal foot (47).

A frequent injury affecting the posterior calf muscle group is the Achilles tendon rupture. Efforts to manage these patients are geared towards restoration of the ability to exert normal plantar flexion torque. There is some evidence that patients post-Achilles tendon rupture can reach comparable levels of torque, as has been shown by the Sjostrom group and the study by Nistor. The former study evaluated patients at about 23 months postoperatively and found that static and dynamic mean peak torque for the injured leg was similar to that for the noninjured leg. However, two of the nine subjects showed torque losses greater than 50 Nm (47). The other study compared two groups: patients postsurgery and those who were nonsurgically treated. In this case only minor differences were noted between the groups that had a mean follow-up time of 2.5 yr. However, patients in both treatment groups generally produced less torque on the injured than on the uninjured side, with the exception of 11 nonsurgical and eight surgically treated patients who generated greater isokinetic torque on the injured side. The surgical treatment group for the uninjured side developed 149 Nm, while the nonsurgical group produced 161 Nm of torque in the neutral position. Surgically treated injured legs produced 124 Nm plantar flexion torque as compared to the 127 Nm for the nonsurgical group. One other study evaluated 32 patients a mean length of 35 months postinjury and noted mean torques of 63 Nm for the injured leg and 75 Nm for the normal leg (35).

Other investigators noted that the closed method of repair resulted in a larger loss of torque (44). In any case, a summary of these data indicates that losses of plantar flexion torques can be avoided with adequate care. Therapists that institute appropriate rehabilitation programs can anticipate achieving the torque that can be produced in the uninjured limb. Surgical procedures necessitating removal of the triceps surae would also be projected to have a devastating effect. Based on theoretical calculations of the torque contributed by the triceps surae, the loss should be approximately 80%. However, it is interesting that Murray and coworkers have reported such a case showing the loss to be only 62% of the total torque (33). Combined paralysis of the invertors and evertors is unusual. Isolated loss of the tibialis posterior may result in a very pronated foot, while loss of the peroneus longus and brevis would lead to supination.

Often, foot and ankle deformity is caused by other conditions, such as cerebral palsy or congenital disorders. In these situations the most likely necessity is to offer the possibility of reestablishing kinetic balance. The most popular procedure for accomplishing this purpose is the tendon transfer. Such a procedure has been successfully used for decades, a sufficient length of time to establish some general principles for its use. Crawford has been among those who have identified the important considerations. First the transfer should involve a muscle that has good to normal strength. In addition, if the muscle has to work against an existing deformity, the likelihood of an unsuccessful transfer is high. The procedure should always allow the tendon to be directed in a straight line and pass through smoothly gliding tissue without restriction. A further criterion is that a patient should be of sufficient age to effectively participate in a program of therapeutic muscle reeducation. Finally, when function is taken into account the phase of activity becomes important. That is, if the muscle transfer requires a plantar flexor to become a dorsiflexor during an activity such as gait, there is a high degree of probability that the transfer will fail (7).

Most frequently the disabilities managed by tendon transfer are for lateral instability and loss of active dorsiflexion. An example would be the lateral transfer of the anterior tibial tendon for treatment of extreme equinovarus (clubfoot) deformity. In this procedure the tendon is released from its attachment and surgically transferred to the cuboid and the base of the fifth metatarsal (15). Another example is the use of the posterior tibial tendon in cases of plantar flexion and inversion deformities. In this procedure Green and associates split the tendon proximal to the medial malleolus and passed the tendon posteriorly and laterally so that the new insertion would lie next to that of the tendon of the peroneus brevis. Although two patients required osteotomies of the calcaneus for fixed deformities, no varus deformity recurred, and the equinus portion occurring during gait was eliminated (16). Numerous other examples of transfers at the foot and ankle could be cited. The principles of the procedures are similar: the primary focus being to locate the new insertion in such a position that the mechanical effect produces the appropriate kinetic balance.

EMG may also be used effectively in the evaluation and treatment of the inappropriate phasic behavior of muscles that affect the ankle and foot. Monitors that can be applied to specific muscles are available for the purpose of determining the timing and degree of activity of the musculature. A muscular contraction pattern may be determined to be inconsistent. Therapeutic interventions may be indicated that will modify the muscles' sequence of activity. That there are abnormal patterns of firing in neurological patients has been demonstrated in the premature firing of the triceps surae and prolonged firing of the tibialis anterior during stance phase (38).

Overuse Syndromes

Conditions that appear commonly in the lower leg and foot, mostly due to sports or other high levels of activity, have been known to produce dysfunction. The injuries most frequently occurring from improper conditioning, training, or biomechanical faults include shin splints, tendinitis, bursitis, and stress fractures. Although some of these disorders have been related to muscle imbalances, leg length discrepancies, and lumbosacral disorders, a majority of the problems are considered to have their derivation from the biomechanics of the foot and ankle. Of primary concern is the altered mechanics of the subtalar joint, because changes at this joint may produce changes in patterns of muscular use. For example, consider that the foot cannot move into supination during the latter stage of the support phase. In this case the normal arthrokinematics of the subtalar and transverse tarsal joints are disrupted and the foot will not have become an effective lever to which muscle and passive forces can be applied (53).

A particular overuse syndrome, known as shin splints, has been analyzed in terms of mechanics of the foot. This condition, characterized by pain in the lower leg, has been variously considered to have its etiology based in bone, vascular or soft tissues. In an attempt to evaluate the biomechanical aspects of the etiology, an assessment was made of lower leg and heel position, the passive range of the subtalar joint, and the angular displacement of the midline of the Achilles tendon. Results demonstrated significantly greater Achilles tendon angles and subtalar mobility of the shin splint subjects. Other differences between the two groups implicate both structural and functional abnormalities in the feet and ankles of those with the shin splint overuse syndrome (55).

Arthrodesis and Arthroplasty

Surgical fusion of the ankle and joints of the foot has been used for decades, primarily for the treatment of painful feet. These arthrodeses have not been limited to any single joint; rather, they have been used according to the location of the pathology. An understanding of the mechanics of the ankle and foot will clarify the significance of fusion of any single joint or collective joints.

Consider arthrodesis of the ankle joint. Any such successful procedure will place additional stress on the subtalar joint, although the magnitude of this stress can be somewhat controlled by the position of the ankle joint. Excessive deviation in either supination or pronation is thought to cause the patient difficulty when the center of gravity of the body passes over the foot. Increased joint loading can also lead to subtalar and midtarsal pain as well as secondary knee and hip pain. Excessive pronation may cause the patient to roll over the medial aspect of the foot, which may in turn lead to hallux valgus deformity or pain on the medial aspect of the knee. Similar considerations can be applied to varus or valgus tilt of the talus and the degree of dorsiflexion or plantar flexion of the ankle. For example, in the latter case the ankle should be placed in the plantar-flexed position in cases where the limb is comparatively shortened. On the other hand, too much plantar flexion will potentially cause a circumstance where genu recurvatum (hyperextended knee) deformity results.

Similar difficulties can readily arise with fusions of other joints of the foot.

Increased stress will occur in surrounding joints, leading to other pathologic situations. Disrupted gait patterns have been blamed on an arthrodesis of the subtalar joint. According to Mann, a valgus (pronation) tilt of 5° in the subtalar joint is preferred because good stability of the ankle is permitted (29).

Ankle arthroplasties have also been performed, sufficiently so that results from clinical trials have been reported. Stauffer and Segal have reported on a group of 102 patients, more than 90% of which reported significant postoperative pain relief. Although ankle range of motion increased by only 6°, 75% of the patients had improved gait (49). In another series Newton reported on 50 patients. In his population, ankle scores that measured pain, range of motion, and function, were improved in patients having osteoarthritis (osteoarthrosis), failed arthroplasties, and rheumatoid arthritis (34). In general, the best results appear to be in cases with rheumatoid arthritis or in posttraumatic arthritis among patients under 60 yr of age (49). In any case rehabilitation involves the restoration of normal arthrokinematics in the ankle and other joints of the foot. As further investigations of the capabilities of the components used in surgical procedures for the ankle are accomplished, the characteristics associated with each of the designs will become more widely known (25, 41).

SUMMARY

In this chapter the pertinent anatomical and biomechanical factors that affect the ankle and foot have been presented. As the segment that makes contact with the supporting surface, the foot and ankle must be flexible enough to accommodate to different surfaces yet stiff enough to provide the torque required. The foot and ankle meet the criteria necessary for effective function by combining a series of joints and controlling forces that interact so that the requirements of both static and dynamic situations can be met. Disruption of the mechanics of the kinetic chain leads to pathological function. Several alterations that produce these disruptions were presented and discussed.

References

1. Ambagtsheer JBT: The function of the muscles of the lower leg in relation to movements of the tarsus. *Acta Orthop Scand [Suppl]* 172:1–196, 1978.
2. Barry RJ, Scranton PE: Flat feet in children. *Clin Orthop* 181:68–75, 1983.
3. Basmajian JV: *Muscles Alive.* Baltimore, Williams & Wilkins, 1979.
4. Black KD, Halverson JL, Majerus KA, Soderberg GL: Alterations in ankle dorsiflexion torque as a result of continuous ultrasound to the anterior tibial compartment. *Phys Ther* 64:910–913, 1984.
5. Campbell KM, Biggs NL, Blanton PL, Lehr RP: Electromyographic investigation of the relative activity among four components of the triceps surae. *Am J Phys Med* 52:30–41, 1973.
6. Collis WJMF, Jayson MIV: Measurement of pedal pressures: an illustration of a method. *Ann Rheum Dis* 31:215–217, 1972.
7. Crawford AH: A discussion of tendon transfers in the paralytic foot. *Arch Podiatr Med Foot Surg* 2:47–60, 1974.
8. D'Amico JC: The pathomechanics of adult rheumatoid arthritis affecting the foot. *J Am Podiatry Assoc* 66:227–236, 1976.
9. DiMonte P, Light H: Pathomechanics, gait deviations, and treatment of the rheumatoid foot: a clinical report. *Phys Ther* 62:1148–1156, 1982.
10. Elftman H: The transverse tarsal joint and its control. *Clin Orthop* 16:41–46, 1960.
11. Falkel J: Plantar flexor strength testing using the cybex isokinetic dynamometer. *Phys Ther* 58:847–850, 1978.
12. Frankel VH, Nordin M: *Basic Biomechanics of the Skeletal System.* Philadelphia, Lea & Febiger, 1980.

13. Fugl-Meyer AR, Sjostrom M, Wahlby L: Human plantar flexion strength and structure. *Acta Physiol Scand* 107:47–56, 1977.
14. Furlani J, Vitti M, Costacurta L: Electromyographic behavior of the gastrocnemius muscle. *Electromyogr Clin Neurophysiol* 18:29–34, 1978.
15. Garceau GJ, Palmer RM: Transfer of the anterior tibial tendon for recurrent club foot. *J Bone Joint Surg [Am]* 49:207–231, 1967.
16. Green NE, Griffin PP, Shiavi R: Split posterior tibial-tendon transfer in spastic cerebral palsy. *J Bone Joint Surg [Am]* 65:748–754, 1983.
17. Hicks JH: The mechanics of the foot. I. The joints. *J Anat* 87:345–357, 1953.
18. Hicks JH: The three weight-bearing mechanisms of the foot. In Evans FG (ed): *Biomechanical Studies of the Musculoskeletal System.* Springfield, IL, Charles C Thomas, 1961.
19. Inman VT: *The Joints of the Ankle.* Baltimore, Williams & Wilkins, 1976.
20. Johnson EE, Markolf KL: The contribution of the anterior talofibular ligament to ankle laxity. *J Bone Joint Surg [Am]* 65:81–88, 1983.
21. Jones RL: The human foot:an experimental study of its mechanics, and the role of its muscle and ligaments in the support of the arch. *Am J Anat* 68:1–39, 1941.
22. Kapandji IA: *The Physiology of the Joints.* New York, Churchill Livingstone, 1970, vol 2.
23. Katoh Y, Chao EYS, Laughman RK, et al: Biomechanical analysis of foot function during gait and clinical applications. *Clin Orthop* 177:23–33, 1983.
24. Kessler RM, Hertling D: *Management of Common Musculoskeletal Disorders.* New York, Harper & Row, 1983.
25. Lachiewicz PF, Inglis AE, Ranawat CS: Total ankle replacement in rheumatoid arthritis. *J Bone Joint Surg [Am]* 66:340–343, 1984.
26. Lehmkuhl LD, Smith LK: *Clinical Kinesiology.* Philadelphia, FA Davis, 1983.
27. MacConaill MA, Basmajian JV: *Muscles and Movements: a Basis for Human Kinesiology.* Baltimore, Williams & Wilkins, 1969.
28. Mann RA: Biomechanics of the foot. In *Atlas of Orthotics: Biomechanical Principles and Application.* American Academy of Orthopedic Surgeons. St. Louis, CV Mosby, 1975, pp 257–266.
29. Mann RA: Surgical implications of biomechanics of the foot and ankle. *Clin Orthop* 146:111–118, 1980.
30. Mann RA: Acquired flatfoot in adults. *Clin Orthop* 181:46–51, 1983.
31. Manter JT: Movements of the subtalar and transverse tarsal joints. *Anat Rec* 80:397–410, 1941.
32. McPoil TG, Brocato RS: The foot and ankle:biomechanical evaluation and treatment. In Gould JA, Davies GJ (eds): *Orthopaedic and Sports Physical Therapy.* St. Louis, CV Mosby, 1985.
33. Murray MP, Guten GN, Baldwin JM, Gardner GM: A comparison of plantar flexion torque with and without the triceps surae. *Acta Orthop Scand* 47:122–124, 1976.
34. Newton SE: Total ankle arthroplasty: clinical study of fifty cases. *J Bone Joint Surg [Am]* 64:104–111, 1982.
35. Nistor L: Surgical and non-surgical treatment of achilles tendon rupture. *J Bone Joint Surg [Am]* 63:394–399, 1981.
36. Nistor L, Markhede G, Grimby G: A technique for measurements of plantar flexion torque with the cybex II dynamometer. *Scand J Rehabil Med* 14:163–166, 1982.
37. Perry J: Anatomy and biomechanics of the hindfoot. *Clin Orthop* 177:9–15, 1983.
38. Perry J, Waters RL, Perrin T: Electromyographic analysis of equinovarus following stroke. *Clin Orthop* 131:47–53, 1978.
39. Procter P, Paul JP: Ankle joint biomechanics. *J Biomech* 15:627–634, 1982.
40. Sammarco GJ, Burstein AH, Frankel VH: Biomechanics of the ankle: a kinematic study. *Orthop Clin North Am* 4:75–96, 1973.
41. Scranton PE, Fu FH, Brown TD: Ankle arthrodesis: a comparative clinical and biomechanical evaluation. *Clin Orthop* 151:234–243, 1980.
42. Seireg A, Arvikar RJ: The prediction of muscular load sharing and joint forces in the lower extremities during walking. *J Biomech* 8:89–102, 1975.
43. Sgarlato TE: *A Compendium of Podiatric Biomechanics.* San Francisco, California College of Podiatric Medicine, 1971, pp 209–225.
44. Shields CL, Kerlan RK, Jobe FW, et al: The cybex II evaluation of surgically repaired

achilles tendon ruptures. *Am J Sports Med* 6:369–372, 1978.

45. Simon SR, Mann RA, Hagy JL, Larsen LJ: Role of the posterior calf muscles in normal gait. *J. Bone Joint Surg [Am]* 60:465–472, 1978.

46. Sims DS: The Effect of a Balanced Foot Orthosis on Muscle Function and Foot Pronation in Compensated Forefoot Varus. Master of Arts thesis, University of Iowa, 1983.

47. Sjostrom M, Fugl-Meyer AR, Wahlby L: Achilles tendon injury: plantar flexion strength and structure of the soleus muscle after surgical repair. *Acta Chir Scand* 144:219–226, 1978.

48. Stauffer RN, Chao EYS, Brewster RC: Force and motion analysis of the normal, diseased, and prosthetic ankle joint. *Clin Orthop* 127:189–196, 1977.

49. Stauffer RN, Segal NM: Total ankle arthroplasty:four years' experience. *Clin Orthop* 160:217–221, 1981.

50. Stokes IAF, Hutton WC, Stott JRR, Lowe LW: Forces under the hallux valgus foot before and after surgery. *Clin Orthop* 142:64–72, 1977.

51. St. Pierre RK, Rosen J, Whitesides TE, et al: The tensile strength of the anterio talofibular ligament. *Foot Ankle* 4:83–85, 1983.

52. Subotnick SI: Biomechanics of the subtalar and midtarsal joints. *J Am Podiatry Assoc* 65:756–764, 1975.

53. Subotnick SI: Lower extremity problems in athletes: a biomechanical approach. *Arch Podiatr Med Foot Surg* 2:23–29, 1978.

54. Sutherland DH: An electromyographic study of the plantar flexors of the ankle in normal walking on the level. *J Bone Joint Surg [Am]* 48:66–71, 1966.

55. Viitasalo JT, Kvist M: Some biomechanical aspects of the foot and ankle in athletes with and without shin splints. *Am J Sports Med* 11:125–130, 1983.

56. Warwick R, Williams PL (eds): *Gray's Anatomy*, ed 36. Philadelphia, WB Saunders, 1980.

57. Wiesseman GJ: Tendon transfers for peripheral nerve injuries of the lower extremity. *Orthop Clin North Am* 12:459–467, 1981.

58. Wright DG, Desai ME, Henderson BS: Action of the subtalar and ankle joint complex during the stance phase of walking. *J Bone Joint Surg [Am]* 46:361–382, 1964.

59. Wynarsky GT, Greenwald AS: Mathematical model of the human ankle joint. *J Biomech* 16:241–252, 1983.

12

Trunk

SPINE

The segment of the body known as the trunk is of interest because often the arms, legs, and head must rotate in relationship to this segment. Although respiratory mechanics are of considerable importance, the biomechanics of the spine are of primary interest. This series of joints, arranged in a column consisting of anteroposterior deviations, produces an incredible array of movement patterns. Yet, this flexibility must be coupled with the capacity to handle significant loads, either as part of regular or imposed activities. These requirements probably predispose the spine to dysfunctions that are often manifested in postural, gait, or other functional disorders. Although entire volumes have been written about the spine, this chapter will discuss aspects of muscular control, arthrology, and arthrokinematics and biomechanics as related to the spine. The pathokinesiology associated with several common disorders will also be presented. A similar topical outline will be followed for respiration.

Muscular Actions

Control of the trunk can be conveniently considered from either the viewpoint of flexors versus extensors or by way of region of the spine. The former provides the ability to categorize the musculature functionally while the latter allows for discussion based on some important regional differences. This section will combine the two approaches and close with some information on the role of the musculature in various exercises.

The extensor musculature is composed of a large amount of muscle that is layered both in depth and breadth. Extensive descriptions are available in classic anatomy texts, and it is not the intention of this volume to reiterate anatomical relationships. Rather, the functional significance of the different portions should be stressed. In general, the deepest may be considered to be responsible for finer movements of intervertebral joints because their attachments extend over a limited number of vertebral segments. Certain sections are also larger in any given area of the spine, such as the multifidus in the lumbar and sacral regions. The contributions of these segments to the overall mass of the erector spinae musculature thus account for the findings of the greatest extensor muscle mass in the lumbar spine. According to some, the deeper portion of the multifidus thins out over the thoracic spine, becoming thicker again in the cervical spine (35). The necessity for increased extensor torque in these two areas may explain the increased mass in these two areas of the spine.

The specific role of each of the segments of the erector spinae has escaped identification because of the difficulties associated with in vivo studies. Isaacson goes so far as to say that the short deep portions of the erector spinae are responsible for maintaining some degree of rigidity in the vertebral column. Because change in the position of one of any of the motion segments with respect to another can produce stretch, passive tension can certainly exist. Further comments on this topic are found in the section of kinetics. Conversely, the superficial and longest layers can be considered the prime movers for vertebral extension, lateral flexion, and rotation (35).

Other descriptive systems of the posterior musculature of the lumbar spine also exist. For example, Kapandji describes the musculature according to three planes: deep, intermediate, and superficial. The deepest is composed of all components of the erector spinae group, the intermediate of the serratus posterior inferior, and the most superficial of the latissimus dorsi. In addition to extension of the lumbar spine, these muscles are also effective in increasing lumbar lordosis (41). For a detailed description of the erector spinae in the lumbar spine, the work of Bogduk would be of considerable interest (8). In considering the extensors of the thoracic spine, no additional comment is necessary because the topography and function of the erector spinae muscle in this area are similar to those of the lumbar segment of the spine.

The posterior muscles of the neck are a far more complex matter because of the increased rotational requirements of this segment of the spine. For purposes of convenience and function, Kapandji has identified four planes. The deepest contains primarily the suboccipital muscles, while the semispinalis plane includes the semispinalis capitis and cervicis and three other small muscles. The splenius and levator scapulae compose the area just deep to the superficial plane, which is made up of the trapezius and the sternocleidomastoid muscles. All but the superficial plane muscles extend, rotate, and laterally flex ipsilaterally. In the case of the trapezius and sternocleidomastoid, the fiber direction of the muscles is such that rotation is in the contralateral direction.

With the extensive musculature in the posterior cervical spine, numerous examples of synergistic and antagonistic action can be cited. For example, contraction of the unilateral suboccipital group causes lateral flexion while bilateral contraction causes extension of the cervical spine. An additional example is provided by considering rotation. Contraction of one splenius capitus muscle causes rotation of the head to the same side. To complement this action the contralateral sternocleidomastoid muscle must be active. Thus, in this case, these two muscles participate as a force couple in producing rotation of the head and the cervical spine. A superior view of the head and trunk, depicting the muscle forces, is shown in Figure 12.1.

The role and responsibility of the erector spinae muscles are unquestionably to hold the trunk erect during postures while also providing the capability of generating sufficient tension required during such tasks as lifting heavy objects from the floor. In cases of standing postures, nonexistent or low levels of activity appear to predominate across subjects and across different levels of the spine, as has been shown by the work of Joseph and McColl. EMG activity was evaluated at 12 vertebral levels and subjectively graded according to pre-established voltage ranges. Their data show rather high degrees of variability from segment to segment and from subject to subject. Presumably the resulting activity is dependent upon the configuration of the spine and the posture assumed during

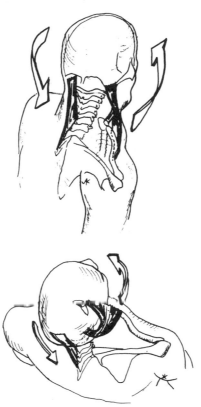

Figure 12.1.   A posterolateral and superior view of the head and upper trunk representing the left splenius capitus and the right sternocleidomastoid muscles depicting use as a force couple for rotation of the head. The approximate location of the axis of rotation is in the cervical spine, as shown in Figure 12.10.

the test (40). Similar results have also been derived from EMG evaluations by placing electrodes at different depths of the erector spinae at one vertebral level. Although there will continue to be some minor debate about the level of activity of the erector spinae in standing and sitting postures, a fair summary would be that the slight EMG activity of the thoracic levels of the muscles is greater than that recorded from the lumbar and cervical regions (39, 57).

As the trunk goes into flexion from the standing position, the activity of the erector spinae increases commensurate with the flexion moment created. That is, as the trunk is inclined anteriorly; the flexion at each motion segment requires greater tension in the extensors at each respective segment. There is a point around 50° of flexion, however, at which erector spinae activity diminishes until, at full flexion, the muscles are inactive. This progressive decrease in muscular tension is due to the fact that as the erector spinae are elongated, sufficient passive tension is generated in elastic elements of the muscle. In fact, Bogduk and MacIntosh have established that erector spinae muscles and the thoracolumbar fascia interact as they function to control the trunk (9). Combined with tension arising in the posterior spinal ligaments, and compression of the anterior aspect of the intervertebral disc, support of the trunk in the fully inclined position becomes a passive mechanism (11). In this position the hamstring muscles are active for purposes of securing the pelvis and the trunk over the feet and legs. If such were not the case, the entire body would fall in an anterior direction.

Lateral flexion and rotation of the trunk also require activity from the back extensors. On lateral flexion there is activity in the muscles contralateral to the side of flexion. Rotation produces a more complex pattern, and there are differences of opinion as to the role of each segment. Most evidence appears to indicate that lumbar rotation is produced by ipsilateral longissimus and iliocostalis muscles in combination with contralateral multifidus and rotator muscles.

Activity of the extensors has been studied during functional activities and exercises. Lifting has been of considerable interest because of the potential role of the musculature in producing and preventing low back injury and pain. In general, lifting style and load are major determinants in the degree of activity required of the extensors. More elaborate consideration will be given to this topic in chapter 14 of this book, Ergonomics. Other functional activities studied have been rising from supine to sitting and rising to standing from a sitting or squatting position. The former case produced intermittent minimal to no activity while the latter caused continuous moderate to maximal activity (21). The properly executed Valsalva maneuver has also been known to produce moderate changes in the intensity of muscle contraction (76). Finally, because of interest in the sit-up exercise as a preventive measure for the back patient, the extensor activity has been monitored during this movement. Recordings from four paraspinal locations from the cervical to the sacral regions established that the levels respond independently of each other during the performance of Williams' flexion exercises. In the event that minimal activity of the extensors is desirable, the pelvic tilt, curl up, knees to chest, and hamstring stretch with posterior tilt should be used. Conversely, higher levels of activity exist in the standing exercises and anterior pelvic tilt positions (6).

Flexor musculature can also be considered from the viewpoint of contributions to the motion of the lumbar and cervical portions of the spine. In the cervical spine a number of muscles are responsible for flexion: the scalenes, sternocleidomastoid, longus colli, and longus capitis. Kapandji adds the longus cervicis to the flexor group. As is true for the posterior neck musculature, the flexors are also capable of performing multiple functions. Because all the musculature are attached to structures (cervical spine and head) that are mobile in three dimensions, contraction of any single muscle will ordinarily produce triplanar motion. Bilateral contraction of muscles results in neutralization of rotation and lateral flexion functions and produces the most effective flexion. Although most authors consider the sternocleidomastoid and scalene muscles to be neck flexors, certain qualifications need to be made regarding their function. For example, if the cervical spine is not held rigid, the bilateral contraction of the sternocleidomastoid muscles will increase the cervical lordosis, in effect causing flexion of the lower cervical spine on the upper thoracic spine and extension of the head. On the other hand, if other prevertebral muscles hold the neck rigid, the sternocleidomastoid and the scalenes can draw the head forward during cervical spine flexion (41). Therefore, contractions of these muscles have different effects depending upon the underlying conditions.

The musculature comprising the abdominal wall is of much interest because of the potential for controlling the lumbar spine. Composed of the transversus and rectus abdominus and the internal and external oblique muscles, an effective syncytium is formed that can protect and support the abdominal viscera as well as produce motions of the lumbar spine. Generally the transversus has been credited with the ability to increase the intraabdominal pressure. The oblique muscles are productive in rotation, the contralateral components being active together. Clearly, the oblique muscles contribute to flexion, as can be seen from the somewhat vertical orientation of the muscle fibers. Primary responsibility for flexion has been credited to the rectus abdominus, however.

Another muscle on the anterior aspect is the psoas muscle, extending from the upper lumbar spine to an insertion at the lesser trochanter of the femur. Much study and speculation have taken place concerning this muscle. The complex function of the muscle is due to multiple-segment attachments. Furthermore, the muscle is draped over the anterior rim of the pelvis, which provides a mechanism for altering the position of the pelvis. Because upward and downward tilting of the anterior rim of the pelvis is directly related to the degree of respective flexion and hyperextension in the lumbar spine, the effect of this muscle on the lumbar spine can be dramatic. To elucidate, consider the patient to have tightness of the psoas muscles. In this case the tension in the muscles will pull the anterior rim inferiorly, referred to as a downward or anterior tilt. Such tilt causes the sacrum to be inclined further forward, which in turn positions the fifth lumbar vertebrae more anteriorly. The result, shown in Figure 12.2, is to increase the lumbar lordosis.

The segmental interaction that occurs is noteworthy. Hip flexion, accomplished by the psoas and other musculature, would shorten the length of the muscle and remove the potential for production of the downward tilt of the pelvis. Hip

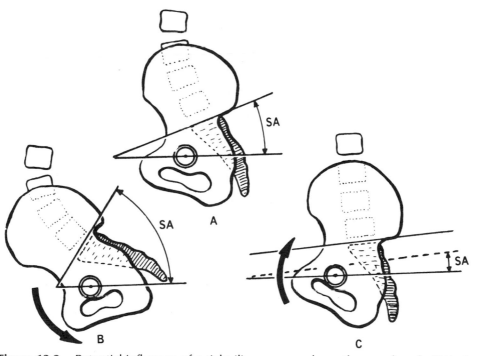

Figure 12.2. Potential influence of a tight iliopsoas muscle on the sacral angle (*SA*), the position of the pelvis, and the degree of lumbar lordosis. Normal attitude is shown in *A* while the effect of a tight iliopsoas muscle is reflected in *B*. Position *C* may result from contraction of the abdominal-gluteal muscle force couple. (From Calliet R: *Low Back Pain Syndrome.* Philadelphia, FA Davis, 1968).

flexion carried through a full range of motion ultimately requires that the pelvis be tipped posteriorly, altering the sacral angle and reducing the lumbar lordosis. Thus, hip flexion, posterior pelvic tilt, and flexion of the lumbar spine are related, as would be hip extension or hyperextension, anterior pelvic tilt, and extension or hyperextension of the lumbar spine. In addition to being a powerful hip flexor then, the psoas can strongly influence the lumbar spine indirectly or through the usual functions of lumbar spine flexion, lateral flexion, or rotation. The importance of this muscle is manifested by an entire volume having been written to describe its function (52).

Evaluation of in vivo function has been completed for the abdominal musculature. Of most interest have been activities intended to strengthen the anterior abdominal wall. Among these exercises is the straight leg raise, which has been shown to require the greatest contraction in the rectus abdominus and external oblique as judged by subjective grading of muscle activity (12). Yet, when compared to conventional, hooklying, and arched back bilateral leg raises, straight leg raises were judged to be less effective in eliciting motor unit activity in the rectus abdominus (48). Analysis of the pelvic tilt has also produced interesting results. In the supine position this motion was apparently performed primarily by the rectus abdominus and the external obliques. In standing, the internal obliques were more active than the external obliques, with little activity in the rectus.

Most commonly assessed have been various versions of the sit-up maneuver. The purpose of attempts to gain insights into the function of the abdominal muscles during these exercises is clearly a search for the most effective means of strengthening the anterior abdominal wall. Methodological differences across studies make comparisons difficult, if not impossible. Some generalizations may be safely made, however. All of the analyses appear to demonstrate that highest levels of rectus abdominus activity occur during the sit-up performed in the hook-lying position. Long-lying positions produced activity in the rectus abdominus and the obliques for an average of 19 to 37% of the total duration of the sit-up maneuver (29), although one investigation states that the sit-up performed quickly in the long-lying position produced the greatest duration of activity (25).

The curl, which is performed until the scapulae clear the floor, is also affected by the abdominals. Compared to EMG produced by maximal voluntary contractions, about 50% of the maximal activity is achieved during a curl to 45° of upper trunk flexion (18). Another comparative study showed the rectus to be active for 93% of the cycle associated with the curl exercise (29). Although suggested that simultaneous plantar flexion of the feet or completion of the exercise with a dorsally extended spine would produce more rectus abdominus activity, results have not supported these arguments (18). In all cases, a more effective contribution will be made by the oblique muscles if rotation is added to the trunk flexion motion.

Arthrology and Arthrokinematics

An analysis of motion in the spine is compounded by the fact that each of the cervical, thoracic, and lumbar segments function differently. In addition, there exist special segments, such as those found at the atlantooccipital, atlantoaxial, and lumbosacral joints. In spite of their functional variation, all of the joints are synovial in nature and enjoy relatively common forms of ligamentous support. In most cases the joints of the spine are essentially planar. Available motion, however, can be considered to consist of 6° of freedom, because rotations and translations can occur in any of the three planes. To consider these joints as less than capable of these motions would not represent an accurate picture. This section of the chapter will describe the arthrology attendant to the motions of the spine and will discuss the influence of passive structures on the achievable range of movement.

Intervertebral Joints

Although the articulation of one vertebral body on an adjacent vertebral body and the interposition of the disc can be considered a joint, most of the significance of this articulation is associated with the mechanical properties of the disc. Some consider that the disc allows relatively unconstrained motion in all 6° of freedom, while the facets serve to constrain motion. However, in this section of the chapter, the focus of the discussion will be on the role of the facet joint in determining the direction and magnitude of the motion in the various spinal segments.

The facet joints, so named because of their bony outgrowths from the vertebral arches, are synovial joints made up of the inferior and superior articular facets of the respective vertebrae. The capsules of these joints are thin and loose, being longer and looser in the cervical than in the thoracic or lumbar spine (90). Each is freely movable yet constrained by its own capsule and the ligaments that support the entire vertebral arch. Primarily important are the ligamenta nuchae, the ligamenta flava, and the supraspinous, interspinous, and intertransverse ligaments. Detailed descriptions can be found in classical anatomic texts, but in essence their names are descriptive of their attachment sites. These ligaments, plus the posterior longitudinal ligament that is located inside the vertebral canal and adherent to the posterior surfaces of the bodies of the vertebrae, compose the posterior elements that appear to be crucial to support of the human spine.

Motion in the spinal segments will be readily understood if some study of the planes of the facets is undertaken. Beginning at the occiput, note that the atlas has bilateral concave superior facets that are tilted somewhat medially and directed such that the axes are of an oblique nature. Such a combination allows for slight lateral flexion and considerable flexion and extension (90). The latter motion has been described as the motion of a ball rolling back and forth, as would occur during repetitive nodding of the head. Because these joints exist bilaterally, rotation is extremely limited. The C1-C2 facet joints are almost circular, but the superior facet of the axis is flattened posteromedially. The C2 facet is convex, sloping posteriorly and laterally (78). Such a horizontal joint configuration is conducive to large amounts of rotation. Perhaps as much as 50% of the cervical spine range of motion exists at this joint. Note that lateral bending at this joint would be markedly limited.

From the C2-C3 facet joint to the lumbosacral junction, the female, or concave surface, is the superior portion of the joint. A gross examination of these joints shows that they follow an orderly change in the transverse and frontal planes. These changes, depicted in Figure 12.3, originate in the upper cervical spine, progressing so that in the lower thoracic spine the joints are quite vertical. Then, in the lower thoracic spine the joints begin to rotate to the sagittal plane, so that throughout the lumbar spine the articulating surfaces have been turned by 90°. Note should also be made that the curvature of the lumbar facets is such that the anterior portion of the joint is in the frontal plane while the posterior portion

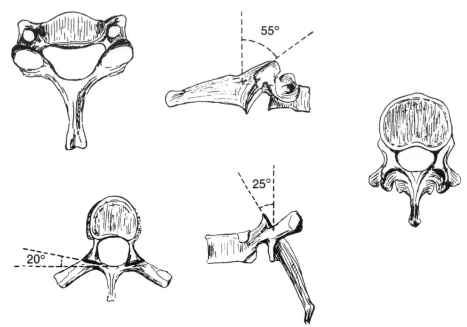

Figure 12.3. Views of cervical (*upper left*), thoracic (*lower left*), and lumbar vertebrae (*right*) to show the plane of the facet joints in each segment of the spine. Note the cupped shape arrangement of the lumbar facets. (From Stoddard A: *Manual of Osteopathic Technique.* London, Hutchinson & Co., Ltd., 1980.)

is in the sagittal plane. At the termination of the lumbar spine an interesting and significant change occurs, in that at the articulation of the fifth lumbar vertebrae with the sacrum, the facet joints have returned to a frontal-plane orientation. This feature will be discussed in the section on pathokinesiology. Of some interest is that modified vertebrae appear at approximately C7-T1, T12-L1, and at L5. In these locations, the joints have superior and inferior facet orientations such that a transition to a different portion of the spinal column is allowed. Clinicians may need to focus specific attention on the evaluation/treatment of these joints.

In addition to the joint orientation and the role that ligamentous structures may play in restraining movement, two other factors should be mentioned. First, bony geometry is important because such factors as length of the spinous process may determine the available range of motion. Second, the disc and its mechanical properties are influential in that they provide a fulcrum upon which the vertebrae can displace. Furthermore, the disc contains a nucleus pulposus that has hydrodynamic properties (44). Although the relative importance of each of the factors involved in spinal motion in unknown, surely each element makes some contribution, particularly if a complete range of motion is attempted.

Sacroiliac Joints

At the base of the lumbar region is a portion of the spine often ignored. The sacrum, considered as five fused vertebrae, does serve an important function in their articulation with the pelvis. These sacroiliac joints are complex in configuration, in spite of the appearance that they have been wedged between two sections of the pelvis. In appearance from the lateral view the joint looks like an "L" that has been turned on its side. The long arm is directed caudally while the short arm is directed cranially (5). The first sacral vertebrae articulates with the caudally directed segment, and the second and third vertebrae have facets associated with the cranial limb (28). According to Weisl, responsible for in depth study of this joint, the surfaces are very complex. In general, the sacral surface of the joints can be described as having a caudal and a cranial elevation, the latter in association with the lateral aspect of the first sacral vertebra. Between these two elevations is a saddle-shaped ilia depression. Furthermore, although the iliac surfaces are reciprocally shaped, the two surfaces forming the joint are not mirror images (83). Covered with 1 to 3 mm of fibrocartilage, the joints are frequently dissimilar (5).

Key structures associated with the function of the sacroiliac joints are two sets of ligaments. The first, the capsular, are primarily responsible for maintaining the integrity of the sacroiliac joint. The other set, the accessory, consists of three separate sets of ligaments that serve to control separation of the iliac bones and rotations in the sacroiliac joints (5). All are exceedingly strong, having high tensile strength for purposes of adequate control of motion in all three planes (28).

Kinematics

Prior to considering the range of motion available in the spine, description of the motion of one segment on another may prove helpful. Consider flexion of the trunk so that the third lumbar vertebra is moved on the fourth. During this movement, the body of the third vertebra slides anteriorly on the intervertebral disc. Simultaneously, tilting of the vertebral body will cause compression of the anterior portion of the disc. At the facet joint, the articular surface of the third vertebra slides superiorly on the surface of the fourth vertebra, causing compression of the facet surfaces face to face while concurrently having a shearing effect. Note also that this movement is potentially unlimited, were it not for restraint imposed by the ligaments of the vertebral arch, the posterior longitudinal ligament, the facet capsules, posterior musculature, the thoracolumbar fascia, and the posterior annulus (41). A corollary sequence of events could be described for extension. Now, however, consider lateral flexion. In this case, compressive disc forces would occur on the side to which the lateral flexion takes place. At the facet joints the motion is more limited, because with this movement, joint compressive forces are increased due to the tendency of the articular surfaces to move only slightly in this plane of motion. Thus, limited lateral flexion may be anticipated in the lumbar spine.

The possibility of completing the motion of flexion followed by lateral flexion raises another interesting phenomenon associated with spinal kinematics. These two motions require the bending of a flexible rod (the spine) in two planes that are perpendicular to each other. To do so requires that the rod also undergo axial rotation (63). This characteristic, provided as an example associated with spinal kinematics, is known as coupling, and involves the consistent association of axial rotation with movement about another axis (85). This coupling will occur in any segment of the spine, but recall that facet planes restrict rotation in the lumbar spine. The cervical and thoracic facets allow much rotation, while in the thoracic spine the rib cage, with its sternal junctions, restricts rotation. This feature will prove to be of importance when the kinematics and kinetics of scoliosis are considered in the section on pathokinesiology.

Various summaries of the ranges of motion available in each of the spinal segments have been published. A useful figure (Fig. 12.4) presented by White and Panjabi, is shown. Several key aspects related to joint orientation should be

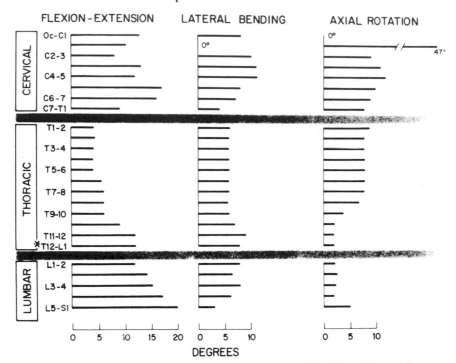

Figure 12.4. Composite of the degrees of rotation in each of the planes of movement for all regions of the spine. (From White AA, Panjabi MM: The basic kinematics of the human spine. *Spine* 3:12–20, 1978.)

emphasized. Lack of axial rotation in the occiput-C1 joint and in the C1–C2 areas for lateral flexion is entirely consistent with the joint geometry. An example of the complexity of the process exists in that some consider the "true" upper cervical articulation to be between the occiput and C2, with C1 functioning as a "washer" interposed between. Upon lateral flexion to the left, C1 translates to the left to adjust the position of the left lateral mass of C1, which otherwise would prevent the left side flexion. The right alar ligament is pulled tight by the left side flexion, and it then pulls on the dens, rotating C2 to the left. This rotation allows the atlas to approximate the axis, as they are no longer riding on the "high point" which occurs in neutral, allowing further slack in the alar ligaments which permits further side flexion. The conjunct right rotation of the occiput relative to C2 also tends to slacken the right alar ligament, allowing further left side flexion to proceed. This process continues until the right occipital rotation has taken up all the slack in the left alar ligament (which was slackened by the approximation of C1-2 and the left side flexion). At this point, all components of the mechanism have reached their limits, and side flexion of about 10° has occurred (37). Note should also be made of the relatively large total excursion of the cervical spine in all of the planes of motion.

Conversely, motion in the thoracic spine is limited in all planes, mostly due to the ribs. Extension is primarily constrained by the spinous processes. The lumbar spine can be characterized by the large excursions in flexion and extension but by markedly limited range in rotation. Finally, attention should be called to the great degree of flexion-extension available at the articulation of the fifth lumbar vertebrae with the sacrum. More detailed analyses of the differences between segments can be determined from Figure 12.4 or from more comprehensive descriptions (44, 87).

Certain coupling patterns have been noted to occur. For example, lateral bending from C2 through C7 is accompanied by axial rotation. Specifically, if lateral bending is to the left, the rotation in the cervical spine is to the left, frequently observed by viewing the spinous processes deviating to the right. Data on coupling in the thoracic spine is less convincing because the results have been somewhat varied, depending on the segments studied (87). Little information exists as to coupling in the lumbar spine (88). Pearcy and Tibrewal have concluded that there is no simple mechanical coupling of the rotations in the lumbar spine. The lumbar lordosis and muscular control have been identified as the two primary factors in determining the relationship between primary and accompanying rotations (60).

More precise analytic work has now been done which enables detailed descriptions of spinal segment motion. One such example is provided by a study evaluating the size of the intervertebral foramen. In the normal spine, as compared to a degenerated cadaver specimen, flexion/extension showed the most change of width in the intervertebral foramen. An example of the changes is shown in Figure 12.5. Of significance is that flexion caused an increase in the foramen area of 30% while extension closed the foramen by about 20%. Note in the figure the difference in what is called the neutral zone. This zone, according to Panjabi and coworkers, represents a discontinuity between flexion and extension flexibility curves and implies that within this zone one vertebra may move with minimum effort with respect to the other vertebra. Furthermore, within this zone there is no appreciable resistance to motion offered by the ligaments, disc, or facets. Outside of this zone the elasticity of various structures will impede further motion (58). Others consider the anteroposterior dimension of the

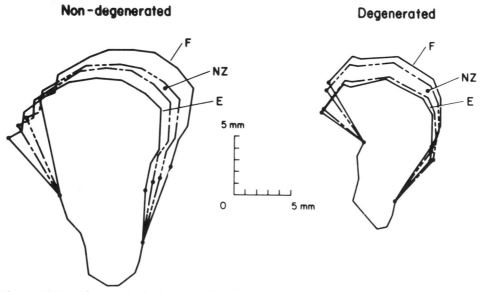

Figure 12.5. Changes in the intervertebral foramen shape for the boundaries of a defined neutral zone (*NZ*). The extremes of flexion (*F*) and extension (*E*) ranges of motion for a moment of 7.5 Nm are also shown. (From Panjabi MM, Takata K, Goel VK: Kinematics of lumbar intervertebral foramen. *Spine* 8:348–357, 1983.)

intervertebral foramen to be critical, rather than the vertical dimension. This is because disc and facet osteophyte trespass usually involve anteroposterior compression rather than vertical. Even in segments having undergone disc thinning and facet overriding, it is the anteroposterior diameter which is affected in much greater proportion than the vertical. Further details of how such motion is restricted follow in the next section.

The impact of vertebral motion upon the foramen is of specific interest because of the potential impact upon the nerve root exiting from the foramen. Isaacson has described the foramen in terms of two compartments. Division of the compartment is by means of a limiting membrane, creating a superior, or conduction, compartment, and an inferior, or motion, compartment. During normal motion of the segments the superior compartment is unperturbed, while in the pathological situation the limiting membrane may be distorted and may subsequently affect the roots and vessels entering and leaving the conduction compartment (35).

Detailed analyses of the various segments of the spine also provide insight into normal kinematics. For example, motion in the cervical spine has been analyzed by means of radiographs, cineradiography, and stereoradiography (20, 32). These studies allow for more precise identification of the geometric relationships and the angular changes occurring with motion and are likely to contribute to a better understanding of normal and pathological motion of vertebral segments. One specific example should suffice. Dimmet et al have shown that in full flexion the upper cervical spine was almost straight (lateral view), remaining so until complete extension. At this time occiput-C1 motion recurred. By comparison, the lower half of the cervical spine demonstrated motion throughout, concave anteriorly in full flexion to convex anteriorly in full extension. Furthermore, there was evidence that the motion in the lower cervical spine was greater than in the upper levels, which showed greater variability of motion between segments (15).

Specific data on rotation in the thoracic and lumbar areas is also available via an early study that mounted pins directly into spinous processes of multiple vertebrae. Various activities were studied. Generalizations are difficult to make because the subjects did not have all the spinous processes marked. However, up to 9° of rotation occurred between the lumbar vertebrae while an average of 6° of rotation was available in all joints above the thoracolumbar junction (27). Implications of this and other information on spinal kinematics will be discussed in the section of pathokinesiology.

Role of Passive Structures

An understanding of the kinematics of the human spine requires knowledge of the role of supporting structures. Included within this category are the intervertebral discs, the joints, and the ligaments. Commonly the assessment of the role of these structures has been completed in cadaver specimens because of inability to study the contribution of each of the factors in vivo.

In sectioning the various structures that offer spinal support, virtually all tissues have been analyzed. Because the posterior structures are relied upon to control the flexion moment, this motion has been used to evaluate the role of individual structures. For two positions of flexion the average results for each of the structures is found in Table 12.1. Note that the supraspinous/interspinous ligaments and the ligamentum flavum have reciprocal roles in the two positions while the capsular ligaments and intervertebral disc do likewise (3). The properties of several tissues have also been reported. In a study detailed by Charzal et

Table 12.1. The Averaged Results[a]

	Supraspinatous/ interspinous ligaments	Ligamentum flavum	Capsular ligaments	Intervertebral disc
Bending moment resisted at full flexion (%)	19 (±7)	13 (±6)	39 (±8)	29 (±12)
Bending moment resisted at half flexion (%)	8 (±5)	28 (±10)	25 (±8)	38 (±13)

[a] From Adams MA, Hutton WC: The resistance to flexion of the lumbar intervertebral joint. *Spine* 5:245–253, 1980.)

al, the spinal ligaments studied exhibited elastic properties, demonstrating a load-deformation response that was sigmoid in shape. The most resistant structures were the intertransverse posterior longitudinal ligament and the ligamentum flavum. These data appear to establish the import of these structures in supporting the spine during the flexed posture (13).

Twomey and Taylor have presented similar data resulting from sectioning of the ligaments of the spine. Their study is interesting because facet joint apposition had a greater restraining influence than the ligamentous factors on the sagittal plane range of motion in the lumbar spine. Apparently the restraining influence of the facet joint is greater than for the ligaments, in extension as well as in flexion. A summary of the contribution of each of the factors is shown in Figure 12.6. Some caution may need to be used in interpreting these data, however, because the pedicles of the vertebrae were cut, allowing the facet joints to slide anteriorly during the flexion motion (79). Similar analyses have also been completed in the cervical spine. In this case the anterior ligaments contributed more to stability of the spine in extension than the posterior ligaments. The converse was true in flexion.

Other work has evaluated the role of spinal structures in resisting and limiting torsion. Adams and Hutton, for example, have performed studies that established that primary resistance is from the apophyseal (facet) joint that is in compression. The intervertebral disc also is a primary limiting factor in resisting torsion, but the capsular ligaments and the supraspinous and interspinous ligaments are unimportant (2). Further work will allow other determinations of the degree of contribution of specific structures. In fact, the work of White and Panjabi has demonstrated progress towards an in-depth understanding of the mechanics of the spine (58, 87, 88).

Total motion of the spine is thus a resultant product of the collective kinematics of multiple joints made up of the multiple segments. Forward inclination of the trunk is a classic example of the collective participation of these segments, the sacroiliac joints and the hip. In the forward-bending position, perhaps 50 to 70 total degrees of flexion are available from the sacrum to the first thoracic vertebrae. Recall that the majority of this motion occurs in the lumbar spine, with little contribution from the thoracic region. The remaining motion is accounted for by interaction of the pelvis with the hip, a large range of motion being available in this joint. The role of the musculature and the passive contribution of the other structures have been previously discussed.

Biomechanics

Spinal column biomechanics are of interest to the practitioner because the joints or the soft tissues of the spine appear to be incapable of tolerating the

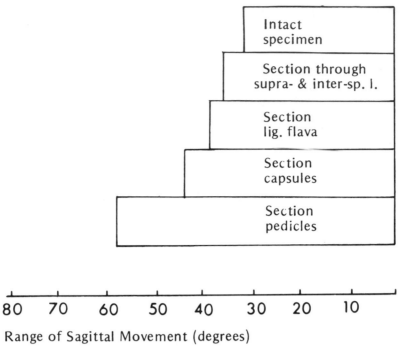

Range of Sagittal Movement (degrees)

Figure 12.6. Mean ranges of sagittal plane movements of the lumbar spine following progressive release of the identified posterior vertebral elements. (From Twomey LT, Taylor JR: Sagittal movements of the human lumbar vertebral column: a quantitative study of the role of the posterior vertebral elements. *Arch Phys Med Rehabil* 64:322–325, 1983.)

mechanical requirements of this multiple-segmented column. Injuries to the low back have become a primary focus of attention due to the considerable monetary compensation paid to persons suffering from probable mechanical faults of the spine. This segment of the chapter will deal with general considerations, will discuss the mechanical properties of the tissues, and will include information on torque and instant centers of rotation.

General Mechanical Requirements

Discussed in the earlier sections of this chapter have been the anatomical structures that support the spine and the associated kinematics that result during motion. Due to the supporting nature and functional requirements of the spine, external loads are imposed in a number of ways. As has been indicated previously, each of the motion segments is capable of 6° of freedom, three translational and three rotational. As a result, the soft tissues are subjected to different effects as the loads and ensuing motions occur at each of the segments. In turn, the mechanical properties of these tissues influence the biomechanics of the spine and the individual motion segments. Before discussing the material properties of the pertinent structures, consideration needs to be given to the various loads imposed upon the spine.

Axial loading in compression is inherent to the spine by virtue of the weight of the trunk, head, and arms. There have been some recent accounts that the facet joints are capable of carrying 18% of the load in compression (61). Primarily responsible for withstanding compressive forces are the intervertebral discs. Another study has established that during axial loading the load is along a direction perpendicular to the facet surfaces. The authors go on to state that this orientation implies that the total load is distributed so as to share axial loading between intervertebral and facet joints and resist anterior and lateral shear (49). Notably larger in the lumbar segment of the spine, these discs are also capable of responding to motion by resisting shear and accommodating to spinal segment rotations.

In contrast with compression loading, another form of axial force is tensile loading. Usually applied only in treatment situations such as traction, tensile loading increases the distance between each segment. The intervertebral disc itself becomes elongated and narrowed as the ligaments become stretched. Because the vertebrae may be guided by surrounding soft tissues, such elongation effects are often instituted as a result of fractures or fracture-dislocations in the spine (63). No matter the direction of the axial load, factors of stress, strain, and elasticity are all to be considered. The resultant effect is dependent on the direction of the load as well as the magnitude and rate of application of the load.

Bending, commonly labeled as flexion, extension, and lateral flexion, creates different demands. In this case moments produce the respective bending. As has been discussed in the section on kinematics, the effects of the soft tissues or the bones may be important limiting factors, the former due primarily to excessive elongation. Note should be taken that the compressive effect due to bending is entirely dependent upon the locus of the center of rotation of the segments undergoing the motion. Thus, for forward flexion the anterior structures are compressed while the supraspinal ligaments are elongated, assuming that the axis of rotation is located in the posterior aspect of the vertebral body-disc-vertebral body (intervertebral) joint. Compressive stress is realized in the anterior structures while tensile stress occurs in the posterior structures. Tissues located along the axis about which the turning is taking place remain relatively unstressed. Further discussion of the effects of various tissues will be offered in the kinetics section.

Two other motions of considerable import are shear and torsion. The former is known to be a problem because the anteroposterior curvatures in the spine, particularly in the lumbar region and at the lumbosacral joint, tend to produce anterior translatory motion of the superior vertebra on the inferior vertebra. In this case shear occurs in the intervertebral joint and also in the facet joints. The magnitude of the shear is increased by the forward leaning of the body because the effect of gravity on the superior vertebra will be more pronounced. Any effects on soft tissue can be specified by means of a free body diagram and the analysis of the tendencies for motion.

In torsion (rotation) about the longitudinal axis of the spine, the effects of movement are dependent on the location of the center of rotation (53). Particularly in the lumbar segments is the shear force at a maximum. Recall also that the plane of the lumbar facet joints differs from that of the thoracic, influencing the resultant kinematics. In any case, torsion produces asymmetrical effects. For example, considering the facet joints during rotation, one joint is compressed. Once rotation has progressed to the point that one lumbar facet engages its joint partner, the center of rotation of further movement must move to a point between those facet surfaces. Since the disc is at some distance from this center, it must necessarily experience shear if further rotation occurs. The contralateral facet is simultaneously further distracted. The soft tissues maintaining the integrity of these joints are shortened and elongated, respectively (37).

After years of debate that was centered on both theoretical and clinical bases, there is now general agreement that motion does exist in the sacroiliac joints. Although constrained in its articulation by the bony and ligamentous elements described in the earlier sections, the force of gravity continually attempts to drive the superior aspect of the sacrum into the pelvic cavity. Because of the frequent asymmetry in the joints, a greater load is created in the ligaments on the side with the narrower lateral mass of the sacrum. The same can be said of the joint whose lateral inclination in the frontal section is smaller than that of the contralateral side (77). However, several studies have confirmed that motion does occur in the sacroiliac joints. Translatory and angular movement have been determined to be of as much as several centimeters (22), and may occur along a number of different axes (89). Weisl has indicated that maximal constant ventral movement of the sacral promontory of 5.6 mm occurs as a result of a change of position from recumbency to standing. The axis of rotation was also identified as being located 5 to 10 cm vertically below the promontory, but so variable, depending on the subject and the movement, that the description could not be considered to comply with typical, more rigid terminology (84). The fact that significant distraction of these relatively "rough" joint surfaces may be required would further compound the identification of the true axis (89). Implications of the normal and abnormal motion of the sacroiliac joint have been more commonly identified in the literature (16). As both purely scientific and clinical means are refined, certainly the true role of this joint will be elucidated.

Mechanical Properties

Of the elements responsible for maintaining the integrity of the spine, the intervertebral discs, ligaments, and vertebrae all have specific mechanical properties that are of some importance. Of these, the properties of the vertebrae will not be discussed at length, partly because the general structure and functions of the facet joints have been presented earlier in the chapter. Bone strength is of import, however, in cases of large and/or sudden axial loads which may readily result in fractures. Furthermore the cartilaginous endplate can be considered an interface with the intervertebral disc, yet this structure is subject to failure such as occurs in an endplate fracture.

Of greatest interest to students of spinal biomechanics is the intervertebral disc, often because the structure has been perceived to be a significant factor in low back pain. In general, the disc serves to absorb loads and distribute the forces applied to the spine. Two constituents assume responsibility for these functions. The most centrally located is the nucleus pulposus. This substance contains a relatively high proportion of glycosaminoglycans which are capable of imbibing (holding) water. As a result, the nucleus is a gelatinous hydrophilic substance that contains as much as 88% water (42). Because of this affinity for water and the contained space in which it resides, the nucleus is always under pressure to expand outwardly. This preexisting tension is known as "preload," and influences the mechanical behavior of the disc (36). With the exception of the lumbar spine, the nucleus can be considered to be centrally located within the disc. In this case the position is somewhat more posterior (87).

A second structure, the annulus fibrosus, surrounds the nucleus. This fibrocartilaginous structure is composed of fibers arranged in a laminated fashion, that is, the fibers run obliquely to each other at an angle of about 30° to the plane of the disc. Centrally the fibers are attached to the cartilaginous endplates while peripherally the attachments are directly into the osseous tissue of the vertebral body. Note should also be made that the fibers are thicker and more numerous anteriorly than posteriorly. In addition, the posterior and posterolateral fibers have a more parallel alignment than do the anterior fibers (34, 59).

As a result of these anatomical features of the intervertebral disc, the structure can be considered to be anisotropic, that is, the mechanical properties vary with different spatial orientations (87). For example, the elastic properties of the annulus vary with the distance from the center of the disc and with the relative orientation of fibers and the applied load (42). Note that the laminated structure in effect "contains" the preloaded nucleus pulposus while simultaneously having the ability to resist tensile and shear forces resulting from movement of the spine.

Because of the role of the discs in spine mechanics, extensive work has been done on behavior during various loading conditions. Axial loading, producing compression of the disc, has been of most interest because of the similarities with the loads imposed on the disc by virtue of the upright posture. In general, compressive loads increase the internal pressure in the disc, stretching the fibers of the annulus and loading the endplates. Therefore, load is transmitted to the adjacent vertebrae and absorbed in the outer layers of the annular fibers (43). With high compressive loads, herniation of the nucleus through the annulus would be expected. However, studies have shown that failure occurs in the body of a vertebra or in the cartilagenous endplates, usually in the form of a fracture (31).

Other tests have evaluated the rate of loading of the disc. Results have demonstrated loading properties in that low loads produced little resistance while at higher loads the disc becomes stiffer. Thus, flexibility is provided at low loads and stability at high loads (87). Consider these events with what Kapandji has called the mechanism of self-stabilization. In this situation when an asymmetrical load applies a moment to a vertebra, the pressure increases in the nucleus on the side towards which the bending occurs. As a result, the tendency is for unbending to occur, equilibrating the stretch on the fibers of both sides of the annulus. Thus, the mechanisms associated with spinal motions are contingent upon the interaction of both the nucleus and the fibers of the annulus (41).

Resistance to tension and shear produced by spinal movement is another important feature of disc mechanics. Again, the angular orientation of the laminated annular fibers assists to resist excessive motions such as those in the posterior fibers during forward bending. Simultaneously with flexion, the anterior, as well as posterolateral, portions of the disc become remarkably compressed and stretched, respectively, and may sustain potentially dangerous injuries. During rotation, both tension and shear are created in the annulus. Shear, of course, takes place in the horizontal plane around which the rotation is occurring. Tension would develop in the fibers oriented in the direction of the rotation and shear would exist between these fibers and the adjacently oriented fibers of the annular laminae. Because motion is greatest in the fibers that are farthest from the center of rotation, the greatest stresses are expected in the peripheral segments of the annular fibers. The effects of these motions are shown in Figures 12.7 and 12.8 (87).

Experimental studies have also evaluated the behavior of the intervertebral joints under conditions of physiological loading. In this type of testing, axial and shear loads have been used in isolation, in combination with each other, and with eccentric (off-center) loading. Such techniques allow the study of disc and

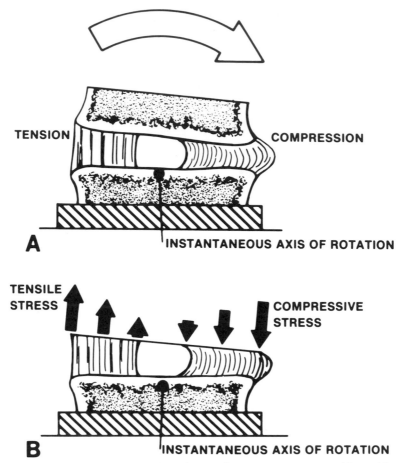

Figure 12.7.   Stress in the disc with bending in flexion, extension, and lateral bending. *A* shows that one portion of the disc is subjected to compression while the opposite side is under tension. Note that in *B* the stresses vary in magnitude in relationship to the location from the instantaneous axis of rotation. (From White AA, Panjabi MM: *Clinical Biomechanics of the Spine.* Philadelphia, JB Lippincott, 1978.)

annulus behavior and the mechanical analysis of the effects of sectioning various structures. One exemplary piece of work has been completed by Lin and coworkers, who established that anterior disc bulging is usually greater than the lateral bulge during axial or eccentric loads. Furthermore, failure occurred in the vertebral body and not in the annulus fibrosus, confirming numerous other studies offering the same finding. Their study also sectioned the posterior elements. Following testing of the specimens, the conclusion was reached that the posterior elements play a minor role in bearing axial loads. However, during complex loading consisting of compressing, bending, and/or shear, a load path through the superior and inferior articular processes is activated. These authors further found that the posterior elements are responsible for increased shear stiffness of the intervertebral joint (47). Other studies have used models of the disc, evaluating the loads that can be tolerated within normal physiological limits. Some of these studies, which primarily concern the annulus, have shown that fiber rupture is not likely to occur because of the tendency for endplate failure to be reached first. In fact, bending, shear or axial rotation does not appear to

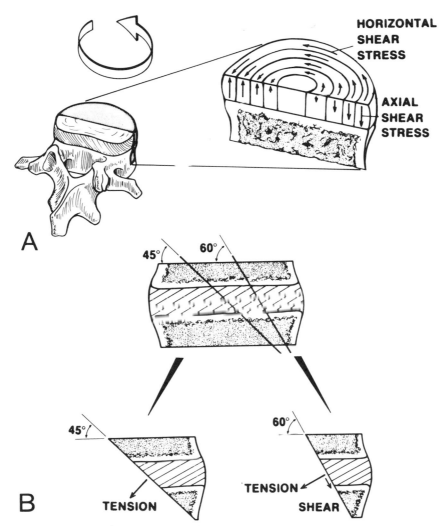

Figure 12.8. Stress in the disc with torsion. Shear is produced in the horizontal plane as well as in the axial direction, both of equal magnitude. The stress varies at different points in the disc in proportion to the distance from the instantaneous axis of rotation (*A*). *B* shows that at 45° to the plane of the disc, there is no shear (because of the orientation of the annular fibers). Note that at 60° both shear and tension stresses would exist. (From White AA, Panjabi MM: *Clinical Biomechanics of the Spine.* Philadelphia, JB Lippincott, 1978.)

produce fiber rupture, except when these loads are combined with very high axial loads (10).

Behavior of the disc is typical of a viscoelastic material. This is demonstrated in the effects of loading rate on the degree of stiffness of the disc. Recall also that the nucleus has a high percentage of water. Furthermore, because of viscoelastic qualities, creep, relaxation and hysteresis are demonstrable. In the case of hysteresis, where energy is lost when a structure is subjected to repetitive loading and unloading cycles, greater loads have been found to produce greater hysteresis. Virgin found that lower lumbar discs had greater hysteresis than the upper lumbar and lower thoracic vertebrae and that younger groups had more than a middle-aged population (80). Each of these factors may eventually play a role in the normal or abnormal mechanics of the spine.

These structures identified above have been evaluated for their material properties because they do appear to have a significant role in both the kinematics and kinetics of the spine. Of most interest are the posterior elements, primarily because of the potential, and apparently real, ability to assist with control or production of extension moments. Recalling the anatomy of the posterior ligamentous system reminds one that some ligamentous structures are located posterior to the spinous processes by as much as 1 to 1.5 cm. Two benefits accrue as a result: the first being that ligamentous tension improves passive extension leverage and reduces the amount of compression at the intervertebral joint due to muscular contraction. The second advantage relates to the orientation of ligament fibers in that they are more perpendicular to the spinous processes, rather than in a superior-inferior direction, as is often depicted. Because of the direction of the supraspinous and interspinous ligaments, the effect is to allow flexion to occur up to a point rather than constrain the motion of one vertebra over the others. Note also that the ligaments span only one joint, because if 30% extensibility were allowed, abnormally large rotations would occur at the intervertebral joints (26).

Another interesting finding is that "pre-tension" apparently exists in spinal ligaments. Based on studies of the ligamentum flavum that have determined the properties of the tissue a stress-strain plot can be produced. Such is shown in Figure 12.9. First, note that the ligament is under 15% pre-tension in the neutral position. This level of tension means that if the ligament were transected, shortening would occur to a new length 15% shorter than the in situ length. If the neck is extended, the strain decreases to 5% but does not allow the ligament to buckle into the spinal canal. Conversely, flexion allows an increase of 35% strain. If force, stiffness and energy absorbed were calculated from the curve, relatively small values for these mechanical parameters would result. However, after the full range of flexion is reached, note that the curve has a very steep slope, indicating a high degree of stiffness. Thus, the cervical spine has the

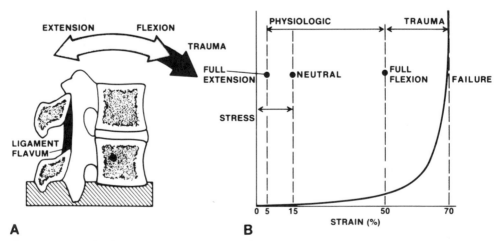

Figure 12.9.   The functional position of the ligamentum flavum preceding the motions of flexion and extension. (A) Specific points in the range of motion are shown in the stress-strain curve shown in B. See text for further details. (From White AA, Panjabi MM: *Clinical Biomechanics of the Spine*. Philadelphia, JB Lippincott, 1978.)

capability of operating effectively within the physiological range as the ligament accomplishes supportive functions. Yet, the ligamentum flavum has the ability to protect the spine by absorbing large amounts of energy before the failure point is reached (54). Although the ligamentum flavum has a uniquely high elastic fiber constituency, similar principles may be applied to other ligaments. Little specific experimental evidence exists as to the function of these ligaments but different tissue constituency will be responsible for differing degrees of mechanical effect.

Instant Centers of Rotation

The various motion segments of the spine are of interest to study because of the distinct relationship to kinematics and kinetics and potential impact on pathomechanics. Study of the axes of motion is complicated, however, by the influence of each of the adjacent motion segments and the difficulties associated with study of multiple motion segments, each possessing 6° of freedom. In spite of these factors, some information is available on the instant centers of rotation.

In the cervical spine the occiput-C1 and C1-C2 joints deserve special consideration. In the former, the sagittal plane (for flexion and extension) is believed to be located 2 to 3 cm above the tip of the dens. For lateral bending the axis appears to be located in the midline slightly more distant from the tip of the dens. Although this information, as reported by White and Panjabi, was published in 1863, no additional information has disputed the findings of Henke (87).

In the C1-C2 joint, the axis for sagittal plane motion is believed to be located in the middle third of the dens. As may be anticipated, rotation occurs about the axis and, because lateral flexion at this joint is small or nonexistent, the location of an axis for this motion may be irrelevant. Details associated with this issue were discussed in the previous section on kinematics. The locations of the axes for the remainder of the cervical spine have been identified for the sagittal and the horizontal planes. The latter is less well agreed upon, but the anterior portion of the subjacent vertebrae is the likely location. Keep in mind the issue of coupling (see section on kinematics) (87).

No specific agreement has been reached on lateral bending axes in the cervical spine. For the thoracic spine locations have been identified for all planes. Compared to the other segments of the spine, the centers in the lumbar spine are located more specifically for the motion taking place in the respective plane (87). These are shown in Figure 12.10.

The locations of these instant centers further the understanding of the kinematics of the spine and assist the study of kinetics because forces can then be related to axes of motion about which the turning effect can be determined. In many activities, whether functional or therapeutic, therapists can apply known mechanics to produce desired effects. The application of these principles will be discussed in a subsequent section on pathokinesiology.

Torque

Despite the professed importance of the trunk musculature in the prevention and/or treatment of low back pain and dysfunction, generally little is known about the ability of the flexors or the extensors to exert torque. The problem is confounded by motion occurring at multiple segments simultaneously, thereby not lending the question to an easy answer because of methodological difficulties.

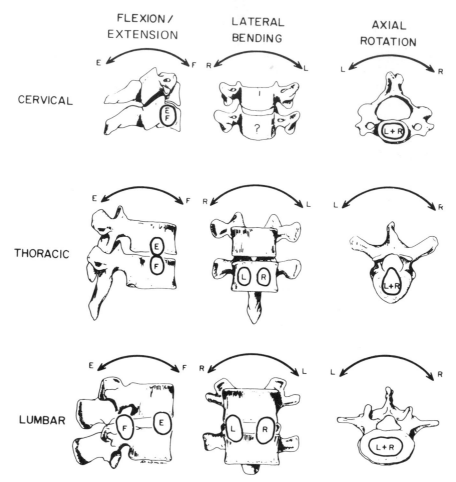

Figure 12.10.   Shown are the approximate locations of the instantaneous axes of rotation for the three cardinal planes of motion for the cervical, thoracic, and lumbar vertebrae. Flexion and extension are indicated by *F* and *E*, respectively. Left (*L*) and right (*R*) are used to designate the direction of motion. (From White AA, Panjabi MM: Spinal kinematics. In *The Research Status of Spinal Manipulative Therapy*. NINCDS Monograph, no. 15. Washington, DC, U.S. Department of Health, Education and Welfare, 1975, p. 93.)

Recently, attempts have been made to determine flexor and extensor torque. However, because of methodological differences, comparisons across studies are difficult at best. One study used the sidelying position to evaluate concentric, isometric, and eccentric torque capabilities. In all cases of dynamic exercise, the velocity was limited to 13°/sec. Peak isometric flexion torque was 194 Nm in the neutral position, increasing to 211 Nm at 20° of trunk extension. Isometric extension torque was 380 Nm at 40° of flexion, diminishing to 312 Nm at 20° of flexion. As anticipated from the force-velocity relationship, the eccentric values were higher than isometric torque and the concentric values were lower. Variation of dynamic torques from the isometric values was relatively small due to the slow velocity used during testing (74).

Shortly thereafter, another study tested subjects ranging in age from 10 to 59 years with a constant velocity dynamometer. In general, the highest torque was produced by the 20 to 29 year olds. The supine abdominal test torque for men averaged about 175 Nm and diminished to 100 Nm by age 50 to 59. Values for females were less than 50% of those generated by male subjects. Extensor torque, measured from the prone position, was approximately 135 Nm for young women and 50% greater for men (30). In the most recent study, a sitting posture was used for concentric and isometric flexion and extension of the trunk. Of interest are the much higher values obtained by this method, such that men exceeded 400 Nm during isometric extension. Women generated 57% of the torque of the male group. In flexion, women produced torque of almost 150 Nm, just over half of that of the male subjects (73). The differences across these studies can serve as primary examples of the importance of testing technique. Although comparison is made possible because of the use of the torque (rather than force) measurements, the large discrepancies probably are due in large part to the methodologies employed. With the advent of developing dynamometers, additional data on both normals and subjects with low back pain-dysfunction will be forthcoming.

Kinetics

For reasons previously cited, the forces associated with motion of individual or collective segments of the spine are difficult to determine. This fact does not negate the importance of these determinations, because the magnitudes and temporal sequencing of the contributions of both the active and passive structures are critical factors for normal movement. Disruptions in normal kinematics may alter kinetic requirements and subsequently alter the ability of the individual to perform either functional or work-related tasks. This section will address the kinetics of the spine, first concentrating on intradiscal pressure, then focusing on muscular and ligamentous forces, and finally on their interaction as related to trunk movement.

Interdiscal Pressure

Measurement of the pressure within the disc has been completed in vitro and in vivo. Under the former conditions, cadaver specimens were used to demonstrate that pressure was 1.3 to 1.6 times the vertical load applied per unit area. Pressure increased linearly for loads up to 2000 Newtons (N). Motion studies on such specimens have become less important since the advent of a special transducer used for direct measurement of the intradiscal pressure. This technique has now been used to collect information on intradiscal pressure during various postures, activities, and exercises. Table 12.2 provides a summary of the approximate loads in the third lumbar disc of a person with a mass of 70 kg. Note specifically that standing at ease and upright sitting without support both result in considerable intradiscal pressure, the latter being about 40% greater than that of standing. All modifications of posture are seen to influence pressure values. One posture not listed but of potential interest is the standing position with one foot placed in front and elevated by 6 to 12 inches. In this case the intradiscal pressure is decreased from the standing value. A summary of the technique and results can be found in a publication by Nachemson (56).

Lifting Mechanisms

Many of the functions of the human body, during either work or everyday activities, require flexion of the spine. As implied by earlier sections of this chapter, this task necessitates the generation of forces in numerous tissues of the spine, primarily those of the lumbar region. To support the weight of the trunk and any object that may be held in front of the body, the spine has to

Table 12.2. Approximate Load on L3 Disc in a Person Weighing 70 kg[a]

	N[b]
Supine, awake	250
Supine, semi-Fowler position	100
Supine, traction 500 N	0
Supine, tilt table 50°	400
Supine, arm exercises	500
Upright sitting, without support	700
Sitting with lumbar support, back rest inclination 110°	400
Standing at ease	500
Coughing	600
Straining	600
Forward bend, 20°	600
Forward bend, 40°	1000
Forward bend, 20° with 20 kg	1200
Forward flexed 20° and rotated 20° with 10 kg	2100
Sit-up exercises	1200
Bilateral leg lift	800
Lifting 10 kg, back straight, knees bent	1700
Lifting 10 kg, back bent	1900
Holding 5 kg, arms extended	1900

[a] From Nachemson AL: Disc pressure measurements. *Spine* 6:93–97, 1981.
[b] Newton (N) is the force unit of the SI system. N is defined as the force necessary to give a mass of 1 kg the acceleration 1 m/sec^2. 1 N = 0.102 kp. For practical purposes 10 N = 1 kp = 2.25 lbf.

develop an adequate extension moment. Although the magnitude of this moment is contingent upon the mass and location of the object being held and the mass and position of the trunk, the tissues responsible for the extension moment are the posterior muscles and ligaments, the anteriorly compressed disc and those other tissues involved in increasing intraabdominal pressure. Any changes in the former parameters affect the latter forces required to maintain the trunk in equilibrium or alter the dynamic state. The magnitude of such changes is based upon the amount of the load variation, the new position assumed, and such factors as the velocity with which the changes occur. Clearly, the greater the loads and/or degree of trunk flexion, the greater the requirements of the structures responsible for the extension moment. In essence, the extension moment required to offset the weight of the trunk would be reflective of the trigonometric functions (see Appendix A). Any additional load would commensurately increase the magnitude of the flexion moment produced and that must conversely be neutralized by the extension moment in order that equilibrium be maintained.

Not to be minimized is the concurrent tendency, in greater angles of forward leaning, for increased shear forces. An appreciation of this fact can be readily gained by drawing a simple diagram of the pelvis and the lumbar vertebrae. In Figure 12.11, the upright posture demonstrates the greatest amount of load in axial compression. As the fully flexed posture is assumed, each of the vertebrae tends to shift anteriorly due to the weight of the trunk and any load supported by the hands. This shifting tendency becomes an important factor, because it determines what forces are needed to counteract an anterior displacement and maintain appropriate kinematics and/or moments.

Much attention has been paid to the role of the musculature in the control of the trunk flexion. Very low levels of erector spinae and lower extremity extensor muscle activity are required during the normal standing posture. As the trunk is

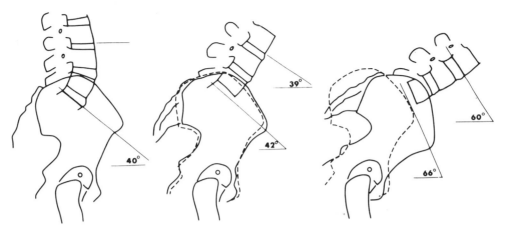

Figure 12.11. Lateral view of pelvis and lumbar spine motion during flexion. Composite angular motions are shown, but particularly note that with increased flexion the shear of each vertebra on adjacent segments is markedly increased. (From Farfan HF: Muscular mechanism of the lumbar spine and the position of power and efficiency, *Orthon Clin North Am 0,133–144, 1975.*)

inclined forward, the degree of activity progressively increases until about 45 to 60° of flexion. At that point, muscle activity rapidly diminishes, even though there is a necessity for large extension moments.

Attempts have been made to determine the amount of force generated in the back extensors so that an assessment could be made of the contribution of these muscles to the total extension moment. Rab and coworkers calculated that the erector spinae group contributed between 37 and 59% of the total extensor moment at the L4-L5 interspace for two different specimens (62). Schultz and assistants determined that the contraction forces of the extensors ranged from 0 to 890 N, the latter for the case of 30° of trunk flexion with the arms out and holding an 8-kg weight (67). In a separate study the extensor muscle force ranged from 100 to 2270 N (bilaterally), with the highest value required during trunk flexion with a load of 80 N held in the hands (66). Large forces such as these point out the significant contribution of the extensor muscle mass. Yet, as the need for the extension moment increases with forward flexion of the trunk from the standing position, active muscle contributions are diminished in favor of reliance upon passive elements. Although elastic tissue in the extensor muscles and tendons are certainly capable of contributing some tension, a major role appears to be played by the ligaments. How much of the moment can be controlled by the posterior ligaments is open to speculation. However, by knowing the cross sectional area of the midline and facet joint ligaments and the thickness of the lumbodorsal fascia, a determination of the support can be made if individual tensile muscle strengths are known. Following this procedure Gracovetsky and Farfan calculated that the posterior structures can support a moment of about 127 kg (1245 Newton meters) (26).

Pathokinesiology

Numerous and extensive injuries to the various segments of the spine are responsible for the production of movement abnormalities. Extensive chapters and entire volumes have been written on the pathologies as they affect the spine. Rather than attempt an exhaustive survey of the possible causes of pathological motion, only selected representative problems will be discussed. A number of problems disrupting cervical spine motion will first be presented. Following a brief discussion of spondylolisthesis, the problem of low back dysfunction and forms of exercise treatment will be considered. Finally, more extensive analysis of the mechanical principles of scoliosis treatment will be provided.

Cervical Spine Pathomechanics

Within the cervical region of the spine, as with the other regions, dislocations can occur between any two motion segments. Such dislocations can be unilateral or bilateral, depending on the type and degree of forces that create the abnormal kinematics. Unilateral dislocation results from a combination of excessive lateral bending and axial rotation such that the superior vertebra is carried anteriorly and superiorly on the inferior surface. Bilateral dislocations cause the unit to lock until reduction is attained. These cases are most likely caused by excessive flexion that forces anterior and superior gliding of the superior surface on the lower vertebra. In either case, capsular integrity may be totally lost, presenting problems with spine stability across the injured segments. Furthermore, bilateral facet joint dislocation can significantly damage the posterior elements, leading to further loss of stability. Ultimately treatment is directed towards correcting alignment, allowing healing, and restoring normal joint kinematics (87).

More complex problems are usually created by extension injuries. Forceable extension, particularly at high velocity, may rupture the anterior longitudinal ligament. Extreme range of motion may even cause the annulus fibrosus to be separated from the upper vertebra. Commonly this hyperextension injury follows some degree of flexion, as seen in the whiplash injury. Often the sixth cervical vertebra is affected relative to adjacent segments because sagittal plane motion is more limited in this portion of the cervical spine. At any rate, the restoration of normal cervical kinematics is difficult because of the apparent myriad of problems associated with this injury. For example, disc narrowing, pain, and muscle spasms are often encountered, leading to compounding of the pathology, even though the problem may be limited to small quantities of soft tissue.

Central to the issue of cervical spine pathology are neck orthoses. Although they are frequently used for the purpose of controlling motion of the spine in both acute and chronic injuries, little assessment of their effects has been completed. One of the most complete attempts in this regard was the work completed by Johnson and coworkers. This group studied the effectiveness of five different braces, ranging from soft collars to a skeletally fixed halo device. The study showed that increasing the rigidity and length of the orthosis improved ability to limit motion. However, lateral bending and rotation of the entire cervical spine, as well as flexion and extension in the upper levels, were not well controlled with any of the orthoses tested. In general, the best conventional means of bracing controlled 45% of flexion and extension while the skeletally attached device restricted 75% of these motions (38). This study and others point out that even judicious use of bracing may not result in limiting motion at the desired spinal level.

Lumbar Spine Dysfunction

Because pain or discomfort in the lower spine has been reported in as high as 80% of the population, the question of causative factors has been the subject of frequent study. Specific attempts have been undertaken to identify the risk factors associated with painful conditions. In a sample of over 1200 patients, those with severe pain were found to hold jobs requiring repetitive heavy lifting, the use of jackhammers and machine tools, or the operation of motor vehicles (23). Fatigue-induced failures have been specifically elucidated (65). It was of some interest that those with moderate pain tended to maintain a higher level of sports activity than those with severe pain, but the explanation for this finding could be due to the fact that severe pain limited participation (23). Clearly the low back dysfunction patient is likely to have a diminished range of motion (51).

Included among the potential causes of low back dysfunction is the problem of spondylolisthesis. This anterior slipping, usually of the fifth lumbar vertebra on the sacrum, may result from several causes, for example, a fracture through the pars interarticularis. In fact, the superior vertebra slides anteriorly because of anterior shear force. Natural lumbar hyperextension is partly at fault but the condition may be worsened by flexion of the lumbar spine because, as discussed earlier, the flexed trunk posture increases the likelihood of anterior shear. Resistance to shear would be available via the facet joints, but such force, applied continuously, leads to plastic deformation of the anterior and posterior ligaments and fibers of the annulus. Restoration of normal biomechanics may require operative intervention for the purpose of stabilizing the joint. Until that time, the joint would be considered unstable from both a clinical and functional point of view. However, a spondylolisthesis may involve a fixed displacement—one that doesn't alter as seen on stress films. Thus, instability may not be present. In contrast, a spondylolisthesis that involves less total displacement may also very easily displace and reduce: this one is symptomatic, while the former may not be at all (37).

A common opinion as to the cause of low back pain is degeneration of the disc. High incidence of narrowing of the intervertebral space has been associated with low back pain. Narrowing also occurs with aging, another factor closely linked to low back pain. However, note should be made that symptomatic lumbar spines often become asymptomatic with advanced age, apparently because dehydration of the disc and stiffness of the ligaments serve to immobilize the spine and prevent aggravation by movement.

An interesting point has been raised by Fahrni. Because disc lesions and chronic back pain are rare in cultures that frequently adopt the full-sqat position, he evaluated the degree of disc narrowing in several groups. Perhaps not surprisingly, the groups assuming the primitive posture had by far the least incidence of disc narrowing. Note in Figure 12.12 that the incidence for a Swedish group involved in heavy labor was as high as 80%. Caution may be necessary, however, because the study does not state that the primitive people were involved in as heavy labor as the Swedish group. If not, this element could be a very significant confounder because it is known that heavy lifting versus light lifting—for groups with consistent postural habits—makes a great difference in the incidence of disc narrowing. Thus, there may still be some question as to the effects of the lordotic posture on disc degeneration (19). Physiological phenomena such as thinning of the cartilaginous plates, loss of nuclear water content, and changes in the annulus are other factors that demonstrate degeneration of the disc. Thus, as expected, degeneration leads to loss of the intrinsic stability of the spine, predisposing the segments or entire regions to injury and/or dysfunction. Providing data to support this concept Seligman and coworkers have determined that centrodes of spinal motion segments were significantly increased, even in the earliest stages of degenerative disc disease. Centrodes for

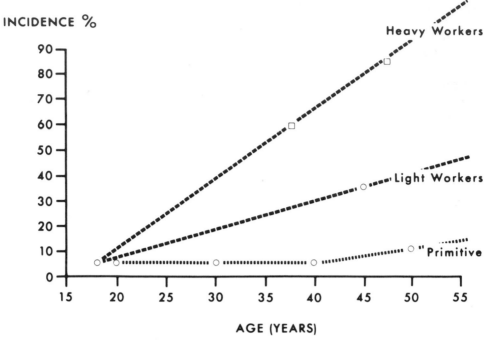

Figure 12.12.   Incidence of disc narrowing, determined by radiograph, plotted versus age. Primitive cultures consistently assume a full crouched position, as opposed to the lordotic position of the working classes. (From Fahrni WH: Conservative treatment of lumbar disc degeneration: our primary responsibility. *Orthop Clin North Am* 6:93–103, 1975.)

normal spines were located in the posterior half of the disc space and averaged 21 mm (69). Clearly, one way to eliminate the unstable segment is through the surgical performance of a fusion. Often criticized for relatively high rates of unsatisfactory results, their use and success has been variable. Often, adjacent stable segments have a postfusion increase in range of motion and added stress on the facet joints. Although all fusions provide increased stiffness, the bilateral-lateral fusion may be the best to use, at least at the lumbosacral joint (46).

Morris and Markolf go so far as to state that disc narrowing and instability tend to cause a posterior displacement of the segment centers of rotation during flexion and extension (53). Further causes of back pain and resulting dysfunction can be related to impingement of a nerve or nerves exiting through the intervertebral foramen (7, 50). Although possibly caused by disc narrowing, pressure on a nerve root could also result from herniation of the nucleus and bulging of the posterior portion of the annulus. Because these and other pathologies, such as acute strains and facet syndromes, are also known to produce low back pain, only when more discriminative tests are available will the more precise cause of low back pain be identified (53).

Therapeutically, practitioners are faced with procedures that should enable the patient to have a more stable lumbar spine for the performance of both functional and lifting activities. Based upon previous information in this chapter, the primary objective of treatment then would be to increase the strength of the extensors and the flexors. The fact that weakness in both of these muscle groups has recently been demonstrated would lend credence to this approach (73).

The form of treatment in terms of strengthening the abdominal musculature may not be as specific as that for the back extensors. Numerous exercises have been suggested for abdominal strengthening, but in all cases selection is based upon several considerations. Of primary concern is the effect on the lumbar spine while the exercise is being performed. In the hooklying position, for example, the degree of lordosis in the lumbar spine is reduced. However, the degree of anterior compression of the disc is probably increased. Longlying may prove to be dangerous from the standpoint of allowing the greatest anterior displacement of the fifth lumbar vertebrae on the sacrum. Bilateral straight leg raising also has a potentially undesirable effect in that iliopsoas muscle tension contributes to the elevation of the legs. In the early portion of the range of motion, the weight of the legs produces a large moment in the direction of hip extension. The resulting effect is that the tension in the iliopsoas muscle causes the anterior lip of the pelvis to move in an inferior direction. Thus, the indirect effect is to increase lordosis, since the angle of inclination between the top of the sacrum and the fifth lumbar vertebra must increase. Another factor to consider is that restraining the feet to the floor so that the patient can complete the exercise may be ill advised on the basis that this maneuver allows the distal attachment of the iliopsoas muscle to be fixed, allowing force to be exerted on the lumbar spine. One alternative that has been commonly used is the hooklying curl exercise. In this exercise, the initial phase is to flex the head, neck, and shoulders forward until the sternum and the crest of the pubis can come no closer together. At this point the scapulae should just clear the supporting surface; further forward movement is stopped; and the person then "uncurls" in reverse sequence. Little lumbar spine motion has occurred, but tension in the abdominal musculature is generally required to be at a high level (75). And, as velocity of muscle contraction has been shown to have an effect on performance, avoiding high-velocity exercise may be well advised.

Also of interest in this regard are intradiscal pressure measurements made while subjects complete therapeutic exercises. Table 12.2 shows that the sit-up exercise creates pressure over twice the value attained during standing at ease. Bilateral leg lifts do not demonstrate such a pronounced effect, perhaps because the transducer measuring the pressure was located in the posterior aspect of the disc. The inference from the Nachemson data is that patients recovering from back pathology should use forms of isometric training on the basis that these exercise forms produce the least increase in intradiscal pressures (55).

One further consideration in treatment would be instruction in the principles of correct lifting technique. These principles have been presented earlier in the chapter. More precise guidelines are also provided in the chapter on ergonomics. As evidence is now surfacing as to the differences in the muscular and other mechanisms used to function, knowing what activities require large moments and what procedures should be followed for control of the kinematics and kinetics of the lumbar spine may effectively prevent further recurrences of injury.

Scoliosis

Abnormal spinal curvatures in the frontal plane have proven difficult to prevent and/or treat. Because the condition is likely to present, clinically effective treatment, usually applied to prevent the progression of the curvature, must be understood and vigorously pursued. Such changes in curvature can be directly related to the principles associated with the treatment applied. This section will discuss the application of these principles to the management of scoliosis.

Before considering the specifics of the mechanisms available to reduce the scoliotic curve, recall that the spine is similar to a flexible rod. If the rod is bent in two planes perpendicular to each other, rotation must occur. So, now consider the case of lateral flexion of the thoracic and lumbar spine. Both of these portions of the spine have sagittal plane deviations, upon which we impose lateral flexion. In the normal circumstances the body of a vertebra rotates towards the side of the concavity of the laterally flexing spine. Because of the location of the center of rotation, each spinous process points to the convexity of the curve. However, in scoliosis, the mechanics are altered so that the resulting motion is opposite that of the normal coupled motion, i.e., the axial rotation, coupled with the lateral bending, is in the wrong direction (86). The result is a clinical presentation in which the spinous processes appear straighter than the vertebrae's real configuration, i.e., the curvature is greater than appears (37).

Now, in order to apply the principles of treatment, consider the case of the simple lateral curvature designated as a C curve. Assuming that movement of the spine is possible, there are two mechanisms that can be used to straighten the curve. One mechanism applies axial loading, i.e., along the long axis of the spine (Fig. 12.13). Note that forces must be applied in the opposite direction so that the entire spine will not be moved in the direction of the force. The tendency to reduce the curve is thus dependent upon two factors: the magnitude of the load and the length of the moment arm between the applied force and the spine. This distance is illustrated in the figure.

Consider that the curve is more extreme than that shown in the figure. Given the same axial load, the tendency to reduce the curvature will be increased. The other mechanism of reducing the curve is by means of the application of

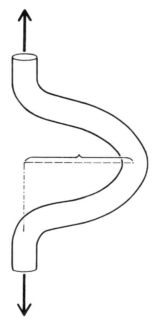

Figure 12.13. A simple C curve to designate the effect of axial loads on scoliosis. The unbending moment would be considered as the force (vectors) multiplied by the distance to the apex of the curve. See text for further details. (From Radin EL, Simon SR, Rose RM, Paul IL: *Practical Biomechanics for the Orthopedic Surgeon.* New York, J Wiley & Sons, 1979.)

transverse load. In the case shown in Figure 12.14, the three-point principle of force application is again demonstrated. The applied force toward the left is equal to the two forces shown directed to the right, the resulting effect being a clockwise rotation of the upper portion of the curve and a counterclockwise rotation of the lower portion. Now consider, as for the axial load, that the curve is more extreme than that shown in Figure 12.14. In this case the resulting effect is to decrease the tendency of the applied moment to reduce the curve.

The net effect of the two mechanisms provides a third alternative for the management of the patient with scoliosis. This form of treatment is the combined approach, used because at all degrees of angular deformity the resultant effect is best. The results of this technique are depicted in Figure 12.15. As indicated, the effect of the axial load increases as the angular deformity increases. For the transverse load technique the maximal corrective moment is for the cases with the mildest degree of curve. Combining the two techniques of reduction results in a corrective moment that is adequate at any degree of angular deformity. Note, however, that at an angle of 53°, the effects of either load are similar (86).

In managing scoliosis with either technique, the effects of tissue creep and relaxation are used. The former is realized by way of additional correction after no additional load is applied. The tissues continue to deform, in this case elongate, without any increase in load. Relaxation, the observed decrease in load with time, is also prevalent since as the deformation remains constant, the tissue accommodates, reducing the load on the supporting device or structure. Manipulation of these factors is responsible for the accommodation seen in the scoliotic curve. As the tissue is loaded there is elongation, allowing reduced curvature. And, as the tissues relax, additional loads can be tolerated that will achieve even further distraction.

Treatment of scoliosis is a classic example of the use of axial and transverse loading systems. Pure axial load can be applied by means of halofemoral or halopelvic traction through fixation of the cranium and the femora or pelvis. Transverse loads can be applied by means of a body jacket, which restrains the

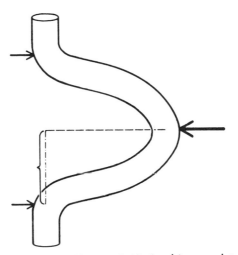

Figure 12.14. Same curve as in Figure 12.13. In this case lateral forces are applied. Because the moment arm is less, there is less effect on straightening of the curve. See text for further description. (From Radin EL, Simon SR, Rose RM, Paul IL: *Practical Biomechanics for the Orthopedic Surgeon.* New York, J Wiley & Sons, 1979.)

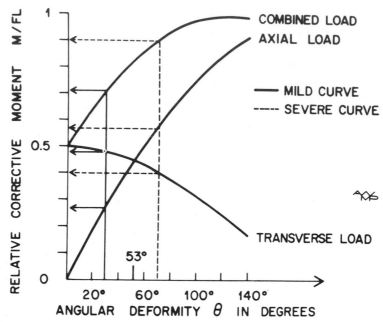

Figure 12.15. Representation of the relative corrective moment plotted versus the angular deformity for each of three methods used to control/alter scoliosis. See text for an explanation, noting that two theoretical patients with mild (30°) and severe (70°) curves are shown. (From White AA, Panjabi MM: The clinical biomechanics of scoliosis. *Clin Orthop* 118:100–112, 1976.)

curve from further deformation. Serial casting can then be used to modify the position of the spine.

Special comment is reserved for the Milwaukee brace and internal means of fixation, particularly the Harrington rod. Figure 12.16 shows a patient in a Milwaukee brace. Note that axial forces are applied by means of supports from the occiput and mandible to the upper rims of the pelvis. Transverse loading is accomplished by means of the pad applied to the lateral aspect of the ribs. Adjustment of the pads and the forces, along with the patient's conscious effort to unload the supports, offers some advantages. On the other hand, the relatively localized application of forces limits the amount of force that can be produced at any one point. Other disadvantages accrue with larger curves; thus, the use of this device is limited to curves of less than 60° (63). There is also evidence that the Milwaukee brace is best for curves in the high thoracic region of the spine, although other body jacket methodologies are starting to produce promising results for cases of scoliosis with the apex of the curve from T7 to T9 (45).

Of several fixation techniques, the most popular has become the insertion of Harrington rods. This surgical method uses rods in which tension can be adjused at the time of the insertion. In effect they apply axial loads through either a compression on the convex side and/or a tension on the concave side of the curve. Figure 12.17 shows the rods in place after they have been secured to the posterior elements of the spine. Note that the distraction rod would be more effective on the basis of greater moment arm but would become less effective as the curve decreases. Disadvantages, however, are that only a moderate force can be applied through the rods, primarily because of the relative weakness of the bony points of attachment. Of interest are the findings of Dunn et al, who

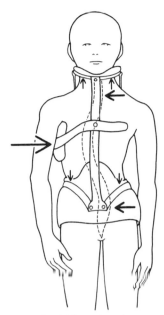

Figure 12.16. Graphic depiction of a Milwaukee brace, including representation of the forces. Note that this is a combined loading system that should allow for maximum control/alteration of the scoliosis. Further description is contained in the text. (From Radin EL, Simon SR, Rose RM, Paul IL: *Practical Biomechanics for the Orthopedic Surgeon*. New York, J Wiley & Sons, 1979.)

showed that the recommended force levels are sometimes exceeded during the insertion procedure. Conversely, too little force may explain some of the results in which less than the desired 40% of minimum correction is achieved (17). Reapplication of the forces after pausing several minutes between distractions, or reoperating 10 to 14 days later, may also take better advantage of tissue relaxation. Although some desirable changes may occur in the sagittal plane, fusion with the rods below the level of L3 is contraindicated on the basis that low back pain may increase (1, 14). In addition, posture and gait are likely to be altered (82).

Finally, some consideration should be given to muscular effects on the reduction of scoliosis. Of at least some relevance is that there are differences in fiber type proportions on the two sides of the scoliotic spine. The convex side of the curve has a higher proportion of type 1 fibers, thus reflecting abilities associated with endurance capabilities (91). To investigate the biomechanics of scoliosis Schultz and coworkers completed a theoretical analysis, stating that the muscles on the convex side of a lateral curvature may be able to correct the curve. Their work also indicated that the bulkiest, most laterally placed musculature would have the greatest effect. Some muscles included for correction of a left lumbar curve were the left lateral erector spinae, the left internal and external obliques, and the rectus abdominus (68). Other potential treatment suggestions were made, some of which were tested in an in vivo study by Axelgaard and assistants. This work is of interest because of their confirmation of Schultz's theoretical work. In this effort, the amount of curvature correction was found to be a linear function of the length of the moment arm between the lateral musculature and the vertebral elements of the spinal column. For example, the unbending moment from electrical stimulation of the lateral musculature was three times

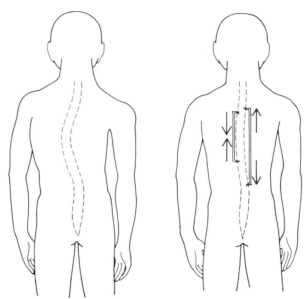

Figure 12.17.   Posterior view of uncorrected scoliosis and the same scoliosis following the surgical insertion of Harrington rods. The combination of tensile and compressive forces, in equal and opposite directions, creates bending moments to control/alter the scoliosis. (From Radin EL, Simon SR, Rose RM, Paul IL: *Practical Biomechanics for the Orthopedic Surgeon.* New York, J Wiley & Sons, 1979.)

that from the stimulation of the paravertebral musculature. These results, that demonstrated that compensatory curves were also reduced, provide a promising method for control or correction of scoliosis and reconfirm the ability of the muscles to effect significant torque (4).

RESPIRATION

Compared to the function of other mechanisms of the body, the mechanics and pathomechanics of respiratory function have received little attention. Although some may claim that care of patients with abnormal kinematics or kinetics of respiration are not within the purview of the therapist, the clinical responsibilities in this area actually have been increasing. This section will discuss the relevant features of the biomechanics of respiration and will conclude with a discussion of the alterations in some of the more common clinical conditions that affect respiration.

Muscular Actions

Function of the muscles producing respiration is somewhat difficult to study because of their size and the anatomical relationships to other muscles. Intramuscular electrodes make EMG study technically and methodologically arduous at best, often yielding results that are not definitive. Thus, much of the function has been derived on the basis of nonexperimental data. In any case, the muscular actions can be considered on the basis of function during the distinct motions leading to either inspiration or expiration.

In the case of inspiration, or expansion of the thorax, one muscle thought to be primarily responsible is the diaphragm. Upon contraction, this dome-shaped muscle moves downward and somewhat forward, enlarging the thorax in the vertical direction. Wade was able to quantitate the movement of the muscle, stating that its movement is about 1.5 cm in quiet respiration. When subjects were placed supine, less reserve diaphragmatic movement was available, perhaps due to pressure exerted by the abdominal contents (81). This idea is supported by the later work of Reid (64). Others, such as Kapandji, describe the diaphragm as descending inferiorly until the central tendon becomes fixed. At this point the muscle can elevate the lower ribs by means of lateral fibers because the origin of these fibers is more superior than their site of attachment to the ribs. In this fashion, the lateral diameter of the thorax is increased (41). In virtually any case the diaphragm has been credited with being the principal, although not essential, muscle of inspiration (70).

Other muscles participating in inspiration are the external intercostals and muscles that could be considered to be accessory. The latter would include the sternocleidomastoid, scalene, serratus posterior superior, and pectoralis minor muscles. Furthermore, if the glenohumeral joint is abducted to at least 90° and fixed in this position, other thoracoscapulohumeral muscles can assist with elevation of the thorax.

Expiration as a result of muscle action has been debated for a considerable length of time. The majority of evidence indicates that the internal intercostal muscles have this responsibility, when indeed such activity is required. Under normal quiet respiration, expiration is thought to be a passive process, controlled by a braking type action through eccentric contraction of the diaphragm and the intercostal muscles (64). Under conditions involving forced expiration, such as during exertion, the expiratory muscles may play an active role in rib depression and diminution of the size of the thorax. Such motions may also be aided by accessory muscles such as the rectus abdominus, serratus posterior inferior, iliocostalis, and quadratus lumborum. Thus, respiration operates as an efficient system, capable of responding to different demands by altering the contraction intensity and timing of the active muscles while simultaneously using the elastic properties inherent within the lungs.

Arthrology and Arthrokinematics

The motion of the ribs can be described by means of the events that occur between the ribs and the vertebrae, and among the ribs, costal cartilages, and sternum. Beginning at the spine each rib has two articulations. As a rib approaches the vertebra, contact is made with each transverse process. This synovial joint has strong ligaments that are restrictive of gross ranges of motion. Each rib articulates proximally with the superior border of the lower vertebra and the inferior border of the upper vertebra, forming the costovertebral joint (41). This is true in all cases except for the singular articulations at T1 and T12. Moving anteriorly, each rib (except the eleventh and twelfth) is contiguous with costal cartilage that articulates with the sternum. Although the first costal cartilage is directly attached to the sternum by means of a synchondrosis, the second through seventh cartilages are attached through fibrocartilagenous expansions (90).

Movement at the costovertebral and costotransverse joints is restrained by ligaments. Furthermore, the arrangement of the two joints dictates a mechanical coupling between them, such that rotation occurs about an axis that passes through each. Study of the axes of these two joints for the various levels of the thoracic vertebrae reveals that the axis for the upper vertebrae is more mediolateral in direction. Thus, rotation about this axis produces an anterior elevation of the rib. For the lower ribs, however, the axis through the two joints is more anteroposterior, causing elevation in the lateral direction. The resultant effect is an increase in the anteroposterior dimension of the upper ribs and an increase in the mediolateral dimension of the inferior ribs. Concurrently, modest gliding-type motions occur at the respective costosternal joints (41).

Other descriptions of the motion of the thorax are also possible. Note, for example, that the anterior aspect of each of the ribs is lower than the posterior aspect. Thus, as the shaft of a rib is elevated, it rises in a forward direction. Movement also is influenced by their anterior attachments. In the case of the superior, or vertebrosternal, ribs, motion is as described for the upper and lower ribs in the previous section. Starting at the anterior attachment of the seventh rib (vertebrochondral), motion of the ribs contributes to enlargement of the upper abdominal space to allow expansion of the organs displaced by contraction of the diaphragm muscle. Furthermore, the costal cartilages of ribs 5 through 10 articulate with each other, in effect causing elevation of the rib superior in location and elevation of the distal sternum. Ribs 11 and 12, called vertebral ribs because of their lack of anterior attachment, have limited motion due to fixation by the quadratus lumborum. Such fixation does, however, provide a fixed point of action of the diaphragm, which inserts on their superior aspects.

The mechanical characteristics of the ribs have been evaluated to some degree. Stiffness measurements have shown variation between ribs, but generally the individual ribs are highly flexible. Although stiffness in each joint may also be measured, there is little impact of these measures upon the mechanics of the thorax (87). An elastic effect may be related to the costal cartilages. In inspiration, the elevation of the thorax causes rotation of the cartilage. Because the costochondral and the sternochondral joints are both articulations that allow little motion, the cartilage becomes twisted. As inspiration is completed, the elasticity within the cartilage tends to untwist the cartilage, completing the process as expiration ensues (41).

Some note of the effect of the ribs upon thoracic spinal motions should also be made. Generally, flexion-extension range of motion of any of the segments does not exceed that of any of the cervical or lumbar motion segments. Lateral bending is limited to less than 10° per segment while rotation is similar to that available in the lower cervical spine. In actuality, were it not for the rib cage, the angulation of the thoracic facets would permit the most motion of any spinal region, except for extension (due to the apposition of spinous processes).

Biomechanics and Kinetics

Information relative to the biomechanics and kinetics of the ribs is scant. The salient features have been covered under the topic of arthrology and arthrokinematics. Further work in this area may be slow in developing because of the persistent technical problems that may preclude definitive data as to the mechanics and kinetics of motion of the ribs.

Pathokinesiology

The effects of respiratory or thoracic spine pathology have not been extensively described. Most information available concerns chronic respiratory problems and the changes that occur secondary to scoliosis. Earlier in this chapter, discussion focused upon the influences of posture as related to the effectiveness of respiratory mechanics and, as stated by Housset et al the goals are to reduce bronchial obstructions and alter the mechanical properties of the chest wall (33). As noted in the supine position, the abdominal organs push the diaphragm superiorly, making inspiration more difficult. Furthermore, as Kapandji indicates, in the sidelying position the diaphragm is pushed upwards much more on the lower side, making this lung less efficient than the other (41). Although loss of abdominal tone may have further effects, the remainder of this section will concentrate on chronic obstructive pulmonary disease (COPD) and scoliosis.

Among the most common COPD is the condition of emphysema. In this case the chest is held in a position of inspiration, partly due to a loss of lung elasticity. As a result, the diaphragm is unable to move superiorly in an attempt to assume its usual dome-shaped position. To compensate for the decreased effectiveness of the diaphragm, the accessory muscles become primary. The result is that the diaphragm only contributes 30% (compared with its usual 65%) of inspiratory force while the accessory muscles play an increased role (24). To respirate effectively, the patient performs a slow, deep, or rapid uncontrolled inspiration, primarily with the accessory muscles, followed by a forced and usually prolonged expiration. Such a pursed lip technique may be facilitated in expiration by contraction of the abdominal muscles.

Evidence exists to support the positioning often employed by therapists in the treatment of COPD. Sharp and coworkers, for example, showed that although the EMG of the accessory inspiratory muscles was greater in standing and erect sitting than in forward leaning, one patient group reported relief of dyspnea in the latter position. The suggestion was made that this position allowed for better fixation of the accessory muscles, so that synergistic action made respiration more efficient (72). Earlier work had also strongly suggested that in COPD, the diaphragm was under two mechanical disadvantages. One is related to the geometry of the muscle, and the other relates to the ability of the muscle to exert tension because of the alterations in length. Similar deficiencies are not likely to occur in the intercostal or accessory muscles of respiration (71).

Orthopaedic disorders of the thoracic spine may also influence respiratory mechanics and function. Some of the most acute effects can result from advanced stages of scoliosis. Lateral curvature and rotation can alter the shape and the spatial relationship of the ribs and can have the potential to severely retard lung function. Figure 12.18 is a graphic depiction of the dimensional alterations that can occur in the thoracic cavity. Obviously, chest wall motion will be distorted at all segments, predisposing the patient to symptoms associated with fatigue, shortness of breath, and chronic respiratory problems. The magnitude of the problems in patients with deformities past 90° has been shown, in that almost two-thirds of the vital capacity and one-half of the total lung capacity are lost (92). Therefore, attention needs to be given to these patients in terms of assurance that respiratory mechanics will not be totally compromised.

SUMMARY

This chapter has considered normal and pathological mechanics of the trunk. This region of the body has an incredibly complex structure, primarily because of the multiple joints of each of the motion segments of the spine. This region of the body is very important, however, because adequate trunk control is essential for effective use of the upper limbs. Any disruption of normal kinematics

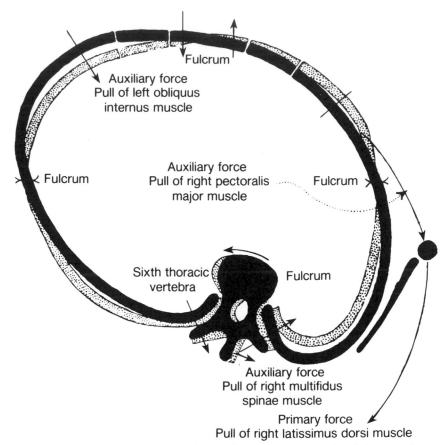

Figure 12.18.   Cross section through the trunk to demonstrate the deformity that can be associated with scoliosis. (From Michele AA: Iliopsoas: Development of Anomalies in Man. Springfield, IL, Charles C Thomas, 1982.)

or kinetics, particularly of the lumbar spine or the respiratory system, can have the ultimate effect of total incapacitation. Recognition of normal and abnormal studies and the location of the pathology often makes the difference in restoring normal motion.

References

1. Aaro S, Ohlen G: The effect of Harrington instrumentation on the sagittal configuration and mobility of the spine in scoliosis. *Spine* 8:570–575, 1983.
2. Adams MA, Hutton WC: The relevance of torsion to the mechanical derangement of the lumbar spine. *Spine* 6:241–248, 1981.
3. Adams MA, Hutton WC, Stott JRR: The resistance to flexion of the lumbar intervertebral joint. *Spine* 5:245–253, 1980.
4. Axelgaard J, Nordwall A, Brown JC: Correction of spinal curvatures by transcutaneous electrical muscle stimulation. *Spine* 8:463–481, 1983.
5. Beal MC: The sacroiliac problem: review of anatomy, mechanics, and diagnosis. *J Am Osteopath Assoc* 81:667–679, 1982.
6. Blackburn SE, Portney LG: Electromyographic activity of back musculature during Williams' flexion exercises. *Phys Ther* 61:878 885, 1981.
7. Bogduk N: The anatomy of the lumbar intervertebral disc syndrome. *Med J Australia* 1:878–881, 1976.
8. Bogduk N: A reappraisal of the anatomy of the human lumbar erector spinae. *J Anat* 131:525–540, 1980.

9. Bogduk N, MacIntosh JE: The applied anatomy of the thoracolumbar fascia. *Spine* 9:164–170, 1984.
10. Broberg KB: On the mechanical behavior of intervertebral discs. *Spine* 8:151–165, 1983.
11. Carlsöö S: *How Man Moves.* London, W. Heinemann Ltd., 1972, p 77.
12. Carmon DJ, Blanton, PL, Biggs NL: Electromyographic study of the anterolateral musculature utilizing indwelling electrodes. *Am J Phys Med* 51:113–129, 1972.
13. Chazal J, Tanguy A, Bourges M, Gaurel G, Escande G, Guillot M, Vanneuville G: Biochemical properties of spinal ligaments and a histological study of the supraspinal ligament in traction. *J Biomech* 18:167–176, 1985.
14. Cochran T, Irstam L, Nachemson A: Long-term anatomic and functional changes in patients with adolescent idiopathic scoliosis treated by Harrington rod fusion. *Spine* 8:576–584, 1983.
15. Dimnet J, Pasquet A, Krag MH, Panjabi MM: Cervical spine motion in the sagittal plane: kinematic and geometric parameters. *J Biomech* 15:959–969, 1982.
16. DonTigny RL: Function and pathomechanics of the sacroiliac joint: a review. *Phys Ther* 65:35–43, 1985.
17. Dunn HK, Daniels AU, McBride GG: Intraoperative force measurements during correction of scoliosis. *Spine* 7:448–455, 1982.
18. Ekholm J, Arborelius U, Fahlcrantz A et al: Activation of abdominal muscles during some physiotherapeutic exercises. *Scand J Rehabil Med* 11:73–84, 1979.
19. Fahrni WH. Conservative treatment of lumbar disc degeneration: our primary responsibility. *Orthop Clin North Am* 6:93–103, 1975.
20. Fielding J: Cineroentgenography of the normal cervical spine. *J Bone Joint Surg [Am]* 39:1280–1288, 1957.
21. Fraser EJ: Extensor muscle of the low back: an electromyographic study. *Phys Ther* 47:200–207, 1967.
22. Frigerio NA, Stowe RR, Howe JW: Movement of the sacroiliac joint. *Clin Orthop* 100:370–377, 1974.
23. Frymoyer JW, Pope MH, Clements JH, et al: Risk factors in low back pain—an epidemiological survey. *J Bone Joint Surg [Am]* 65:213–218, 1983.
24. Garodz Y: Rehabilitation of the patient with chronic obstructive pulmonary disease. *Geisinger Med Bull* 31:10–16, 1971.
25. Godfrey KE, Kindig LE, Windell EJ: Electromyographic study of duration of muscle activity in sit-up variations. *Arch Phys Med Rehabil* 58:132–135, 1977.
26. Gracovetsky S, Farfan HF, Lamy C: The mechanism of the lumbar spine. *Spine* 6:249–262, 1981.
27. Gregersen GG, Lucas DB: An in vivo study of the axial rotation of the human thoracolumbar spine. *J Bone Joint Surg [Am]* 49:247–262, 1967.
28. Grieve GP: The sacro-iliac joint. *Physiotherapy* 62:384–400, 1976.
29. Halpern AA, Bleck EE: Sit-up exercises: an electromyographic study. *Clin Orthop* 145:172–178, 1979.
30. Hasue M, Fujiwara M, Kikuchi S: A new method of quantitative measurement of abdominal and back muscle strength. *Spine* 5:143–148, 1980.
31. Hirsch C: The reaction of intervertebral discs to compression forces. *J Bone Joint Surg [Am]* 37:1188–1191, 1955.
32. Hohl M: Normal motions in the upper portion of the cervical spine. *J Bone Joint Surg [Am]* 46:1777–1779, 1964.
33. Housset B, Tetard C, Derenne JP: Kinésithérapie respiratoire et mecanique respiratore des insuffisants respiratoires chroniques. *Rev Fr Mal Respir* 11:915–921, 1983.
34. Inoue H, Takeda T: Three-dimensional observation of the collagen framework of lumbar intervertebral discs. *Acta Orthop Scand* 46:949–956, 1975.
35. Isaacson PR: Living anatomy: an anatomic basis for the osteopathic concept. *J Am Osteopath Assoc* 79:745–759, 1980.
36. Jensen GM: Biomechanics of the lumbar intervertebral disk: a review. *Phys Ther* 60:765–773, 1980.
37. Johnson D: Personal communication. Iowa City, Iowa, 1985.
38. Johnson RM, Hart DL, Simmons EF, et al: Cervical orthoses—a study comparing their effectiveness in restricting cervical motion in normal subjects. *J Bone Joint Surg [Am]* 59:332–339, 1977.

39. Jonsson B: The function of individual muscles in the lumbar part of the spinae muscle. *Electromyography* 10:5–21, 1970.

40. Joseph J, McColl I: Electromyography of muscles of posture: posterior vertebral muscles in males. *J Physiol (Lond)* 157:33–37, 1961.

41. Kapandji IA: *The Physiology of the Joints.* In *The Trunk and the Vertebral Column.* New York, Churchill Livingstone, 1974, vol 3.

42. Koreska J, Robertson D, Mills RH, Gibson DA, Albisser AM: Biomechanics of the lumbar spine and its clinical significance. *Orthop Clin North Am* 8:121–133, 1977.

43. Kulak RF, Belytschko TB, Schultz AB, et al: Non-linear behavior of the human intervertebral disc under axial load. *J Biomech* 9:377–386, 1976.

44. La Rocca H: Biomechanics of the Cervical Spine. In *Atlas of Orthotics: Biomechanical Principles and Application.* St. Louis, CV Mosby, 1975.

45. Laurnen EL, Tupper JW, Mullen MP: The Boston brace in thoracic scoliosis—a preliminary report. *Spine* 8:388–395, 1983.

46. Lee CK, Langrana NA: Lumbosacral spinal fusion: a biomechanical study. *Spine* 9:574–581, 1984.

47. Lin HS, Liu YK, Adams KH: Mechanical response of the lumbar intervertebral joint under physiological (complex) loading. *J Bone Joint Surg [Am]* 60:41–55, 1978.

48. Lipetz S, Gutin B: An electromyographic study of four abdominal exercises. *Med Sci Sports* 2:35–38, 1970.

49. Lorenz M, Patwardhan A, Vanderby R: Load-bearing characteristics of lumbar facets in normal and surgically altered spinal segments. *Spine* 8:122–130, 1983.

50. Macnab I: Negative disc exploration. *J Bone Joint Surg [Am]* 53:891–903, 1971.

51. Mayer TG, Tencer AF, Kristoferson S, Mooney V: Use of noninvasive techniques for quantification of spinal range-of-motion in normal subjects and chronic low-back dysfunction patients. *Spine* 9:588–595, 1984.

52. Michele AA: *Iliopsoas: Development of Anomalies in Man.* Springfield, IL, Charles C Thomas, 1962.

53. Morris JM, Markolf KL: Biomechanics of the lumbosacral spine. In *Atlas of Orthotics: Biomechanical Principles and Application.* St. Louis, CV Mosby, 1975.

54. Nachemson A, Evans J: Some mechanical properties of the third human lumbar interlaminar ligament (ligamentum flavum). *J Biomech* 1:211–220, 1968.

55. Nachemson AL: The lumbar spine—an orthopedic challenge. *Spine* 1:59–71, 1976.

56. Nachemson AL: Disc pressure measurements. *Spine* 6:93–97, 1981.

57. Ortengren R, Andersson GBJ: Electromyographic studies of trunk muscles, with special reference to the functional anatomy of the lumbar spine. *Spine* 2:44–52, 1977.

58. Panjabi MM, Takata K, Goel VK: Kinematics of lumbar intervertebral foramen. *Spine* 8:348–357, 1983.

59. Parke W, Schift D: The applied anatomy of the intervertebral disc. *Orthop Clin North Am* 2:309–324, 1977.

60. Pearcy MJ, Tibrewal SB: Axial rotation and lateral bending in the normal lumbar spine measured by three-dimensional radiography. *Spine* 9:582–587, 1984.

61. Pope M: AAOS Symposium on the Spine, Miami, 1981.

62. Rab GT, Chao EYS, Stauffer RN: Muscle force analysis of the lumbar spine. *Orthop Clin North Am* 8:193–199, 1977.

63. Radin EL, Simon SR, Rose RM, Paul IL: *Practical Biomechanics for the Orthopedic Surgeon.* New York, J Wiley & Sons, 1979.

64. Reid DC: Electromyographic studies of respiration: a review of current concepts. *Physiotherapy* 56:534–540, 1970.

65. Sandover J: Dynamic loading as a possible source of low-back disorders. *Spine* 8:652–658, 1983.

66. Schultz A, Andersson G, Ortengren R, et al: Analysis and quantitative myoelectric measurements of loads on the lumbar spine when holding weights in standing postures. *Spine* 7:390–397, 1982.

67. Schultz A, Andersson G, Ortengren R, et al: Loads on the lumbar spine: validation of a biomechanical analysis by measurements of intradiscal pressures and myoelectric signals. *J Bone Joint Surg [Am]* 64:713–720, 1982.

68. Schultz A, Haderspeck K, Takashima S: Correction of scoliosis by muscle stimulation-biochemical analyses. *Spine* 6:468–476, 1981.

69. Seligman JV, Gertzbein SD, Kapasouri A: Computer analysis of spinal segment motion in degenerative disc disease with and without axial loading. *Spine* 9:566–573, 1984.
70. Shaffer TH, Wolfson MR, Bhutani VK: Respiratory muscle function, assessment, and training. *Phys Ther* 61:1711–1723, 1981.
71. Sharp JT, Danon J, Druz WS, et al: Respiratory muscle function in patients with chronic obstructive pulmonary disease: its relationship to disability and to respiratory therapy. *Am Rev Respir Dis* 110:154–167, 1974.
72. Sharp JT, Druz WS, Moisan T, et al: Postural relief of dyspnea in severe chronic obstructive pulmonary disease. *Am Rev Respir Dis* 122:201–211, 1980.
73. Smidt G, Herring T, Amundsen L, et al: Assessment of abdominal and back extensor function: a quantitative approach and results for chronic low-back patients. *Spine* 8:211–219, 1983.
74. Smidt GL, Amundsen LR, Dostal WF: Muscle strength at the trunk. *J Orthop Sports Phys Ther* 1:165–170, 1980.
75. Soderberg GL: Exercises for the abdominal muscles. *J Health Phys Ed Rec* 37:67–70, 1966.
76. Soderberg GL, Barr JO: Muscular function in chronic low-back dysfunction. *Spine* 8:79–85, 1983.
77. Solonen KA: The sacroiliac joint in the light of anatomical, roentgenological and clinical studies. *Acta Orthop Scand Suppl* 27: 1957.
78. Stoddard A: Manual of Osteopathic Technique. London, Hutchinson & Co, 1960.
79. Twomey LT, Taylor JR: Sagittal movements of the human lumbar vertebral column: a quantitative study of the role of the posterior vertebral elements. *Arch Phys Med Rehabil* 64:322–325, 1983.
80. Virgin W: Experimental investigations into physical properties of intervertebral disc. *J Bone Joint Surg [Br]* 33:607–611, 1951.
81. Wade OL: Movements of the thoracic cage and diaphragm in respiration. *J Physiol* 124:193–212, 1954.
82. Wasylenko M, Skinner SR, Perry J, Antonelli DJ: An analysis of posture and gait following spinal fusion with Harrington instrumentation. *Spine* 8:840–845, 1983.
83. Weisl H: The articular surfaces of the sacro-iliac joint and their relation to the movement of the sacrum. *Acta Anat* 22:1–14, 1954.
84. Weisl H: The movements of the sacro-iliac joint. *Acta Anat* 23:80–91, 1955.
85. White AA, Johnson RM, Panjabi MM, Southwick WO: Biomechanical analysis of clinical stability in the cervical spine. *Clin Orthop* 109:85–96, 1975.
86. White AA, Panjabi MM: The clinical biomechanics of scoliosis. *Clin Orthop* 118:100–112, 1976.
87. White AA, Panjabi MM: *Clinical Biomechanics of the Spine*. Philadelphia, JB Lippincott, 1978.
88. White AA, Panjabi MM: The basic kinematics of the human spine: a review of past and current knowledge. *Spine* 3:12–20, 1978.
89. Wilder DG, Pope MH, Frymoyer JW: The functional topography of the sacroiliac joint. *Spine* 5:575–579, 1980.
90. Williams PL, Warwick R (eds): *Gray's Anatomy—36th British Edition*. Edinburgh, Churchill Livingstone, 1980.
91. Zetterberg C, Aniansson A, Brimby G: Morphology of the paravertebral muscles in adolescent idiopathic scoliosis. *Spine* 8:457–462, 1983.
92. Zorab PA: Respiratory function in scoliosis. In Zorab PA (ed): *Scoliosis*. Springfield, IL, Charles C Thomas, 1969.

13

Posture and Gait

POSTURE

The arrangement of the body segments relative to each other determines the posture assumed. Although the positions that could be assumed are essentially infinite in number, only a few erect and sitting postures are frequently used by any individual. Any posture necessitates specific joint positions and forces necessary to maintain the selected posture. Thus, an analysis of kinematics and kinetics can be completed from a description of the posture. Many consider posture to be a static phenomenon and make reasonable assumptions that allow such a description. In fact, even relatively gross analysis has shown that the whole body and individual segments are in motion. The influence of body posture on joints and the tissues responsible for maintaining the joints in the desired position has to be considered.

Human postures have largely been derived from our necessity to free the hand for use. Accommodations have been made by bony and soft tissues in order to enable the performance of the tasks now required of a "modern" society. For example, as suspensory postures (hanging by upper limbs) were assumed, the lower limbs became extended in line with the body and the shoulder girdle required greater mobility. Increased supination and pronation also developed, and the prehensile hand found even greater use. Other changes were seen in the thorax, in that flattening developed anteroposteriorly and the scapula moved posteriorly. The lower limb was not free from modification. The foot lost most of its grasping ability, bony articulations were altered, and muscles changed attachment sites. More proximally, the mass of the gluteus maximus developed to a size unique to man, probably forcing a concurrent increase in the size of the quadriceps femoris.

Perhaps most important have been the changes to occur in the spine. Because of an approximately 30° anteroinferior tilt of the sacrum in the upright posture, the lumbar spine has been forced into the commonly known position of hyper-extension, or lordosis (38). Often blamed, either justly or unjustly, for predispos-ing man to low back pain and dysfunction, the sagittal plane configuration will continue to be of interest to clinicians and scientists alike. Regardless of these and other effects produced by human postures, dramatic changes are unlikely to occur in the near future. Therefore, therapists need to understand the implications of the postures that are commonly assumed and how the postures or their determinants can be altered to produce desired results.

Standing

Requirements

For maintenance of the upright posture, multiple joints need to be controlled in each of three planes of motion. In general, such control will be determined by a number of factors. One is the relationship of the body's line of gravity with respect to the joint. Fortunately, for the sake of efficiency, the verticle line through the center of gravity of the body is located just anterior to the second sacral level, passing close to or through the sagittal plane axis of many of the joints of the lower limb. This line of gravity (force) multiplied by the distance (moment arm) to the center of the joint determines the moment required to control the position of the joint under consideration. Because the distance to any relevant joint axis is small, the moment is minimized. Another factor is the position of the joint. Often, the posture chosen approximates the close-packed position of the joint. In these cases, with minor modification in the posture assumed, the joints can be placed in positions which require minimal muscle force because ligaments and joint capsules can be used to control joint torque rather than muscle contraction. Because postures are frequently altered and force requirements are modified on a regular basis at all of the joints, such events as venous stasis and fatigue are avoided. Finally, realize that postures such as standing are asymmetric (45). The result is that different requirements exist for different joints. The effects of these and other factors are to produce different joint positions, resultant forces, and torques at the respective joints. The remainder of this section will describe such results in terms of the requirements of the joints of the lower limb and the spine.

The foot and ankle are of import because these joints provide the basis for the position of the remaining joints. As pointed out in the chapter on the foot and ankle, the bony makeup of the foot allows flexibility in conforming to a wide variety of supporting surfaces. However, the most important situation is the consideration of the requirements at the ankle as seen in the sagittal plane. In standing, the line of gravity falls anterior to the axis of the ankle. Thus, the muscles of the posterior calf must have active or passive tension so that the body will not fall anteriorly. Although muscles such as the gastrocnemius, tibialis anterior, peroneals, and tibialis posterior are all available to produce the tension required to maintain relative equilibrium, most accounts agree that the soleus muscle is primarily responsible (11, 32). Functionally, this is the most logical selection, because the others either are two-joint muscles or are required for the control of foot motion. Physiologically, as a slow twitch muscle, the soleus is also well prepared to exert long durations of relatively low tensions. Note that in this case the moment of the body is taken about the mediolateral axis of the ankle. Sway in a posterior direction may involve sufficient displacement of the line of gravity, such that the musculature of the anterior compartment would contract, pulling the body anteriorly. If such was required an anterior counteracting moment is produced so that equilibrium can be maintained.

As stated in the chapter on the knee, the center of rotation of the knee in the sagittal plane is located within the femoral condyles. Because the line of gravity falls anterior to the axis of rotation of the knee, an extended position results, requiring little force from the quadriceps. In fact, during standing, manual movement of the patella is accomplished easily because of the lack of tension in the quadriceps muscles. If the knee is allowed to assume full extension, the close-packed position has been achieved and probably diminishes the need for great amounts of muscular tension. Complete hyperextension of the knee, commonly assumed in standing posture adopted for long durations, involves reliance upon the posterior capsule. This practice probably should be avoided, even though there is little or no evidence that it has a negative effect.

Carlsöö provides an extensive discussion of the knee during the standing posture, relating events to the principles of a closed kinetic chain. That is, because the distal segment is fixed and because the pelvis and trunk are carried over the knee and essentially fixed, the knee can be affected by any force that tends to pull the distal femur or proximal tibia posteriorly. Such is the possible action of the hamstring and soleus muscles, both of which are active during standing posture (11, 37). As could be implied by this analysis, musculature that has been credited with control of the hip or ankle may directly affect the knee. Therefore, as has been pointed out previously, therapists should be cognizant of the functional changes that may occur when a closed kinetic chain is used during the movement.

Posture assumed by the hip has been debated, and currently there is no consensus as to the position most commonly adopted. In fact, the collective line of gravity from the head, arms, and trunk segments fall either directly through, just anterior, or slightly posterior to the center of the hip joint when the upright body is viewed sagittally. As the line of gravity shifts, the moment requirements vary, but in any case the muscular tension requirements are minimal. This fact appears to have been confirmed with EMG by Basmajian and Portnoy and Morin (3, 37). In most cases the posture assumed will not place the hip joint in a position of complete extension; rather, about 10 or 15° of motion is allowed (11). If, however, the hyperextended position is assumed, the person can rely on the anteriorly located iliofemoral ligament. Such a condition may be energy-efficient, but for reasons cited for the posterior capsule of the knee, the regular assumption of this position may be harmful.

The sacroiliac joints are responsible for transposing the weight transmitted between the spinal column and the two lower limbs. The sacrum, essentially wedged between the two ilia, ordinarily experiences little movement. Upright posture, however, has a tendency to rotate the sacrum forward and downwards (11). Constraint is provided, however, by the tension produced in the sacrotuberous and sacrospinous ligaments (17). Another important consideration related to the sacrum is the role that the pelvic girdle components play in establishing the position of the spine as viewed laterally. This is because the angle of inclination of the sacrum, depicted in Figure 13.1, determines the position of the fifth lumbar vertebra relative to the sacrum. The greater the degree of inclination, the greater the tendency for additional lordosis in the whole of the lumbar spine. The effect of large degrees of inclination has been discussed in the chapter on the trunk, but the implications for postural control of the trunk and head segments are also noteworthy.

The posture of the spinal column is thus a matter of balance among the anteroposterior curvatures of the various segments. That is, greater lumbar lordosis will necessitate greater thoracic kyphosis and perhaps cervical lordosis in order to balance the vertebrae on each other. Although there have been attempts to specify the respective locations of the lines of gravity for the trunk and the individual vertebrae, the only practical analyses are those that can be formulated on the basis of easily accessible body landmarks.

Generally the trunk is well balanced relative to the line of gravity. Thus, in the upright posture there is little requirement for large muscular tensions and

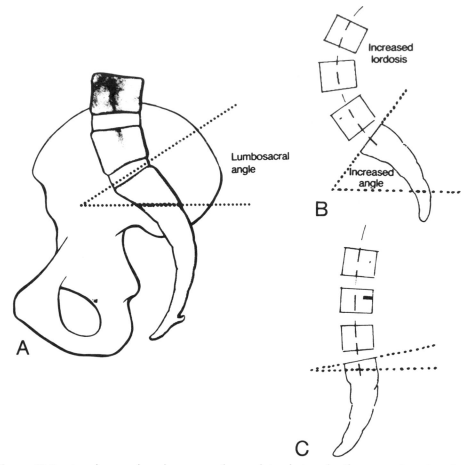

Figure 13.1.   Lumbosacral angle as seen from a lateral view for the normal posture in *A*. In *B* and *C* the angle of inclination of the sacrum has been increased and decreased, respectively, leading to changes in the amount of lordosis in the lumbar spine. (From Cailliet R: *Soft Tissue Pain and Disability*. Philadelphia, FA Davis, 1977.)

moments. There is clear evidence, however, that low levels of EMG activity exist in the majority of persons in the erector spinae muscles (21, 33, 37). The posterior musculature of the neck also is active because of the flexion moment produced by the weight of the head. More detailed descriptions of the postural requirements can be completed by analyzing the motion or potential motion between individual vertebral segments. Such procedures are usually reserved for more sophisticated works, but this type of analytic procedure may soon offer significant information about spinal kinematics.

Forces in the joints are primarily the result of two factors: superincumbent body weight and the level of contraction of the musculature controlling a specific joint. Only in unusual cases would tightness of structures around a joint be a significant factor in increasing such forces. As has been noted, when viewed in the sagittal plane, the line of gravity falls through or relatively close to all of the joints about which moments would have to be considered. Subsequently, there is little need for large muscular forces that increase joint forces. In fact, most joints are at or near their close-packed position, which offers maximal surface area over which to disperse force. Thus, the greater the amount of superincumbent weight, the greater is the amount of compressive force in the joint. Because the force at the joints is directly dependent on body weight, one must resort to body segment parameter information to determine the relative proportion distributed to each of the segments, followed by an appropriate mathematical procedure.

Evaluation

Postural evaluations have been widely used, particularly for the young and in situations such as scoliosis, when therapeutic outcome is dependent on proper alignment. Although there is probably not one posture that all should conform to, a view of the line of gravity, sagittally, should probably fall anterior to the ankle and knee and through the hip joint, acromion process, and tragus of the ear. From an anterior or posterior view the body is dissected into two halves: the line of gravity falls through such centrally located landmarks as the spinous processes posteriorly and the pubic symphysis and nose anteriorly. In either case the position assumed should have a base of support that compromises neither stability nor mobility. Finally, although evaluation in a third plane may be desirable, deviations noted in the lateral, anterior, or posterior views can adequately describe any abnormalities.

Sitting

Trunk Position

Most volumes addressing kinesiology do not discuss sitting as a posture. This position is extremely relevant, however, since many people spend a great amount of time sitting. Furthermore, there is conflicting evidence that those who assume a sitting posture for work incur an increased risk of low back pain (26, 50). Finally, there is distinct evidence that the mechanics of the pelvis and spine changes as soon as sitting is achieved. For example, Carlsöö states that of the 90° between the trunk and thigh, about 40° are in the posterior tilting of the pelvis and 50° in flexion of the hip (11). Assuming this degree of motion, the angle of sacral inclination is also altered, resulting in a less lordotic posture of the lumbar spine.

Another factor that deserves notice is that during sitting, the position of the pelvis can be altered. This change is achieved by positioning of the trunk. Consider the forward leaning posture and the slumped position. Although these postures may produce similar configurations of the lumbar spine, the spinal extensor musculature is required to actively control the forward moment in the former position (assuming the arms are not supporting the weight of the trunk). In contrast, the upright sitting posture demands more lordosis, simulating more closely the lumbosacral position assumed during standing.

That the position of the pelvis and spine is important is partly demonstrated by the amount of study dedicated to alternative postures. One such alternative is a posture that involves direct support of the lumbar spine. Design of office furniture and the manufacture of various sizes and styles of lumbar "support cushions" are ready evidence of the attention paid to this posture. Perhaps at least some of this impetus has been provided by the work of Nachemson, who has stated that unsupported sitting reduces lumbar lordosis and increases the load on the intervertebral discs and posterior structures of the back (31). To combat this criticism of the standard sitting posture there has been some interest in using a seat with a downward inclination of the anterior portion of the supporting surface (Fig. 13.2). In order to evaluate the orthopedic considerations

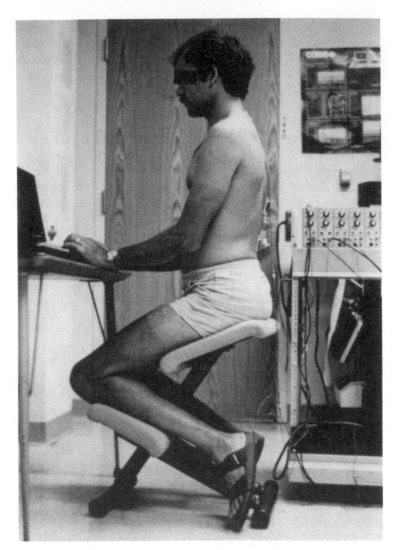

Figure 13.2. Posture of a subject seated on a downwardly inclined supporting surface while EMG data is collected from three levels of erector spinae muscles. Although with this seating device a portion of the weight can be borne on the lower leg, the subject also can position the lower limbs so that the feet are flat on the floor.

associated with this type of seated posture, Keegan used a radiographic approach. Of some interest was that a normal lumbar curve is possible with a thigh-trunk angle of 135° (22). Schlegel also recommended tilting the whole seat forwards (41).

The existing information on the seated posture demonstrates that there are significant differences between standing and sitting, and even between the different sitting postures assumed. As the pelvis changes to a configuration different from that of standing, the spine is required to change its configuration. Thus, force requirements of the supporting musculature are altered, as are intradiscal pressure and tension in passive tissues such as ligaments. In fact, how a patient is positioned may have significant influence on the intended therapeutic outcome. An upright, unsupported posture is distinctly different from a supported posture with a backward trunk inclination. In the latter case Andersson and Ortengren have shown the smallest intradiscal pressures and EMG values with an inclination of 120°. All other seated postures require larger magnitudes of intradiscal pressure and/or EMG (1).

Specifically, the upright posture produces the highest levels of EMG activity in the erector spinae muscles. Slumping diminishes the activity, while more extreme forward bending, even without anterior support mechanisms such as resting the forearms on the thighs, decreases or abolishes the activity. Flexion to approximately 50° eliminates the erector spinae activity in favor of passive tension in the musculature and the posterior elements of the spine.

Two other works have evaluated the sitting posture. The first evaluated the use of an anteriorly inclined seat in altering the magnitude of EMG produced by the erector spinae. While subjects performed a typing task for 15 min, the activity of the musculature was evaluated as the angle of the supporting surface was varied among 0, 10 and 20° of anterior inclination. Results showed statistically significant differences between postures, such that EMG activity decreased as the inclination of the chair increased (46). In other work, the influence of a lumbar roll on the EMG of the erector spinae was evaluated. Test conditions were similar to those described in the previous study. Results showed that both a lumbar roll and a lumbar cushion afforded small decreases in EMG activity at the tested erector spinae levels adjacent to T10, L1, and L3 (Soderberg GL, Venhuizen JK, Reeves DK, Hartness RA: An EMG analysis of the erector spinae muscles during sitting with three lumbar support conditions, unpublished data, University of Iowa, 1984). These studies have possible application to patient care, but further data are needed before definitive conclusions can be reached.

Pathokinesiology

Numerous conditions affect posture. Pain or discomfort frequently is a causative factor in the attitude that a patient may assume, but the key feature will be to attempt to remove the cause so that normal position and function can be assumed. A classic example is a patient suffering from low back dysfunction. If spinal musculature is in asymmetrical spasm, functional scoliosis can be produced. In addition, the pelvis may be unilaterally elevated, causing discrepancy of leg length and forcing modification of posture. Until the condition resolves, normal kinematics and kinetics will not be available, impeding normal motion.

In discussing how pathologies affect posture, there are two helpful principles that should be remembered. First, recognize that distal involvement may have effects at proximal joints. Consider a patient with cerebral palsy that has developed a plantar flexion contracture of the ankle. Such unilateral plantar flexion requires that the hip and knee of the same limb be placed into flexion so that the pelvis can remain level. Thus, the distal joint has determined the position of two other joints, providing a demonstration of the closed kinetic chain in a practical situation.

The second principle to realize is that alterations from an ideal postural configuration usually require greater forces in muscles during functional activities because greater moments need to be generated for control of body segments. Returning to the cerebral palsy case cited above, visualize the patient in the sagittal plane. Note that compared to the normal posture and the close approximation of the line of gravity to joint centers, the location of the centers of rotation have been displaced. The greater the distance from the line of gravity the greater the moment required to maintain a joint in the desired position. In fact, Perry et al have determined that, compared to full knee extension, 51% of the maximal quadriceps force is necessary to maintain the body in an upright position (35). Stress resulting from long-term postures in such positions could ultimately lead to altered structure and function.

Lower Limb Injuries

Virtually any injury of the lower limb has the potential for producing alterations in a patient's posture. Previously in this section the plantar flexion contracture was detailed. Note that similar events would occur if a knee injury resulted in a flexion contracture of this joint. The result would be a concomitant flexion of the hip and dorsiflexion at the ankle, assuming that a level pelvis is maintained. Moment requirements at all joints would be increased.

Deviations in the mediolateral direction are less common. Any unilateral involvement would produce asymmetry and tend to distort optimal postural alignment. Pain arising from any number of foot conditions, an ankle or knee sprain, degenerative joint disease, or other conditions is capable of producing such a distortion. The knee is rather frequently the focus of degeneration, and, being located at the end of two long levers, may be displaced either medially (valgus) or laterally (varus). No matter the direction, stress concentration is likely to develop at one area of the joint, while tension is likely to occur in the elongated soft tissue structures. If the deviation is great enough, the limb can be shortened sufficiently to produce a leg-length difference and ultimately a postural discrepancy.

Muscular deficiencies also can produce deficits that have postural implications. Although most any muscular involvement can have implications, the most serious deficiencies are those that involve the posterior calf muscles, the quadriceps, and the hip extensors. Fortunately such losses do not often involve entire groups, resulting only in weakness rather than major loss. If the plantar flexors are lost, however, maintaining balance becomes a problem. It is more difficult to keep the line of gravity within its anteroposterior limits, since the primary means of shifting it posteriorly toward the ankle axis has been lost. Frequently patients compensate by adjusting their base of support or shifting their weight to the sounder limb (25).

Quadriceps insufficiency creates little difficulty during standing because, as noted previously, the center of rotation of the knee is posterior to the line of gravity. Precautions may need to be taken against hyperextension of the knee. Hip extensor loss can be difficult for a patient, depending on the location of the axis of rotation relative to the line of gravity. The most common compensation is demonstrated by the patient with a spinal cord lesion who assumes a position of hip hyperextension. As noted earlier this allows the load to be borne by the iliofemoral ligament, thus offering sufficient control of the hip extension moment. Caution that the line of gravity is maintained anterior to the hip is extremely important; otherwise, sudden flexion of the trunk on the lower limbs may result in a fall.

Earlier parts of this section have made reference to the fact that the lower limb operates as a closed kinetic chain. In paralytic cases it is important for the clinician to remember that there is interaction among the three joints of the lower limb. One example, the above knee amputee, should suffice. In this situation there is loss of active control of the knee. Subsequently, the patient must stand with the hip short of complete extension so that postural sway can be controlled at the hip. Absence of this technique, or a backward tilt of the pelvis that would create hip flexion, would not allow the upright posture (25).

As has been noted in the chapter on the trunk, the anteroposterior tilting of the pelvis exerts significant influence on the primary curves of the spinal column. Excessive downward tilting is seen in some cases of contracture of the iliopsoas muscles, creating the need for increased curvature of the thoracic spine as a compensatory mechanism. The other primary deviation of the spine, scoliosis, has been detailed in the chapter on the trunk.

GAIT

The act of walking, fundamental to the performance of man, has been described as a series of prevented catastrophies. Yet, when analyzed, the activity known also as gait is carried out with remarkable efficiency. Numerous pieces of literature have described the movement patterns and mechanics of gait (29, 30, 34). Others have focused on the initiation of gait or the development of gait during childhood (27, 49). Still others have completed more complex analyses of the kinematics of human gait through use of the computer (57). However, some of the more useful forms of analysis use systems that are designed for clinical practice settings (4, 53). Although a normal pattern assumes a wide variety of forms, disruptions in the sequence of actions are easily identified. The clinician must be prepared to recognize these alterations in the normal pattern with knowledge of kinematics and kinetics as applied to the gait pattern. This section will discuss biomechanics as applied to gait and then present the common pathologies that produce changes in the gait pattern.

Definitions

In order to adequately describe the gait pattern some system of terminology must be adopted. Many attempts have been made to standardize the descriptors, yet there is currently no one system that is universally accepted. Although the most common systems will be presented in this volume, the reader is advised to be prepared to interpret and make applications to other systems that may appear in the literature.

Fundamental to any description of walking is the term gait cycle, meaning the beginning of an event by one limb and continuing until the event is repeated again with that same limb. One complete gait cycle is known as a stride, while a step is considered to be the beginning of an event by one limb until the beginning of the same event with the contralateral limb (2). Other important terms are swing, stance, and double support, the latter being the period when both feet are in contact with the supporting surface. In general, stance accounts for about 60% of the gait cycle for each limb when walking velocity is normal (Fig. 13.3). Methods are available for describing various parts of these phases of the gait cycle, the most useful being shown in Figure 13.4. Note that heel strike is synonymous with initial contact, and that foot flat is part of the loading response. Heel-off and toe-off are other commonly used events specifying points in the gait cycle. In addition, time can be used to measure any of the events; thus, a temporal sequence can also be ascribed to the events of the gait cycle. Cadence, the number of steps per minute, can also be a descriptor.

Caution must be exercised in strict adherence to this system or any proposed terminology, because in some instances all phases are not discernible. This is

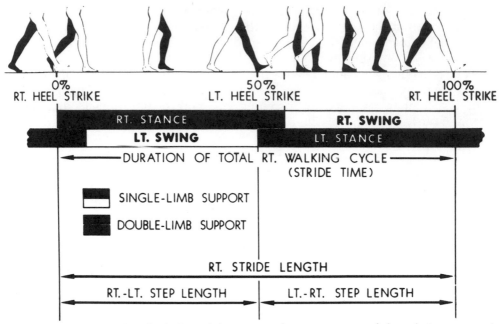

Figure 13.3. A graphic depiction of the temporal components and the relative step and stride lengths that occur during the gait cycle. (From Murray MP: Gait as a total pattern of movement. *Am J Phys Med* 46:290–333, 1967.)

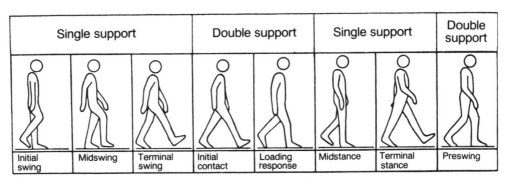

Figure 13.4. Diagrammatic representation of the end points of each phase of the gait cycle. Using this system enables the description of all phases in reasonably equal intervals. (From Bampton S: A Guide to the Visual Examination of Pathological Gait. Temple University Rehabilitation and Research Training Center No. 8. Philadelphia, Moss Rehabilitation Hospital, 1979.)

particularly true when pathology affects the pattern. Regardless of the system or the terminology, successful locomotion requires the ability to support the body, maintain balance, and in some manner execute the stepping movement. Or, as Murray has stated, restraint, support, and propulsion must occur in logical sequence for forward motion to progress (29).

Center of Gravity Displacement

The efficiency of the movement of the total body during gait is produced by the respective kinematics of the segments of the lower limb. One way to describe the efficiency of movement during locomotion is by approximating the location of the center of body mass and plotting its movement during the gait cycle.

Although it is possible, and perhaps important, to evaluate the movement of the center of mass in all three planes, a discussion of motion in the sagittal plane shall suffice. In this case the center essentially moves in a sinusoidal pattern. There are three key points to remember. First, vertical displacement of the center of mass is minimal over the gait cycle and involves little loss of energy, i.e., there is little resistance to the desired forward motion. Second, the pattern is repeated ad infinitum as the various cycles recur with forward progression. Finally, the velocity of the center's forward movement varies considerably. For example, following heelstrike the velocity is decreased. During the propulsive phase in late stance the velocity is increased. All of these events, dependent upon the kinematics and kinetics of the joints of the lower limb, occur in a pattern that results in smooth coordinated movement. Similar descriptions of the paths for the centers of mass for the other planes are available, but in general they are more ellipsoid in shape (11).

Kinematics

Angular rotations of each of the lower limb joints occur predominantly in the sagittal plane. A summary of these movements for the entire gait cycle is shown in Figure 13.5 (20). Each of the respective ranges of motion can be correlated with the various phases of the gait cycle. Particularly note the total ranges of motion required for each of the joints, because the therapist should usually seek to attain these ranges to achieve nonpathological gait.

For the hip, Smidt used electrogoniometry to analyze triplanar motion during gait. A sample of his results are shown in Figure 13.6. Note that only small ranges of motion are required for both abduction-adduction and axial rotation (44). For the knee, virtually no abduction-adduction range would either exist or be desirable. Rotation occurs as part of the screw-home mechanism associated with terminal extension. These features were discussed in Chapter 10. The ankle-foot complex has been more difficult to analyze because of the multiple joints involved in its positioning. Root et al have extensively reviewed and described the motions at each of the joints in the foot. They state that the subtalar joint pronates to allow internal rotation of the leg, while supination allows external rotation. During support phase the foot pronates, and it begins to supinate as the midstance period starts. Supination continues and reaches a maximum shortly before toe-off. Similar types of analysis are available for the midtarsal joint (39).

Motion of the pelvis is critical to normal locomotion. Movement in the sagittal plane is slight, as depicted by Figure 13.5. In the transverse plane the pelvis has been shown to rotate approximately 11.5°, advancing anteriorly on the side of the limb swinging forward (29). Rotation in the frontal plane (abduction and adduction) is critical. This is a direct application of the abductor mechanism described in Chapter 9. Recall that during stance phase the abductors must be active in order to prevent the opposite side of the pelvis from dropping. Thus, in effect, the pelvis on the side of the swinging leg is elevated. According to Eberhart, an average of 8° of motion exists in this plane (14). Attention should also be called to the fact that the upper trunk rotates in the opposite direction of the pelvis. This is apparently a balance mechanism, but the combination of motions requires that rotation occur throughout the spinal column.

Not to be excluded in the kinematics of gait is the motion of the upper limbs. Their motion is correlated with the movement of the upper trunk; therefore, as a lower limb is advanced, the contralateral arm moves forward. Murray has shown that the total amplitude of shoulder flexion and extension is 32° and that

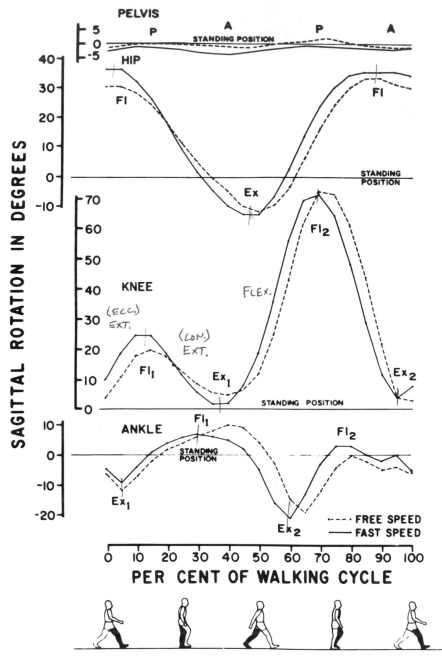

Figure 13.5.   Mean sagittal plane kinematics for the pelvis, hip, knee, and ankle for 30 normal men walking at two speeds. The zero was a reference provided by the joint when the subject was standing. For the pelvis an upward deflection represents posterior tilting (*P*), while a downward deflection represents anterior tilting (*A*). For the other joints flexions are designated with an *Fl* and extensions with an *Ex*. (From Murray MP: Gait as a total pattern of movement. *Am J Phys Med* 46:290–333, 1967.)

the extension range required is considerably greater than that of flexion. The elbow also participates and experiences a total flexion-extension range of about 64 degrees (29).

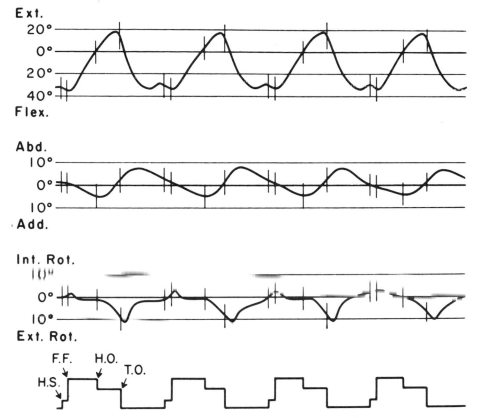

Figure 13.6. Three dimensional electrogoniometric recording of hip motion during gait. Foot switch patterns are used to locate heel strike (*H.S.*), foot flat (*F.F.*), heel off (*H.O.*), and toe off (*T.O.*). (From Smidt GL: Hip motion and related factors in walking. *Phys Ther* 51:9–21, 1971.)

Kinetics

The kinetics associated with gait is an interesting topic because it allows the opportunity to integrate and apply virtually all of biomechanics to a functional activity. The kinematics just discussed are produced by timely and appropriate levels of muscle contraction required by the interplay of gravitational and inertial forces. These contractions are responsible for the generation of joint torque and forces. Thus, this section will discuss each of these aspects as applied to human locomotion.

Muscular Actions

In general, knowing the kinematics will allow a ready understanding of the musculature involved in producing the joint actions. For example, a limb in swing or stance phase indicates whether a muscle will be required to shorten or lengthen and at what velocity it will have to exert tension.

Now, with a review of the sagittal plane motion shown in Figure 13.5, consider the ankle joint throughout the gait cycle. Note that from 5 to 35% of the cycle the ankle is dorsiflexing as the lower leg passes over the foot fixed to the supporting surface. During this time the muscles of the anterior tibial compartment are minimally active or inactive because there is little or no moment requirement (Fig. 13.7). Then, the ankle is plantar-flexed during the propulsive phase. Note the activity of the plantar flexors in the late support phase in Figure 13.7. At toe-off, dorsiflexion begins so that the foot will clear the ground during the swing phase. The EMG data indicate that activity starts just prior to the liftoff of the foot from the surface. This activity is probably timed so that sufficient tension is developed prior to the foot clearing the ground.

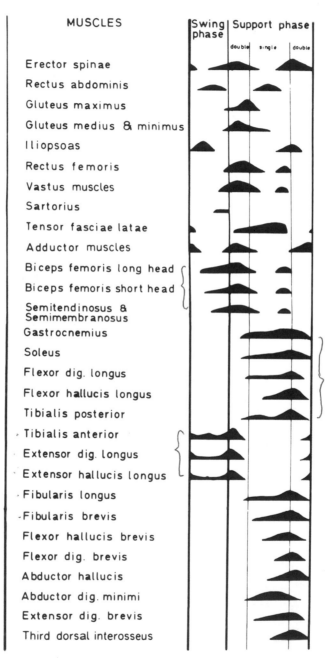

Figure 13.7.   Representation of the "average" electrical activity produced by the muscles of the lower limb during gait. (From Carlsöö S: *How Man Moves: Kinesiological Studies and Methods.* London, William Heinemann, 1972.)

Similar analyses can be completed for each motion of all the other joints required to participate in the gait cycle. For example, consider how the muscular activity shown in Figure 13.7 for the gluteus maximus, rectus femoris, vastus muscles, and hamstrings act to control the extension moments required at the hip and knee. Review of the EMG data would confirm that the muscles affect appropriate moments in each of the planes for each of the joints in the temporal sequence required for the normal gait pattern. Correlation of EMG data with moment data will be possible when joint torque data during gait is presented in the next section.

A number of other features associated with the muscular control of gait should be discussed. Evaluation of the EMG records shows that muscles that are not required to control moments are also active during the gait cycle. The adductor group provides a ready example. Explanation can be offered for activity in early support and early swing phases, in that the former provides stability, while the latter assists with flexion at the hip. Based on the anatomical location of the large mass of the adductors, both of these functions can be postulated. Also, in general, activity in the muscles is initiated prior to the time when tension is actually needed. This preliminary tension occurs for two possible reasons. The first is that the muscle may contribute to deceleration of a segment. Second, because of the physiological characteristics of muscle, the contractile component must be activated early to compensate for its elastic properties (see Chapter 2).

Other information about the role of musculature is also of interest. One classic work was completed by Morrison, in which he studied the mechanics of muscle function during locomotion, taking into account active and passive properties and other physiological characteristics. In studying walking at different velocities on both level and ramped surfaces, he was able to determine tension values associated with changes in muscle length. For example, the maximal muscle force, 540 lbs, was generated during a lengthening contraction of the quadriceps muscle. Forces of up to 400 lbs were recorded at contraction rates of up to 6 inches/sec. Similar values were achieved for quadriceps lengthening contractions of approximately 9 inches/sec. Some import should be ascribed to his conclusion that the mechanism of muscle function normally contained a period of muscle lengthening as force increased, followed by an interval of concentric contraction under a decreasing load. In observing that the muscles studied had an excursion range of 3 to 4 inches, Morrison noted that most forces were produced between a mean and maximal operating length. The muscle was normally inactive at shorter lengths (28). That muscle length and type of contraction must be taken into account has frequently been ignored. Cappozzo et al have been among the few who have considered these factors when relating the contribution of muscle tension to the forces in the joints of the lower limb during gait (10).

Some work has also been accomplished that has evaluated the specific role of certain muscular components during gait. Two corollary studies have assessed the role of the ankle plantar flexors during normal locomotion. The results are interesting, in that they reinforce the points made in the previous paragraph regarding the necessity of considering all of the physiological and functional characteristics of muscle. One of the studies evaluated the posterior compartment musculature during the entire support phase of the gait cycle, concluding that the demands in the first half of support are minimal and not required for normal function. During the second half of support, however, the mechanics of gait are such that the muscles act as a controlling force on the forward momentum of the tibia. Subsequently the group actually serves to restrain forward movement of the body (43). Similar findings were independently produced 2 yr later by Sutherland and coworkers, who concluded that the role of the ankle plantar flexors was to contribute to knee and ankle stability, restrain forward rotation of the tibia on the talus, and minimize vertical oscillations of the body's center of mass, with the latter contributing to energy conservation (48). A further discussion of the mechanics of the posterior compartment muscles will be presented in the following section of this chapter on applications of mechanics.

Joint Torques

During walking the torques of interest are those in the ankle, knee, and hip. Although swing phase torques are of some interest, they are of less import than those during stance phase because they are of less magnitude. This is apparent, as shown in Figure 13.8, for all three joints in all three planes. Of the requirements for extension moments at the three joints during early support, those for the hip are greatest, and those for the ankle the least. All moments progress to flexion moments, but their magnitudes vary considerably. Extension moments for the knee and ankle are produced between heel-off and toe-off, apparently for propulsion.

For abduction and adduction the most significant moment involves hip abduction, required for almost the entirety of the support phase. This moment is consistent with the contraction of the gluteus medius and minimus muscles in the institution of the abductor mechanism that accomplishes elevation of the contralateral side of the pelvis. The other feature that should be noted from Figure 13.8 is the magnitude of the moments. The hip abduction and ankle extension moments are the greatest: each reaches approximately 70 ft lbs (94.9 Nm) (9). More recent work has also generated moment data for the lower limb during gait. There are some differences in the magnitudes compared to those shown in the figure, but the general configuration of the curves are the same. For example, Winter has reported peak ankle moments of 150 Nm and knee moments of about 140 Nm (55). The data of Crowninshield, however, agree rather closely with those of Bresler and Frankel. Peak values for some of the trials were reported to be as high as 80 Nm in abduction (13).

Joint Forces

Using engineering methodology in the determination of joint torque, one then may calculate joint forces. Because direct measures of these forces have not generally been possible, indirect means such as those discussed in Chapter 5 have been used. In general, these techniques use a force plate to determine the reaction forces at the foot. Kinematic data are collected simultaneously so that segmental velocities and accelerations can be calculated. Body segment parameter information, specifically the mass, mass center locations, and mass moments of inertia, are estimated via mathematical techniques. Solutions to equations of motion provide forces and moments for the prediction of muscle forces that are then used in the determination of joint contact forces (13). These contact forces (bone-on-bone forces) include joint reaction force and the effect of active forces due to muscle contraction (54).

These analyses involve relatively complex data collection and analysis procedures. Therefore, the amount of data on contact forces during gait is not extensive. The early work of Bresler and Frankel established, as expected, that the greatest component of joint force acts vertically. Essentially similar patterns

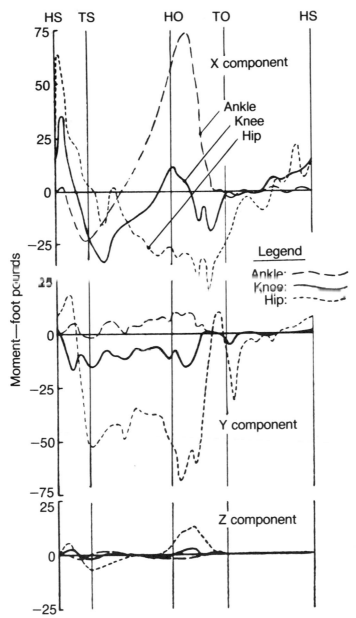

Figure 13.8. Moments at each of the joints of the lower limb during the gait cycle. The X component is for flexion extension, the Y for abduction and adduction, and Z for rotations. See text for further description. (From Bresler B, Frankel JP: The forces and moments in the leg during level walking. *ASME Trans* 72:27–36, 1950.)

exist for all lower limb joints. Forces in the other two directions are considerably less and similar in shape over the duration of the gait cycle (9). Since then, Brand et al and Seireg and Arvikar have performed experiments that show the contact force at the hip to be higher than five times body weight (7, 42). An example of the forces on the femoral head is shown in Figure 13.9. Thus, by using such a complete process, all gravitational, inertial, and muscle forces have been included in the analysis.

These results are remarkably consistent with Rydell's in vivo information

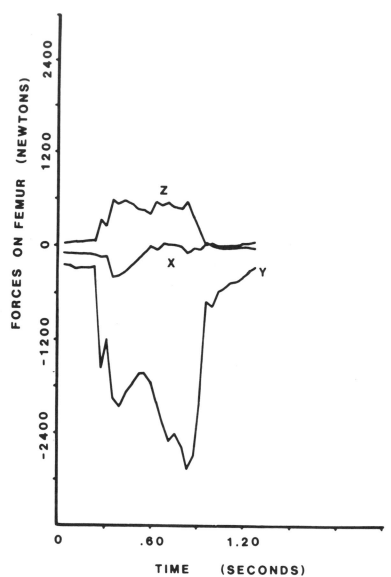

Figure 13.9. Forces on the femoral head during a cycle of level walking in three orthogonal directions. *Y* is vertical, *X* is anteroposterior, and *Z* is mediolateral. (From Brand RA, Crowninshield RD, Johnston RC, Pedersen DR: Forces on the femoral head during activities of daily living. *Iowa Orthop J* 2:43–49, 1982.)

gathered by inserting an instrumented prosthesis into two patients for the specific purpose of measuring hip contact forces. Although the subjects walked with significant perturbances in kinetics and kinematics, the contact forces were reported to be from 1.6 to 3.3 times body weight (40). In view of the differences between the subjects, there thus seems to be reasonable agreement between in vivo and indirect measurement techniques.

Therapists should realize that forces in the lower limb joints are significant during walking. Only a small part of the load is due to body weight; yet, this factor influences the mechanics required for function. Major loading is due to the compressive effect of muscle contraction, so in treatment programs an attempt frequently is made to decrease the muscular requirements. One way is to provide assistive devices so that full weight is not borne on the limb. Peak forces have been shown to be diminished to about 60% of usual upon using a cane (6). Another method to minimize contact forces would be to decrease the velocity of walking. This has the effect of distributing the loading over a longer time interval, avoiding what is known as impulse loading. In addition, decreased velocity lessens the muscular tension requirements, in terms of both the rate of tension development and the total magnitude.

All things considered it is remarkable that the success rates of joint replacements are as high as they are. Not only is the magnitude of loading an important factor, but the number of repetitions required for any semblance of normal function is very high. Thus, considerations related to properties such as material strength and fatigue characteristics must be applied. Surely, further work will help both the surgeon and therapist in the description of the limits that will produce the most effective care.

Applications of Mechanics

Analysis of human locomotion provides an excellent opportunity to discuss principles of mechanical energy. Defined as the ability to perform work or exert force on another body, mechanical energy becomes important in that it is a measure of the efficiency of human function. Although all of the principles to be discussed can be applied to motion of the individual segments, the example used will be the displacements associated with the body's center of mass during the gait cycle.

There are several forms of energy that must be considered. Potential energy is the energy due to gravity, as reflected in the formula PE = mgh, where mass and height are the other important factors. Kinetic energy can be in two forms; translational and rotational. The former is the product of one-half the mass and the square of the velocity. In the latter, mass is replaced with inertia and velocity with angular velocity (54). Given these definitions consider a roller coaster perched at its track's point of maximal elevation. By virtue of position the roller coaster has PE, but by descending to the bottom it has no more (zero height). Rather, kinetic energy now exists so that the coaster can be elevated to the next peak.

These factors, whereby mechanical energy exists either by virtue of position or of motion, allow us to have efficient locomotion. In fact, analysis of the displacement of the center of mass during gait shows similarities with the roller coaster. Refer to Figure 13.10 and note the displacement of the center of mass. Peaks of displacement are reached during single support, while the lowest points are reached during periods of double support. These alternating events using potential and kinetic energy are responsible for our efficiency. Greater and/or more abrupt changes in the displacement of the center of mass would decrease efficiency because more energy expenditure would be required. Caution must be exerted in generalizing these conditions to the center of mass because, as has been pointed out by Winter, energy exchange takes place between body segments. Thus, a more extensive analysis that includes a segment by segment calculation should be performed in order to accurately assess mechanical efficiency (55, 56).

Another application of mechanics to gait can be found in the use of power. Winter has effectively used mechanical principles in analyzing the role of the

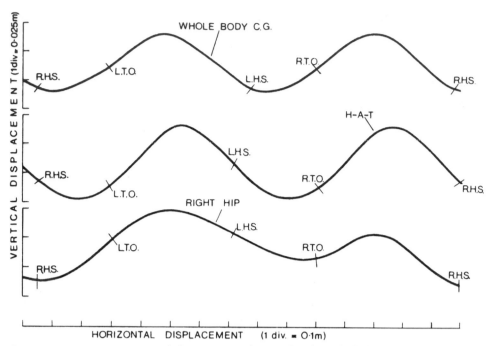

Figure 13.10. Trajectories of the centers of mass for the whole body, the head-arms-trunk (*H-A-T*) segment, and the right hip in the sagittal plane for the gait cycle. (From Cappozzo A, Figura F, Marchetti M: The interplay of muscular and external forces in human ambulation. *J Biomech* 9:35–43, 1976.)

ankle in providing propulsive energy. Figure 13.11 shows power, the product of moment and angular velocity, in the lowest trace. After the foot is flat, a large moment is generated as the leg rotates over the foot, but the product of dorsiflexion velocity and plantar flexion moment is small and negative (A1). Later, however, plantar flexion velocity is rapid and its moment large, resulting in power of 430 W (A2). These facts, coupled with the position of the limb during the terminal phase of support, provide evidence that the plantar flexors are contributing to the potential (upward) and kinetic (forward) energy of the limbs and the upper part of the body.

A clinical note of some import can also be identified by this work. Negative work has been shown to exist throughout the gait cycle, the only exception being when the knee extends slightly during midstance. As a result of these findings, the quadriceps appears to be functioning primarily via eccentric contractions. The therapeutic implications are that perhaps more consideration should be given to eccentric training for the quadriceps muscle. Conversely, because of the concentric role of the ankle plantar flexors, attention should be directed to concentric forms of exercise (55).

Pathokinesiology

Virtually any pathology affecting the lower limbs will have an effect on walking. Both kinematics and kinetics can be slightly to severely modified, although the former is usually far easier to discern clinically. This section will discuss the effects of some pathologies on gait.

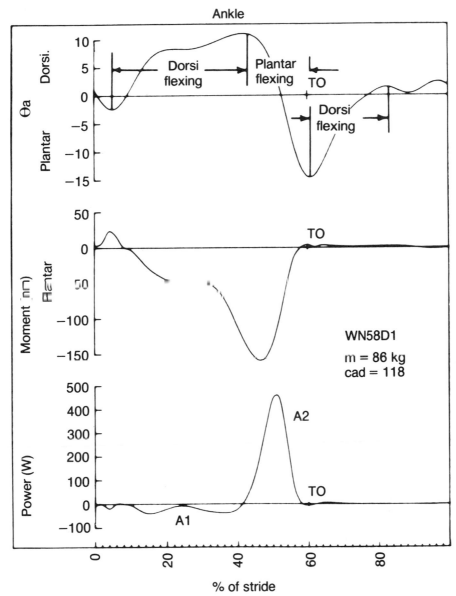

Figure 13.11. Ankle angle, moment, and power for a gait cycle. *TO* is toe off. See text for further description. (From Winter DA: Energy generation and absorption at the ankle and knee during fast, natural, and slow cadences. *Clin Orthop* 175:147–154, 1983.)

Neurological Disorders

Central. One condition that has received considerable attention is cerebral palsy. Numerous reports are available in the literature as to the gait abnormalities produced by this condition. The exact perturbances are related to the nature of involvement. For example, the 25 patients evaluated by Bleck showed patterns of either hip flexion-internal rotation with flexed, hyperextended, or normal knees (5). Sutherland and Cooper reported on the crouch gait of four patients with spastic diplegia. Their kinematic and kinetic analysis demonstrated the effects of exaggerated knee flexion and the requirement of increased dorsiflexion of the ankle. Extensive arm swinging and increased vertical trunk displacements were seen in all subjects. A representation of the patterns of normal and diplegic subjects is shown in Figure 13.12. Note the distinct differences in the line of application of the floor reaction force, such that efficiency of the cerebral palsied individual would be severely hampered. Also, the line of force application is markedly displaced from the centers of rotation of the hip and the knee, particularly early in the stance phase for the hip and late in stance for the knee. An abnormality of knee kinematics is shown in Figure 13.13. For the patients included in this analysis, knee torque was more than six times the value recorded for normals and never approached the normal extension moment occurring during part of the gait cycle (47).

Because of the pathology or the moment requirement, these patients would also produce abnormal EMG patterns. Both level and duration of pattern of muscle activity are distorted. Frequently, EMG data are a primary focus of gait studies of those with cerebral palsy. The foot and ankle complex has drawn much attention, apparently because of the effect on the remainder of the limb and the potential for correction of the kinematics and kinetics of gait. Hoffer and Perry have been very active in pursuing this approach with the cerebral palsied patient and have identified abnormal muscular patterns associated with pes equinus, varus, valgus, and calcaneus. For example, equinus results from premature or prolonged activity of either the gastrocnemius or soleus. Varus can be caused by continuous activity of the anterior or posterior tibialis or phase reversal of the posterior tibialis to swing (19).

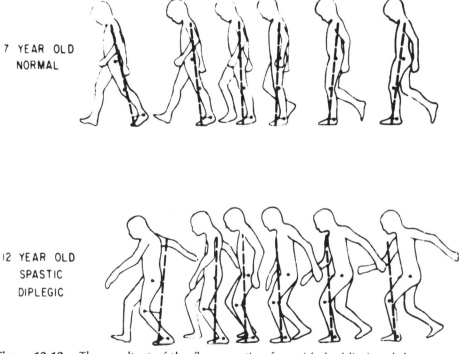

7 YEAR OLD
NORMAL

12 YEAR OLD
SPASTIC
DIPLEGIC

Figure 13.12. The resultant of the floor reaction force (*dashed line*) and the associated kinematics for the two specified subjects. See text for further description. (From Sutherland DH, Cooper L: The pathomechanics of progressive crouch gait in spastic diplegia. *Orthop Clin North Am* 9:143–154, 1978.)

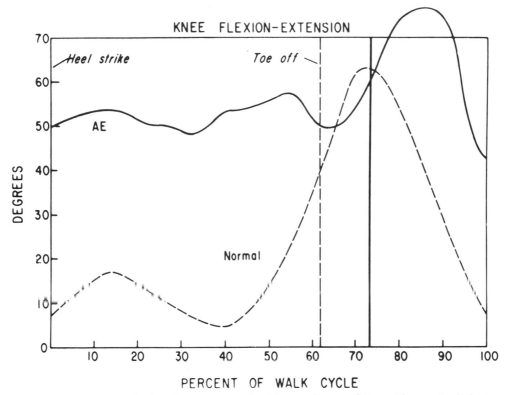

Figure 13.13. Knee flexion for one normal subject and one subject with spastic diplegia. Note that knee flexion of 50 to 60° is maintained throughout the gait cycle of the patient. (From Sutherland DH, Cooper L: The pathomechanics of progressive crouch gait in spastic diplegia. *Orthop Clin North Am* 9:143–154, 1978.) Has limited extension ability.

Using the information derived from EMG, success can be achieved with modifying the gait pattern by means of surgical transfer of the distal muscle attachment. The literature supports the use of these transfers, particularly in the ankle and foot, as a means of improving both the temporal and distance factors associated with gait kinematics. For example, one of the transfers that has been effective for varus is the anterior transposition of the posterior tibialis muscle. However, a key element in the success of a muscle transfer is that the muscle should be active during the appropriate phase of the gait cycle. Otherwise the muscle has to be retrained to function during a different temporal sequence, and in this case, the transfer does not always meet with success (36).

Improved knowledge of the disrupted kinematic and kinetic parameters has been of significant assistance in facilitating effective treatment of the patient with cerebral palsy. As more efficient systems become available to the kinesiologist/ investigator/clinician, even further improvements in the walking patterns of these patients can be anticipated (15).

Another common pathology that has pronounced effects on gait is hemiplegia. As for cerebral palsy, numerous studies have been made of the alterations in both the kinematics and kinetics of gait. As anticipated, because of the variability associated with the location and magnitude of the lesion, the effects on gait cannot be easily categorized. One of the most complete analyses, however, included kinematics and multiple channels of EMG for hemiparetic patients. In nine of the patients, the calf muscles were prematurely activated during stance.

In another nine, the EMG was absent or extremely low for two or more of the muscles examined. Although in four others no common pattern could be identified, the remaining four demonstrated coactivation of several or all of the muscles (24).

These results point out the difficulty with generalizing changes across patients. Rather, the most appropriate mechanism would be to determine which muscles were involved for each patient and attempt to alter the temporal sequencing and/or level of activation by some therapeutic means. An attempt to do so has been accomplished by Waters and associates. EMG was recorded during gait and used as a criterion measure for determining the appropriateness of muscle transfers in equinus or equinovarus deformities of hemiplegic patients. In their sample of 27 patients, preoperative activation patterns almost always were found to be abnormal in the gastrocnemius, soleus, tibialis posterior, flexor hallucis longus, flexor digitorum longus, peroneus brevis, and anterior tibialis. As might have been anticipated, the phase of activity was not altered after the surgery; thus, similar cautions as for cerebral palsied patients are important, i.e., alter only the muscles that are in phase with the desired movements (52).

Other work has evaluated the kinetic and temporal features associated with the gait pattern of the hemiplegic. Findings indicated that the support times of the two limbs were asymmetrical, with those of the affected limb being 10 to 15% percent shorter. As measured by the vertical component, floor reaction force patterns were distinctly different across patients. Finding that the magnitudes of the forces for the two legs were different is important because it represents a deviation from the normal pattern (12). In regard to temporal variables, Brandstater et al have shown that hemiplegic gait is best characterized by the symmetry of single limb support times rather than by the values for each limb. The best indicators of motor recovery are the symmetry of swing phases and walking speed (8).

Other analyses have been applied to those with disturbed motor control, including the parkinsonian gait. In patients with Parkinson's disease, the mean velocity and stride length are markedly reduced, while mean cycle time is increased when compared to normals. Stride length is about one-half of that for normals, and velocity only 0.56 as opposed to 1.36 m/sec for normals. Double stance time is also significantly increased: 25% of the cycle as compared to only 11% for normals. These findings may be expected on the basis of the perceived need for an adequate base of support. Decreased range of motion has also been noted, as may be seen with slower velocities of walking (23).

Peripheral. Finally, other paralytic conditions can alter gait. The gluteus medius gait has been previously discussed. Loss of the gluteus maximus produces a trunk lurch in a posterior direction during weight bearing. The necessity for such a lurch is due to the patient's insufficient hip extensor power used to control pelvic flexion moment created by trunk weight over the fixed lower limb. In order to influence mechanics, a patient throws the trunk posteriorly so that the line of gravity, during receipt of body weight by the supporting surface, falls posterior to the hip. As a result, the moment due to trunk weight produces pelvic extension and is controlled by the anterior capsule or flexor musculature of the hip joint.

Complete or partial quadriceps paralysis is relatively rare and usually does not have a great effect on gait. This is because the knee can be maintained in complete extension or hyperextension during weight bearing by relying upon tension in the posterior capsule. Loss of both hip and knee extensors is a different matter, however, because the line of gravity cannot simultaneously fall posterior to the hip and anterior to the knee. A frequent modification made by patients with combined losses is to press posteriorly on the thigh with the hand during the weight-bearing phase of the gait cycle.

One other loss that is of import is the gait alteration required by paralysis of the anterior compartment of the lower leg. Because the only available dorsiflexors of the ankle reside here, paralysis in a patient will result in the inability to clear the foot from the ground during the swing phase. Complete paralysis can be devastating, but assists by means of functional electrical stimulation or ankle foot orthoses are usually extremely helpful.

Musculoskeletal Dysfunction

Antalgic Patterns. Orthopedic and/or musculoskeletal dysfunction can also have a distinct effect in modifying the gait pattern of any given patient. Witness the effect of pain in any of the joints of the lower limb, noticing in particular the changes in kinematics as well as in stride parameters and temporal sequences (51). Compare, for example, the sagittal plane motion in Figure 13.14 with the normal pattern shown in Figure 13.6. Generally the severity of the kinematic, kinetic, and temporal sequences of events can be related to the degree of involvement of an individual joint. Such changes are typical of the patient with degenerative joint disease. Range of motion usually is limited in all directions. One interesting finding of potential import is that a study of patients with pathological knees revealed no correlation between passive motion available and the amount of motion used during gait (18).

Rate of loading will also be decreased among patients with limb pain during gait in order to avoid further discomfort. Assistive devices may also be advocated by both therapist and patient to decrease the magnitude of loading. Assessment of the deviation from the normal pattern will need to be determined on an individual basis, and therapeutic recommendations should be based on a patient's clinical circumstances.

Amputees. Other clinical entities have been known to alter gait characteristics. Any lower limb amputee in the early stages of rehabilitation will demonstrate

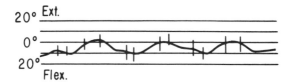

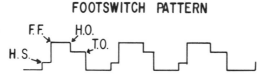

Figure 13.14. Sagittal plane electrogoniogram for a patient with hip pathology. Compared to Figure 13.6 the range of motion is extremely limited. Footswitch events are the same as those for Figure 13.6. (From Wadsworth JB, Smidt GL, Johnston RC: Gait characteristics of subjects with hip disease. *Phys Ther* 52:829–837, 1972.)

asymmetries and other modifications. Different problems will be associated with each level of amputation, but generally such a patient will have to learn to control a new mass (body segment parameter) with appropriate forces (kinetics) in an appropriate temporal sequence to arrive at a pattern (kinematics) perceived to be correct. Walking velocity will also be a factor, as has been demonstrated by Hoy et al in a study of children with lower limb amputations (20). Although it is encouraging that normal EMG patterns are possible with the use of patellar tendon-bearing prostheses, other forms have produced abnormal patterns, such as simultaneous contractions of antagonistic muscles (16).

Finally, mention should be made that orthoses can be extremely important in modifying gait characteristics. Those that use a posterior stop at the ankle can compensate for the inability to actively dorsiflex the ankle during swing phase. Mediolateral stability can also be provided by T straps that are attached to the medial or lateral upright. Other ankle foot orthoses (AFO) are made of plastics or laminates with material properties that can be used to control ankle dorsiflexion and mediolateral shifts in the foot. Furthermore, these materials are appropriate in terms of mass because they provide little change in the total mass of the body segment to which they are applied. No matter the material or the application of the orthosis, the intention is to assist the patient with the control or exertion of appropriate moments during the gait cycle. Design, evaluation, and reevaluation of an orthosis should be based on this intention.

Numerous other deviations from normal gait will be encountered in the clinic. Regardless of cause, the responsibility of the therapist is to determine which characteristics are altered. For example, is decreased stance time due to joint pain, a lack of range of motion, inability of the patient to generate an adequate torque for control of the desired position, or other factors? Finally, logical, scientifically based treatments can be implemented for purposes of modifying the altered characteristics and of returning the patient to a more normal pattern. Sufficient attention to all of the factors involved, and their potential interaction, will be necessary to assure the best and most efficient results.

SUMMARY

This chapter has discussed kinesiological factors associated with posture and gait. Relevant mechanics have been applied while using principles presented in earlier sections of this volume. Selected pathologies and their effects on gait have been discussed and implications for evaluation and treatment reviewed.

References

1. Andersson BJG, Ortengren R, Nachemson AL: The sitting posture: An electromyographic and discometric study. *Orthop Clin North Am* 6:105–120, 1975.
2. Bampton S: A Guide to the Visual Examination of Pathological Gait. Temple University Rehabilitation Research and Training Center No. 8. Philadelphia, Moss Rehabilitation Hospital, 1979.
3. Basmajian JV: *Muscles Alive: Their Functions Revealed by Electromyography*, ed 4. Baltimore, Williams & Wilkins, 1979.
4. Baumann JU, Hanggi EL: A. A method of gait analysis for daily orthopaedic practice. *J Med Eng Technol* 1:86–91, 1977.
5. Bleck EE: Postural and gait abnormalities caused by hip-flexion deformity in spastic cerebral palsy. *J Bone Joint Surg [Am]* 53:1468–1488, 1971.
6. Brand RA, Crowninshield RD: The effect of cane use on hip contact force. *Clin Orthop* 147:181–184, 1980.
7. Brand RA, Crowninshield RD, Johnston RC, Pedersen DR: Forces on the femoral head during activities of daily living. *Iowa Orthop J* 2:43–49, 1982.

8. Brandstater ME, de Bruin H, Gowland C, Clark BM: Hemiplegic gait: analysis of temporal variables. *Arch Phys Med Rehabil* 54:583–587, 1983.
9. Bresler B, Frankel JP: The forces and moments in the leg during level walking. *ASME Trans* 72:27–36, 1950.
10. Cappozzo A, Figura F, Marchetti M: The interplay of muscular and external forces in human ambulation. *J Biomech* 9:35–43, 1976.
11. Carlsöö S: *How Man Moves: Kinesiological Studies and Methods.* London, William Heinemann, 1972.
12. Carlsöö S, Dahllof A-G, Holm J: Kinetic analysis of the gait in patients with hemiparesis and in patients with intermittent claudication. *Scand J Rehabil Med* 6:166–179, 1974.
13. Crowninshield RD, Johnston RC, Andrews RG, Brand RA: A biomechanical investigation of the human hip. *J Biomech* 11:75–85, 1978.
14. Eberhart H, Inman V, Bresler B: The principal elements in human locomotion. In: Klopsteg P, Wilson PD, et al (eds): *Human Limbs and Their Substitutes.* New York, McGraw-Hill, 1974 (reprinted with bibliography. New York, Hafner Publishing Co, 1968).
15. Gage JR: Gait analysis for decision-making in cerebral palsy. *Bull Hosp Joint Dis Orthop Inst* 43:147–163, 1983.
16. Grevsten S, Stalberg E: Electromyographic study of muscular activity in the amputation stump while walking with PTB- and PTB-suction prosthesis. *Upsala J Med Sci* 80:103–112, 1975.
17. Grieve GP: The sacroiliac joint. *Physiotherapy* 62:384–100, 1976.
18. Gyory AN, Chao EYS, Stauffer RN: Functional evaluation of normal and pathologic knees during gait. *Arch Phys Med Rehabil* 57:571–577, 1976.
19. Hoffer MM, Perry J: Pathodynamics of gait alterations in cerebral palsy and the significance of kinetic electromyography in evaluating foot and ankle problems. *Foot Ankle* 4:128–134, 1983.
20. Hoy MG, Whiting WC, Zernicke RF: Stride kinematics and knee joint kinetics of child amputee gait. *Arch Phys Med Rehabil* 63:74–82, 1982.
21. Joseph J, McColl I: Electromyography of muscles of posture: posterior vertebral muscles in males. *J Physiol* 157:33–37, 1961.
22. Keegan JJ: Alterations to the lumbar curve related to posture and seating. *J Bone Joint Surg [Am]* 35:567–589, 1953.
23. Knutsson E: An analysis of parkinsonian gait. *Brain* 95:475–486, 1972.
24. Knutsson E, Richards C: Different types of disturbed motor control in gait of hemiparetic patients. *Brain* 102:405–430, 1979.
25. Lehmkuhl LD, Smith LK: *Brunnstrom's Clinical Kinesiology*, ed 4. Philadelphia, FA Davis, 1983.
26. Magora A: Investigation of the relation between low back pain and occupation. 3. Physical requirements: sitting, standing and weight lifting. *Industr Med Surg* 41:5–9, 1972.
27. Mann RA, Hagy JL, White V, Liddell D: The initiation of gait. *J Bone Joint Surg [Am]* 61:232–239, 1979.
28. Morrison JB: The mechanics of muscle function in locomotion. *J Biomech* 3:431–451, 1970.
29. Murray MP: Gait as a total pattern of movement. *Am J Phys Med* 46:290–333, 1967.
30. Murray MP, Kory RC, Clarkson BH, Sepic SB: A comparison of free and fast speed walking patterns of normal men. *Am J Phys Med* 45:8–24, 1966.
31. Nachemson AL: Lumbar intradiscal pressure. In: Jayson MIV (ed): *The Lumbar Spine and Back Pain.* Kent, England, Pitman Medical, 1980.
32. Norkin CC, Levangie PK: *Joint Structure and Function: A Comprehensive Analysis.* Philadelphia, FA Davis, 1983.
33. Okada M: An electromyographic estimation of the relative muscular load in different human postures. *J Hum Ergol* 1:75–93, 1972.
34. Perry J: The mechanics of walking: a clinical interpretation. *Phys Ther* 47:778–801, 1964.
35. Perry J, Antonelli MS, Ford W: Analysis of knee joint forces during flexed-knee stance. *J Bone Joint Surg [Am]* 57:961–967, 1975.
36. Perry J, Hoffer MM: Preoperative and postoperative dynamic electromyography as an aid in planning tendon transfers in children with cerebral palsy. *J Bone Joint Surg [Am]* 59:531–537, 1977.

37. Portnoy H, Morin F: Electromyographic study of postural muscles in various positions and movements. *Am J Physiol* 186:122–126, 1956.
38. Rasch PJ, Burke RK: *Kinesiology and Applied Anatomy: The Science of Human Movement,* ed 6. Philadelphia, Lea & Febiger, 1978.
39. Root ML, Orien WP, Weed JH: *Normal and Abnormal Function of the Foot.* Los Angeles, Clinical Biomechanics Corp., 1977.
40. Rydell N: Biomechanics of the hip joint. *Clin Orthop* 92:6–15, 1973.
41. Schlegel KF: Sitzschaden und deren Vermeidung durch eine neuartig Sitzkonstruction. *Med Klin* 51:1940–1942, 1956.
42. Seireg A, Arvikar RJ: The prediction of muscular load sharing and joint forces in the lower extremities during walking. *J Biomech* 8:89–102, 1975.
43. Simon SR, Mann RA, Hagy JL, Larsen LJ: Role of the posterior calf muscles in normal gait. *J Bone Joint Surg [Am]* 60:465–472, 1978.
44. Smidt GL: Hip motion and related factors in walking. *Phys Ther* 51:9–21, 1971.
45. Smith JW: The act of standing. *Acta Orthop Scand* 23:159–168, 1953.
46. Soderberg GL, Blanco MK, Cosentino TL, Kurdelmeier KA: An EMG analysis of posterior trunk musculature during flat and anteriorly inclined sitting. Human Factors (submitted for publication).
47. Sutherland DH, Cooper L: The pathomechanics of progressive crouch gait in spastic diplegia. *Orthop Clin North Am* 9:143–154, 1978.
48. Sutherland DH, Cooper L, Daniel D: The role of the ankle plantar flexors in normal walking. *J Bone Joint Surg [Am]* 62:354–363, 1980.
49. Sutherland DH, Olshen R, Cooper L, Woo SL-Y: The development of mature gait. *J Bone Joint Surg [Am]* 62:336–353, 1980.
50. Svenssen HO, Andersson GBJ: Low back pain in 40–47 year old men: Work history and work environment factors. *Spine* 8:272–276, 1983.
51. Wadsworth JB, Smidt GL, Johnston RC: Gait characteristics of subjects with hip disease. *Phys Ther* 52:829–837, 1972.
52. Waters RL, Frazier J, Garland DE, Jordan C, Perry J: Electromyographic gait analysis before and after operative treatment for hemiplegic equinus and equinovarus deformity. *J Bone Joint Surg [Am]* 64:284–288, 1982.
53. Winter DA: The locomotion laboratory as a clinical assessment system. *Med Prog Technol* 4:95–106, 1976.
54. Winter DA: *Biomechanics of Human Movement.* New York, Wiley, 1979.
55. Winter DA: Energy generation and absorption at the ankle and knee during fast, natural, and slow cadences. *Clin Orthop* 175:147–154, 1983.
56. Winter DA, Quanbury AO, Reimer GD: Analysis of instantaneous energy of normal gait. *J Biomech* 9:253–257, 1976.
57. Zarrugh MY, Radcliffe CW: Computer generation of human gait kinematics. *J Biomech* 12:99–111, 1979.

14

Ergonomics

Some individuals, industries, and countries have had a longstanding interest in the effect of the work environment on the individual. Now, agencies such as the National Institute for Occupational Safety and Health (NIOSH) are playing a more active role, and ergonomics has begun to receive considerable emphasis. Furthermore, unions and workers have become more cognizant of the work environment, demanding greater attention to the effects of the workplace on the employees. According to Meister the need for human factors should increase in the future (38).

The workplace is important because of the great amount of time spent there. The greatest implications are probably for those persons who are required to handle objects or materials, particularly if lifting is performed. Specific implications exist for therapists in that the focus of the treatment should take into account the patient's intention to return to work. In fact, the clinical education of Danish physical therapists now includes a training period studying postures and work methods in a factory environment (8). In addition, rehabilitation will probably be considered successful only if work can be adequately performed. This chapter does not intend to discuss all aspects of ergonomics. Rather, selected aspects that have implication for the therapist are presented.

DEFINITIONS AND SCOPE

Several different terms are associated with the performance of human work. Ergonomics, a term which originated over 120 years ago, means the laws of work (15). More broadly interpreted as the study of work, this area includes the application of knowledge of the life sciences to well-being and work performance (51). To apply ergonomics, the variability associated with human form and function must be taken into account. Some factors to include are height, weight, skills, strength, and age. These factors need to be related to work requirements such as sitting height, arm reach, mass of an object to be moved, visual field, and other such considerations. Thus, the focus of ergonomics is on the interaction of work and people, i.e., physiologic and environmental stresses, and such things as complex psychomotor tasks. The primary intent is to establish ways to reduce injuries, accidents, and fatigue and to improve work performance (15).

Human factors and ergonomics are terms often used interchangeably. Both describe the interaction between the operator and the job demands, and both attempt to reduce the stress in the workplace. Human factors, however, has sometimes focused more on the man-machine interface. Frequently called human engineering, the primary goal is to reduce human error. For practical purposes, all of these terms can be considered synonymous.

Others have chosen to use different terminology. According to Chaffin and Andersson the discipline of occupational biomechanics can be defined as "the study of the physical interaction of workers with their tools, machines and materials so as to enhance the worker's performance while minimizing the risk of future musculoskeletal disorders." As a part of the general field of biomechanics, this specialized area requires the application of the laws of physics and engineering to the human body when in the work environment. Thus, ergonomics or human factors tends to be a much broader area than occupational biomechanics, yet the two are highly complementary (11). The text entitled *The Biomechanical Basis of Ergonomics* is perhaps evidence of this fact (50).

WORKSPACE AND ENVIRONMENT

There are a number of approaches possible when applying design to workspace. In this volume general considerations will be presented, followed by more specific guidelines.

In general, body segment parameters serve as the basis for defining the needs of the workspace. Therefore, segment length, weight, location of the mass center, and moment of inertia and radius of gyration are of interest. These properties and the sources for data relative to the body segments have been discussed in Chapter 1. Although little data is available, enough material exists for use in analyses using models of the human body and in estimating the requirements of the workspace.

The design of the workspace must take into account numerous factors. Design should not be used on the average but rather for one extreme or another. Ideally, the workspace should be adjustable, for purposes of accommodating for differences in body height and individual segment length. Most frequent examples are accommodations for short and long legs and allowances necessary for gripping of instruments or tools by individuals with markedly different size hands. Reaching should all be ahead of the shoulder line, and work height should be modified so that the viewing angle is directed slightly downward. Webb suggests that to assess any workspace, determine what the task involves, measure the reach and height conditions, and compare these measurements to existing standards (51). A sample of the guidelines is shown in Figure 14.1.

No matter the workplace or workspace, the working height is of great importance. This is true for both sitting and standing work postures. Concern should be on the position of the head and neck, the lumbar spine, and the shoulder. Each of these segments will be considered in the following paragraphs.

For either the standing or the seated work posture, the best height for performance of work with the hands is a few centimeters below elbow level. Grandjean is rather specific about the dimensions, stating 5 to 10 cm for standing and a few centimeters for sitting. If at all possible, work stations that can accommodate for individual needs are most desirable. Examples are adjustable chairs and the provision of various sizes of stools or boxes to elevate the standing worker so that the shorter person can reach the working surface (22).

Alterations also need to be made, depending upon the task. Use of a typewriter, for example, should be done with the work surface about 10% lower than that used for writing (22). Another modification of the workspace that should be considered is the inclination of the work surface towards the subject. For standardly assumed postures such as in a school and office, inclinations of 10 to 30° are recommended. This modification purportedly has positive effects on the lumbar spine, brings the line of vision into a better position, and eases

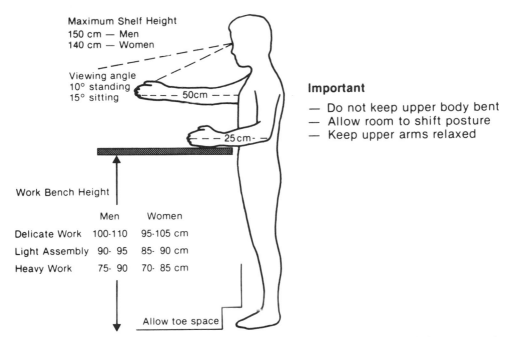

Maximum Shelf Height
150 cm — Men
140 cm — Women

Viewing angle
10° standing
15° sitting   — — 50cm — —

— — 25 cm- —

Important

— Do not keep upper body bent
— Allow room to shift posture
— Keep upper arms relaxed

Work Bench Height

	Men	Women
Delicate Work	100-110	95-105 cm
Light Assembly	90- 95	85- 90 cm
Heavy Work	75- 90	70- 85 cm

Allow toe space

Figure 14.1. An example of the dimensions of the workspace required for men and women. (From Webb RDG: *Industrial Ergonomics*. Ontario, The Industrial Accident Prevention Association, 1982.)

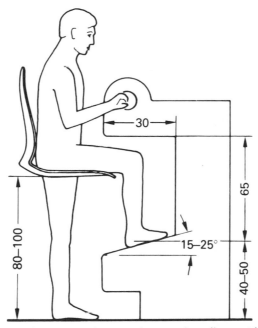

30

65

80–100

15–25°

40–50

Figure 14.2. Suggested dimensions for a workspace that allows either sitting or standing. (From Grandjean E: *Fitting the Task to the Man: An Ergonomic Approach.* London, Taylor and Francis Ltd., 1982.)

tension in the supporting musculature of the cervical spine (36). In support of this concept Eastman and Kamon also found less fatigue and discomfort when the surface was slanted at angles of 12 and 24°, the latter producing the most effect (14). Angles of up to 75° are considered advisable when such things as

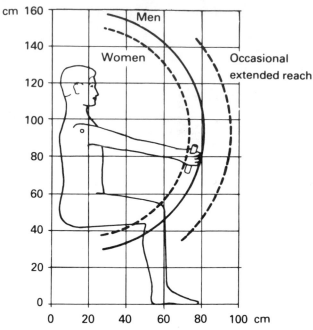

Figure 14.3. Suggested arc in which vertical grasp can be performed. Included here are the extreme percentiles, and therefore the data pertain to even small men and women. (From Grandjean E: *Fitting the Task to the Man: An Ergonomic Approach.* London, Taylor and Francis Ltd., 1982.)

technical drawing are attempted (22). One other alternative that is advisable to consider is a workspace that allows either sitting or standing. Such an arrangement is shown in Figure 14.2. Although allowances for varying postures are created by this arrangement, the appearance of many work stations of this nature does not seem likely in the near future.

Considerations in design and use of workspace should also take into account the reach requirements. In general, work should usually be done within a distance of 25 cm of the body. Occasional work is acceptable up to a distance of 50 cm. More complete information is provided if an arc of movement is described that will indicate the positions in which grasp can be capably performed, as shown in Figure 14.3. Note that the average reach is about 7 cm greater for men than for women. As indicated earlier, extension of the shoulders should be avoided, even though it is satisfactory to allow occasional reaching beyond the normal arc of movement. Other more specific information on height of reach and operating space for the legs is available in the text of Grandjean (22).

In any workspace, other factors such as lighting, noise, and air quality must be appropriate. Because they have little impact on considerations for the therapist, they will not be discussed in this volume. The other issues discussed in this section are, however, well within the purview of the therapist. Yet, they are frequently not considered in either the plan of patient management or in the treatment. Effective discharge planning should include inquiries as to the work environment and, as necessary, recommendations should be developed and forwarded to the person or agency responsible. If workspace is inappropriately designed, the positive effects garnered from therapy may be reversed in a very short time.

POSTURES AND SEATING
Work Position

The most common positions for work are standing and sitting. Many jobs require, however, some degree of movement, either aperiodic or of a repetitive nature. Standing postures that require movement should adhere to the guidelines in the previous section and in the materials handling section of this chapter. When standing is more static, fatigue can be a potential problem, particularly in the lower extremity. Allowing for movement but avoiding stressful situations for body parts is a common recommendation. Other suggestions are to provide armrests and/or provide for sitting, at least occasionally. Efficiency will be increased, and awkward or fatiguing postures will be avoided if properly designed tools are used.

Specific joints are especially susceptible to injury because of work postures. The most commonly affected are the cervical and lumbar spines and the shoulder. The cervical spine is often subjected to poor positioning because of improper workspace design. The location of the work surface is most commonly too low, requiring a flexion moment of the head and cervical spine. Seat height and distance from the work surface are also influencing factors, as is a table that is too low.

Chaffin and Andersson have determined the effect of the angle of forward inclination on the force required in the neck extensors. Considering this force in relation to the neck extension "strength," they have determined that for 30° of flexion, the muscle force is at 50% of the force value necessary to hold the neck at an inclination of 90° (11) (Fig. 14.4). The tension required to support the head and neck at any inclination thus may be a major factor in subjective reports of discomfort. Surely these problems are frequently encountered by therapists evaluating and treating musculoskeletal disorders.

The low back is probably the area of the body most frequently subjected to disorders, many of which arise from improper work positions or job requirements. Any posture requiring the maintenance of a trunk flexion moment should be modified. This can usually be accomplished by elevating the work height. However, according to Chaffin and Andersson, most men and 85 to 90% of women should be capable of tolerating, without adverse effects, forward flexion of the trunk to 20° (11). Further flexion to 30° increases the moment markedly, in turn increasing the tension requirement, and affecting the potential endurance time. Thus, the time that workers are able to hold the posture is dramatically decreased from about 13 min at 25% of their exertion level to less than 4 min at approximately 35% of their exertion level (28).

Another area subjected to musculoskeletal dysfunction is the shoulder. Degenerative tendinitis in biceps brachii and supraspinatus muscles has been reported in subjects in which arm elevation is required (25). Acute tendinitis is also a possibility. Furthermore, fatigue has been shown to be significant when elevated arm work is required. For example, at 30° of abduction, more than an hour of work can be performed without significant fatigue. At 90° only about 10 minutes is tolerable before the onset of severe pain (10). An additional factor is the reach requirement of the task. The greater the mass to be manipulated and the greater the frequency of the task, the more difficulty the shoulder is likely to encounter. One mechanism to counteract potentially harmful effects is to allow support at the elbow, reducing the moment requirement at the shoulder. This procedure usually drastically limits the mobility of the total arm, making this a

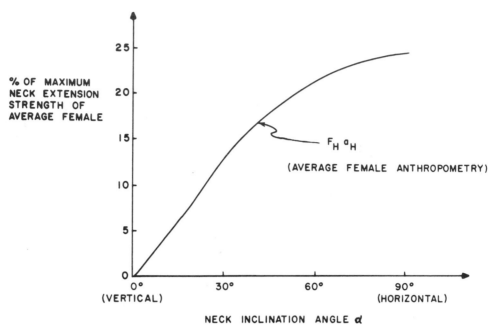

Figure 14.4. Predicted proportion of neck muscle strength to support the head of an average female at varied inclination angles. (From Chaffin DB, Andersson GBJ: *Occupational Biomechanics*. New York, J Wiley & Sons, 1984.)

potentially unacceptable alternative. Other adjustments in the work posture may be necessitated by the specific task involved, for example, if rotation of the forearm is required. In this case elbow flexion may be used to facilitate the ability of the subject to exert a rotational moment. Another example of a modification may be during push-pull operations, when trunk fixation may be helpful.

Seating

Assumption of a seated posture has been thought to be desirable in the work situation because of the ability of this posture to reduce fatigue and improve efficiency. Surely the physiological demands are less when compared to standing. Thus the question arose as to the best sitting posture to assume while performing work. Several advantages, in addition to energy considerations, have been attached to the sitting posture. First is that load bearing is removed from the joints of the lower limb. Simultaneously, greater stability is provided, particularly while performing tasks requiring greater degrees of visual and motor control. Furthermore, fewer demands are made on the vascular system because the lower limbs are placed in a more favorable position (11). Conversely, prolonged slackening of the abdominal musculature and the purported ill effect of flexion of the lumbar spine, affecting digestion and breathing, could be considered as disadvantages (22).

In comparison with standing, the other most frequent posture assumed, the primary impact appears to be on the changes in the lumbar spine. According to Nachemson et al, sitting with the back unsupported causes kyphosis of the lumbar spine, placing stress on the posterior structures of the back (39). Evidence exists that changes do occur in the kinematics of the lumbar spine. In one study the lumbar lordosis decreased by an average of 38°. Although some changes did occur intervertebrally, the majority were due to a posterior rotation of the pelvis (2). As a result, several techniques have been used to alter the spine configuration so that lordosis is maintained during sitting. One of these is the addition of a lumbar support, which has been shown by Majeske and Buchanan to tilt the pelvis anteriorly and the trunk posteriorly (35). Thus, the lumbar spine moves from a position of lesser lordosis toward one of greater lordosis. Andersson et al found that the lumbar spine curve resembled the standing curve when a support 4 cm thick was added between the spine and the supporting surface (2).

Keegan also evaluated changes in the lumbar curve in relationship to sitting postures. Using radiographs he was able to establish the interactions of the thigh and pelvic segments and to study the effects on the lumbar spine. Of some interest was that the normal curve of the lumbar spine is at thigh-trunk and knee angles of 135° (29). Schlegel, as cited by Brunswic, also recommended tilting the whole seat forward (9). Developing a more unique solution, Kroemer suggested that the posteriormost portion of the seat be wedged up by 30° tilting the pelvis forwards and allowing maintenance of lumbar lordosis (31). More recently, Mandal reinforced these concepts, stating that the sitting posture in which reading and writing is done causes 4.8 cm of "extension of the back muscles. Tilting the chair surface 15° anteriorly and inclining the work surface diminishes this extension to only 0.7 cm (36). However, many subjects have found comfort, entry, and egress from one particular chair brand less than optimal (12). Bendix and Biering-Sorenson also evaluated the posture of the trunk when subjects sat on forward inclining seats. Changes, measured by means of bony landmarks, were evaluated at inclinations of 5°, 10°, and 15°. With increased seat angles, the lumbar spine moved towards more lordosis, one-third of the change occurring in the spine and two-thirds in the hip joints. However, the posture of the cervical spine appeared unaffected by the changes in seat angles, and no systematic changes in the back occurred over the 1-h test interval (7). Most recently, Brunswic analyzed the impact of seat design during unsupported sitting. In essence, a linear relationship between the percentage of lumbar flexion and the angles of the hip and knees was established (9).

Two results from the changes in the kinematics of the lumbar spine deserve comment. The first is the effect of sitting postures upon interdiscal pressure. These pressures have been discussed to some degree in the chapter on the trunk. Among the most interesting work is that of Andersson et al. A graphic depiction of their results is shown in Figure 14.5. Note that all of the sitting posture pressures exceed those recorded during standing. The results are most probably due to an increase in the moment produced by the trunk as the pelvis is rotated posteriorly and the lumbar spine and trunk are rotated forward, and by deformation in the disc due to the decrease in lordosis. Although not shown in the figure, pressures can be markedly decreased by the use of a backrest, particularly if the backrest is posteriorly inclined 10° or more from the vertical (4). The use of armrests, and, as commented earlier, lumbar support cushions, also decrease interdiscal pressures (3).

The other primary effect of the change in spine kinematics induced by sitting is manifested in changes in the EMG activity of the erector spinae musculature. EMG studies such as those by Fountain et al and Lundervold evaluated specific segments of the musculature or evaluated the level of EMG activity when subjects were performing in the work environment (18, 34). The latter investigator found that extensor activity increased up to the maximum test time of ½ hour. The study also established that with angular changes of the knee the activity stopped,

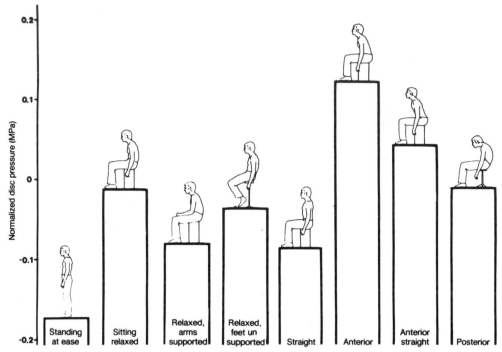

Figure 14.5.   Mean values for normalized interdiscal pressure for various postures. (From Andersson GBJ, Ortengren R, Nachemson A, Elfstrom G: Lumbar disc pressure and myoelectric back muscle activity during sitting. I. Studies on an experimental chair. *Scand J Rehabil Med* 3:104–114, 1974.)

provided that the foot was flat on the floor. In general, however, the level of muscle activity, as measured by EMG, is similar when standing is compared to sitting. Relative to activity produced by maximal isometric contraction the levels are in the range of 2 to 10%. Although relatively low, the long durations of activity required to maintain postures indicate that the levels are of some import when efficiency and energy are considered. Any method that will decrease the flexion moment will decrease the need for active muscle tension. Included would be "slumping," so that passive posterior elements or the discs would assume a supportive role. Anterior arm support or backrests would be two other means of minimizing the flexion moment.

Most EMG data have been derived during studies of the influence of a lumbar support and/or degree of backrest inclination. Knutsson et al analyzed the mechanics and collected intramuscular EMG data from the T12-L1 erector spinae. In asymptomatic subjects 20 to 46 years of age a backrest angle at 110° with the seat was found to give lower EMG than backrests at either 90 or 100° (30). Andersson et al investigated the optimal parameters for sitting posture in a car driver's seat, showing that, as a general rule, the EMG was lowest when the backrest inclination, the lumbar support, and the seat inclination were all as large as possible.

Based upon the mechanics elucidated earlier, sitting on an anteriorly inclined surface should reduce activity levels in the erector spinae. Such was the result of work done by Soderberg et al in evaluating level and 10° and 20° of inclination of the sitting surface. A summary of the results is shown in Figure 14.6 (49).

Other considerations applied to the sitting posture are related to the upper

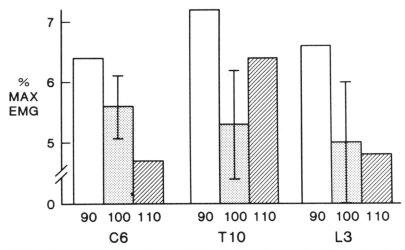

Figure 14.6. Percentage of maximum EMG produced at each of three levels of erector spinae for the three different positions of anterior angulation of the seat. Note the decrease in level of activity as the angulation increased, except for T10 at 110°. Standard error, pooled for all positions, is given in 100° bar. (From Soderberg GL, Blanco MK, Cosentino TL, Kurdelmeier KA: An EMG analysis of posterior trunk musculature during flat and anteriorly inclined sitting. *Human Factors*, submitted for publication, 1985.)

and lower limbs. The height of the work surface has already been discussed relative to implications for the shoulders, head, and neck. Height of the chair is also important because too low a chair places inordinate loads on the ischial tuberosities. Too high a chair does not equitably distribute load under the thigh, potentially causing discomfort in the posterior thigh. Seat area is also a factor, suggesting that movement should be allowed in order to relieve pressure. Suggested dimensions are shown in Figure 14.7. More detailed figures, for specific work circumstances, can be located in volumes intended for that purpose (11, 22, 51).

MATERIALS HANDLING

Virtually all jobs require the direct handling of materials or the manipulation of objects. Approximately one-third of all industrial jobs in the United States involve some form of manual materials handling, namely, lifting, holding, carrying, pushing, and others. These tasks result in 20 to 25% of all compensable industrial injuries and illnesses (5, 20). Thus, there are implications for the therapist, particularly in the management of the low back dysfunction patient. This section of the chapter will discuss the most important considerations associated with the manual handling of materials and will focus on the implications for the patient with real or potential lumbar spine pathology or dysfunction.

Object

Although guidelines for objects to be handled have been generated, we often encounter circumstances in which compliance has been ignored. Witness, for example, the management of an 80-lb bag of water softener salt lifted from a pallet lying on the ground, into and out of a car trunk, and then transported to the softener. The weight exceeds the maximum limit of 25 kg (55 lbs) for men and 15 kg (33 lbs) for women. Neither are there any handles or handholds, as are recommended. Lopsided and loose contents are also possible, a condition

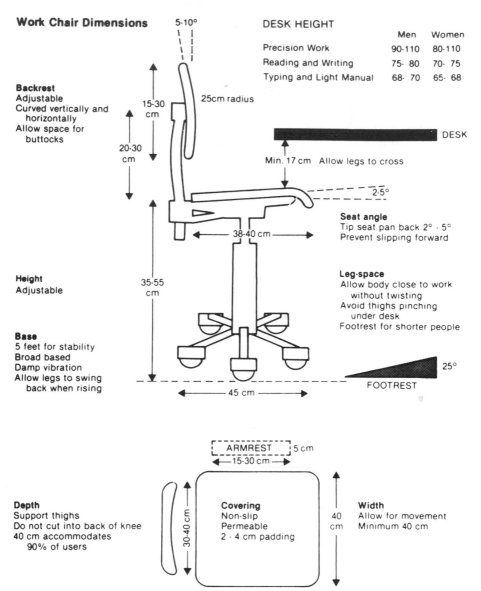

Work Chair Dimensions

5-10°

DESK HEIGHT

	Men	Women
Precision Work	90-110	80-110
Reading and Writing	75- 80	70- 75
Typing and Light Manual	68- 70	65- 68

Backrest
Adjustable
Curved vertically and
    horizontally
Allow space for
    buttocks

15-30 cm

25cm radius

20-30 cm

DESK

Min. 17 cm   Allow legs to cross

2-5°

Seat angle
Tip seat pan back 2° - 5°
Prevent slipping forward

38-40 cm

Height
Adjustable

35-55 cm

Leg-space
Allow body close to work
    without twisting
Avoid thighs pinching
    under desk
Footrest for shorter people

Base
5 feet for stability
Broad based
Damp vibration
Allow legs to swing
    back when rising

45 cm

25°

FOOTREST

ARMREST   5 cm

15-30 cm

Depth
Support thighs
Do not cut into back of knee
40 cm accommodates
    90% of users

30-40 cm

Covering
Non-slip
Permeable
2 - 4 cm padding

40 cm

Width
Allow for movement
Minimum 40 cm

Figure 14.7. Suggested dimensions for the chair of the seated worker. (From Webb RDG: *Industrial Ergonomics.* Ontario, The Industrial Accident Prevention Association, 1982.)

that should always be avoided. Criteria that are fulfilled are that the weight is clearly marked and that the load can be carried close to the body. The latter hardly offset the need for the former. Whenever any object is to be handled, make sure that an accurate assessment of the object's characteristics has been performed. Particularly dangerous are those objects that are likely to produce a sudden change in the body's torque-generating requirements, such as object movement or failure of the container holding the object (51).

Task and Environment

Other requirements exist for the task and the environment. Specifically, all repetitive lifting should be kept between the height of the knuckle and the shoulder of the standing subject. Adjustable platforms appear to be the easiest way to ensure that condition. Limitations imposed on rate should be dependent on the load handled and other factors. Carrying should be minimized, as should upper body movement. As we are aware, the need for accuracy will probably increase muscular effort and perhaps be a significant precursor to the early onset of fatigue.

Environmental factors such as avoidance of constricting spaces and inadequate space for foot location are also of import. The surface should also be uniform throughout the work area so that no differences in constituency or degree of stickiness are encountered. An adequate visual field is also critical, exemplified by the lack of such when a large object carried anteriorly blocks the view of the supporting surface or intended location of object placement (51). Note should also be made that temperature and humidity are compounding environmental factors (27).

Operator/Patient

Often neglected are the worker characteristics. In addition to general health status, such things as age and motor ability should be assessed. Anthropomorphic measures, as compared to the work requirements, are necessary, as are considerations relative to the postures assumed. For example, would you recommend or expect that a patient with low back dysfunction stand all day during work, even without the option to at least periodically elevate one foot onto a stool? Certainly some avoidance of work conditions that could assist with preventing reinjury would be appropriate. Education of the subject should also be required. The importance of this area is now manifested in the number of "schools" for the patient with low back pain or dysfunction. Finally, be sure that all modifications have been made that will make the job the safest and least demanding. This factor, when combined with proper instruction in technique, should minimize the risk of original or recurring injury (51).

Implications for the Lumbar Spine

By far, the most important applications of manual material handling are to the lumbar spine. This is evidenced by the high rate of injury associated with materials handling. Several approaches have been utilized to address the problem of low back injuries and impairments. In 1974 the National Institute of Occupational Safety and Health (NIOSH) convened a panel of experts who reviewed all the available information on the hazards of manual materials handling, establishing a taxonomy to catalog relevant literature (26). In 1981, NIOSH published a document entitled "Work Practices Guide for Manual Lifting" which summarized and synthesized all the available research on overexertion injuries in manual materials handling (52).

This guide, although somewhat limited, does define six variables, such as location of object center of mass and frequency of lifting, that best define hazardous lifts. Furthermore, in developing the guide, epidemiological, psychophysical, physiological, and biomechanical criteria were used. Using these criteria, two levels of hazard were established. The first, called the action limit (AL), is based on facts associated with the four criteria listed above. The second is a maximal permissible limit (MPL), based on other known facts associated with the same four criteria. One example is extracted from the biomechanical criteria: that L5/S1 disc compression force over the 6400 N level cannot be tolerated in most workers. As a result, lifting tasks could be categorized. The categories are shown in Figure 14.8 for occasional lifting of objects. Three distinct areas are established. In the upper righthand portion, the MPL is exceeded, and the lifting conditions in this area are untolerable, necessitating redesign of the task. The *stippled section* labeled with administrative controls required indicates that appropriate employee selection, placement, and training should exist and/or job redesign should take place. The area to the *lower left* is considered to contain the conditions in which nominal risk exists for most workers. It is important to realize that muscle strength and compression forces at L5/S1 define the limits and that fatigue is not an issue in these occasional lifts.

Others have evaluated the maximum load that can be lifted. Poulsen produced data from 50 male and 50 female subjects, proposing that the maximum loads for men should be 1.1 times the isometric muscle "strength." For women the formula is 0.95 times the back muscle "strength" minus 8 kg (43). It is of some interest to compare the material in Figure 14.8 with data referenced in the volume by Grandjean. Using the 50-kp limit for adult men and 20 kp for women, the upper limits of permissible weight are shown as 18 and 12 kp, respectively,

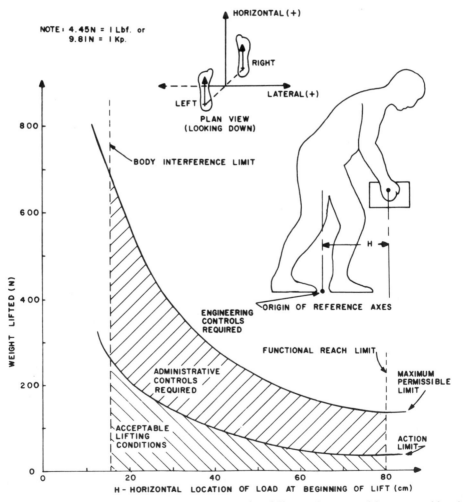

Figure 14.8. The action and permissible limits for different horizontal location of loads lifted from the floor to knuckle height, as described in the text, are shown. (From Chaffin DB, Andersson GBJ: *Occupational Biomechanics.* New York, J Wiley & Sons, 1984.)

when manual lifts are performed frequently. Note is made, however, that these values can only be used as a rough guide (22). Although thought to be a significant feature in low back injuries, fatigue has been investigated little.

Because it is clear that either the muscular force or the tensile capabilities of the passive structures can support the weight of the trunk in any position of forward inclination, there is import as to how these mechanisms interact, particularly in the lowering and lifting of loads. In the lowering phase the muscles can control the movement, as is shown by EMG studies. In the early phases of this movement the posterior ligaments are not in a position to exert any control since they are not in a position of elongation. However, as trunk flexion proceeds, the ligaments are progressively stretched, assuming a position of tension. Thus, it appears that muscle force increases as the requirement for an extensor moment increases until the ligament tension is sufficient to assume control. However, Gracovetsky and coworkers postulate that tension in ligaments should be under active control of muscle at all times, essentially for preventing ligamentous injury (21). Note should also be taken that achieving the fully flexed posture has also required motion of the pelvis on the femur, i.e., hip flexion.

Now consider the converse, the lift of the load. This movement requires concentric action of the muscles, and, based upon the known force-velocity relationship for the two types of contraction, less tension is available in the contractile unit than during the lowering or eccentric phase of the motion. Some investigators, such as Farfan, state that the lumbar spine remains flexed so that the tension in the ligaments and the muscles is maintained. Thus the pelvis must be rotated posteriorly, at least initially, on the hips by the strong hip extensors that can act through a large moment arm (16). As the pelvis rotates, the trunk is lifted, helping to reduce the moment that the extensor musculature has to overcome in order to return the trunk to the upright position. Because the entire maneuver must be completed as a result of muscle shortening, there is no contribution from the passive structures, such as the ligaments. If in fact muscular contributions are not used to protect the ligaments, by way of controlling the motion, soft tissue damage can certainly result.

The most common recommendation given for limiting the need for high extensor moments is that the lift be carried out with the knees bent. Tacit approval of this procedure can only be made if the load can be lifted between the knees because only in this posture can the moment through the lumbar spine be sufficiently reduced to warrant this procedure. That these fundamental rules are important has been verified in the analysis by Lindh. In this case, comparative forward bending moments were calculated for three conditions. In forward bending with the knees straight, the moment was 191.5 Nm. Lifting the same load to the same position with the knees bent and the load between the knees decreased the forward bending moment to 151 Nm. However, if the bent knee lift was used but the object was large enough in size to require lifting in front of the knees, the moment increased to just over 212 Nm (33).

Other work has analyzed four different lifting methods relative to the effect on spinal compression. The conventional bent and straight knee lifts were compared to a trunk kinetic lift and a load kinetic lift. In the former the hips were first extended, followed by the shoulders and the load. In the latter the load was pulled towards the trunk and swung upwards. Results showed that bent knee lifts produced the least peak compression at L5/S1. The trunk kinetic lift was decisively the most stressful. The authors specificially caution that the bent knee lift is of value only for the lumbar spine if lifting the load in front of or beside the knees is avoided. Assurance should also be provided that the knee extensors are of sufficient strength to generate the necessary moment (32). These data reinforce the necessity to consider not only the posture of the spine, but also the size, mass, and location of the object being manipulated.

An additional factor to consider is the effects of contraction of other musculature during the lift. Farfan maintains that the psoas and multifidus are responsible for producing considerable anterior shear in the lumbar spine. Resistance to this shear probably arises in the facet joints, but further contribution to control probably results from the contraction of the internal oblique muscles. This may offer at least a partial explanation as to the activity from this muscle with the lifting of loads greater than body weight (16).

The third factor that contributes to trunk stability during lifting is the increase in intraabdominal pressure. Such pressurization is thought to be reflexive in nature and caused by contraction of the internal and external oblique and transversus muscles. The effect is to provide a distending force between the diaphragm and the rib cage and the pelvic floor, producing an extensor moment for the spine. Studies have shown definitive increases in the intraabdominal pressures during lifting. However, some caution against full contraction of the abdominal muscles must be offered on the basis that the flexor moment created by such a contraction would potentially cancel any extension effect produced by the increase in the intraabdominal pressure (44). A sample of typical results is shown in Figure 14.9 (23). Note that the very large increase occurs at the moment of the lift, returning to levels just over the prelift value for the static condition. Thus, the amount of the load and the degree of acceleration applied appear to be critical factors in determining the degree of increase in the intraabdominal pressure. How important this factor is to the reduction of the extensor moment and the load on the spine has yet to be precisely determined. However, Eie and Wehn, as cited by Lindh, have shown that the pressures in athletes reduced the loads on the spine by up to 40% (33).

Perhaps the important element in the ability of the human to effectively lift loads is the interaction of the active and passive elements of the abdomen and spine, along with the motion of the pelvis on the femur. Clearly, for loads to be lifted, considerable extensor moments of the spine must be generated. Using mechanisms that can ensure the accomplishment of these feats while minimizing the risk of injury to the lumbar spine should be invoked for all, regardless of whether or not low back dysfunction exists. To generalize, as lifting ensues, intraabdominal pressure increases, probably by contraction of the transversus abdominus muscle of the abdomen. Movement of the pelvis on the femur is initiated and, finally, the active muscle contraction of the back extensors contributes to elevation of the trunk to the upright position. It is difficult to believe Farfan's statement that extensor muscle power is not needed for larger lifts or high rates of acceleration on the basis that these muscle forces must be required at some point in the effort. Although the contraction of the abdominal muscles may indeed prevent potential shear in the spine while concurrently increasing intraabdominal pressure, sufficient extensor moments still need to be produced to elevate the trunk to neutral (16). Even then, there is some evidence that activity in the obliques is not a decisive factor in increasing the intraabdominal pressure (24).

Another factor that cannot be ignored is the effect of the lift upon interdiscal pressure. Numerous demonstrations of the effects of different styles of lift and

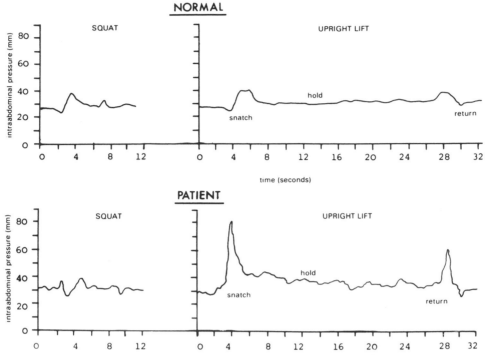

Figure 14.9. Intraabdominal pressures measured during lifting of a 15-kg mass by a normal subject and a patient. (From Grew ND: Intraabdominal pressure response to loads applied to the torso in normal subjects. *Spine* 5:149–154, 1980.)

load lifted have been provided. Larger increases associated with lifts performed in the straight leg position essentially confirm that the degree of activity in the extensor musculature contributes to the increased interdiscal pressure (42). An example of this is provided in the work of Nachemson, who showed that during slight anterior inclination of the trunk while standing, the pressure in the third lumbar disc increased to more than two times the pressure recorded in erect standing. The same degree of load and inclination while sitting increased the pressure to almost three times the standing measurement (40).

Relative to the vertebral disc, the other feature to consider is the asymmetric loading that occurs with forward bending. Instead of the relatively equal distribution of the load, as in standing, trunk flexion significantly increases the pressure on the anterior aspect of the disc. These asymmetries have been thought by some to cause a posterior avulsion, hence, the "ruptured disc" in a posterolateral direction. The magnitude of these forces that has been detailed by Chaffin and Andersson is a multisegment link model of the body. Their calculations show that for the lift of a 450 N load, the compressive force at the L5/S1 disc is 4319 N. Shear reaches a peak value of 400 N (11). Other procedures to determine the amount of load on the lumbar spine have been advocated by Schultz and Andersson (45). In fact, virtually all of the mechanisms associated with lifting increase the compression on the disc and the vertebrae. The remarkable ability of these structures to manage these loads probably enables the lumbar spine to avoid many injuries.

Several generalizations regarding lifting, in relation to the lumbar spine, may be made. Based on mechanics and the literature, the spine should be as straight as possible, maintaining the body in an upright position. With the knees bent, the load should be as close to the body as possible. Furthermore, the load should be 40 to 50 cm above the ground level, which may require the use of ramps and or elevating pallets. Then, if the load is to be transferred to a new location, the spine should be maintained in as straight a posture as possible (22). However, some still say that rules regarding the posture of the lumbar spine to be used in lifting can only be "speculative" (11). Some would say that the lordotic position should be maintained, even though lifting "with the legs" does not preclude this event. Maintenance of lordosis by the back extensors, for example, would allow a stronger contraction of the abdominals so that intraabdominal pressure could be increased. Surely the debate as to the most advised form of lifting will continue until convincing evidence has been presented.

Other implications for the lumbar spine arise from tasks requiring carrying, pushing, and pulling. Regarding carrying, the best solution is to use a yoke across the shoulders. In this fashion the load is closest to the body's center of gravity, minimizing moments. Little information is present in the literature regarding pushing and pulling. Chaffin and Andersson summarize what is available, reporting that for men the limit in either direction is between 200 and 400 N. In the case of either of the activities, a key factor is foot placement and support. Having a firm base of support allowed by advancement of one foot and a surface that will not allow slipping are the two factors that should receive most attention (11).

Although little data exists to support recommendations to not perform asymmetric load handling, enough information is available that indicates that these techniques are more hazardous. For example, Schultz et al. found torsion to significantly increase loads on the lumbar spine (46). Farfan reported that the lumbar spine, designed to support compression force, may incur injury with as little as 2° of axial rotation (17). Because completion of dynamic tasks loads the lumbar spine up to 40% more than static loads (19), and because muscles have been reported to respond differently under isometric and isokinetic conditions (37), Bell and coworkers monitored EMG activity of the L3-L4 erector spinae muscles during dynamic execution of sagittal plane symmetric and asymmetric lifting tasks. Results indicated that EMG activity was significantly greater for asymmetric than symmetric lifting tasks. Activity was also greater on the side away from the rotation, as compared to the side toward the rotation (6). Relating these findings to loading of the lumbar spine is indirect at best. However, in view of the Drury finding that more than 80% of industrial lifting tasks include a twisted position at the start of the task, the ramifications relative to therapeutic recommendations for patients are becoming more clear (13).

MANIPULATION

In most work situations the management of objects is required. In these situations the object itself and the position of the arm and hand are important because of the potential influence on fatigue and musculoskeletal injuries. In general, it is best to mechanize any repetitive task. If not possible, high rates of repetition and extremes of ranges of motion are to be avoided. Another factor that may precipitate fatigue or injury is long duration static contractions that require isometric contractions. For example, one volume on industrial ergonomics recommends a rest/contraction ratio of 10/1 and an avoidance of all contractions in excess of 50% of maximum. Another recommendation is to never exceed 20% of the operator's maximal force in positions requiring prolonged or repetitive work (51).

Because of the attention given to the manipulation of objects, hand tools have undergone considerable design changes. Several factors are of specific concern. The first is that static positioning and/or muscle loading will lead to a fatigue and soreness. To prevent these occurrences the shoulders should be at the sides, and the hand and wrist should be positioned in front of the elbow that is in 90° of flexion. The device being manipulated should allow for easy gripping, perhaps through the provision of an angulated handle. The grip surface should also be of a material that will minimize the likelihood of slippage (51).

Another critical factor is the position of the wrist. The neutral position is highly recommended and is shown in the correct positions in Figure 14.10. Specific examples can be provided by noting that standard pliers and cutting knives have been redesigned to match the neutral position of the wrist. In the former the handle of the pliers was bent to conform to the hand. In the latter case the handle was modified to include a wrap-around restraint with a pistol grip configuration. Decreased incidences of both trauma and chronic problems resulted (11).

A final consideration in use of hand tools is that design should avoid pressures on nerves and blood vessels susceptible to injury. Of specific interest is the area on the palmar surface of the wrist known as the carpal tunnel. To avoid chronic pressures, wrist positions should be monitored. Hand tools should also be manufactured such that the handles for tools do not end in the palm (15).

To avoid problems caused by the manipulation of objects, extensive information is available as to handle length, diameter, and span. Shape, such as the commonly recommended oval and circular grips, also has a set of criteria that can be applied to work settings. Factors such as weight and suspension are important because the operator should not be required to resist a large moment

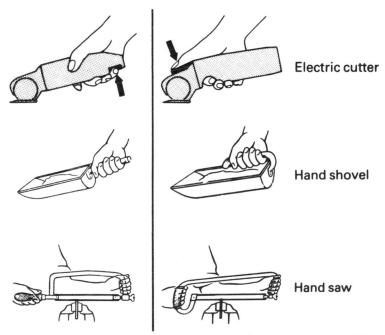

Figure 14.10. Shaping of handgrips should be according to anatomy and function. Poor designs are on the left, good on the right. (From Grandjean E: *Fitting the Task to the Man: An Ergonomic Approach.* London, Taylor and Francis Ltd., 1982.)

caused by the distribution of the mass within the object. Even the location of any triggering mechanism should be given forethought (15). Grip triggers rather than thumb or finger triggers are thought to be the better designs. These and other considerations should allow the worker to perform with maximum efficiency (22).

WORKSITE ANALYSIS

Analysis of the worksite may also be appropriate for the therapist to complete, even though they are not now commonly done. A variety of forms for use during assessment are available, including those for upper extremity and overall posture. Much attention has also been given to the analysis of lifting. In these cases the weight, position of load, frequency, and duration of lift are all factors that are taken into account. Reference to the Chaffin and Andersson volume, or to the reports of the original research, is recommended (11).

Certainly in all site analyses the postures required to perform the task, and the force, duration, and required repetitions are all important factors. Tools, particularly those that require manipulative skills, should be viewed with consideration given to joint positioning and fatigue. Analysis of injury records may also reveal areas in which improvements in work conditions can be suggested. Grandjean has developed a comprehensive checklist that is applicable to the analysis of the work place (22).

APPLICATIONS TO PATIENTS

There is a great deal of evidence that conditions of the work environment can precurse or exacerbate injuries. Direct relationships have been shown for at least the shoulder and wrist, as well as for the joints of the lumbar spine. The role of the therapist could be a preventive one, but more practically the function will be to advise and attempt to control the work situation so that rehabilitation will not be hampered. This section will focus on considerations as they apply to the shoulder, wrist, and spine.

In regards to the shoulder, the position required for work is important. As pointed out in previous sections, work height above the position of the elbow creates the necessity for elevation of the shoulder, increasing the likelihood for injury. This very problem was studied by Chaffin, who reported that fatigue occurred three times faster in 60° of abduction and six times faster in 90° of abduction than when the maintained angle was only 30° (20). Other shoulder injuries can occur as a result of work requirements. Particularly conducive to producing tendinitis, either acute, chronic, or degenerative, is overhead work that requires repetitive and/or high forces. Apparently the biceps brachii and supraspinatus tendons are most susceptible. Patients that have had histories of injury and/or pathology of the shoulder complex should be carefully evaluated for deficiencies in strength and range of motion before return to work in jobs that may demand stress levels that are too high is suggested. Our ability to make these determinations is predicated on the collection of additional information so that we know which of the clinical cases are most likely to succeed with rehabilitative efforts.

The most common predisposing mechanism for injury to the wrist is repetitive exertion by the hand. In most cases improper tool design or tool use can be directly implicated in the onset of impingement of the median nerve in the carpal tunnel. The primary result is manifested in the hand, commonly as pain into the thenar eminence. Losses may also include sensory deficits over the thumb in accordance with the distribution of the median nerve. Although the surgical relief is usually easily accomplished, the cost and lost time from work make prevention the most desirable means of managing this form of disability.

Other hand problems usually focus on tenosynovitis of the long tendons. Again the primary cause is a high repetition rate, often by an individual unaccustomed to that work. Unusual or extreme positions may also account for the pathology. In any of these cases, and in the hand traumatized in the industrial accident, the intention is to return the patient to the same kind of work. Although transfers to different jobs are sometimes practical, the amelioration of the patient's complaints is the immediate goal of effective treatment. Many of these original complaints become chronic, making the circumstances more difficult for the patient, the employer, and the therapist involved. Effective long-term treatment of these cases is probably contingent on consideration given to the work to be resumed by the patient.

Injuries of the lumbar spine are of such prevalence that the clinical conditions manifested by the in-patients returning [injury] by the therapist as to working conditions. Those persons in environments that require either repetitive and/or high load lifting are definitely more prone to original or recurring injury. Muscular strains, ligamentous sprains, disc pathology, or other bony or soft tissue injuries have all claimed a significant toll in patient dysfunction and inability to perform at work. Controlling for the conditions to be encountered demands that the therapist take into account numerous factors before the suggestion can be made that return to work is plausible.

One consideration for the therapist is the overall status of the lumbar spine. Many believe that instability, whether in single or multiple segments, may be critical to the effective function of the lumbar spine. If any patient is determined to have instability from any possible cause, treatment should address that cause. Strengthening of the extensor musculature may be indicated, although definitive data is yet lacking. Reports are beginning to appear in the literature, however, as to the capabilities for trunk control by the low back dysfunction patient (1, 47). It has also been established that the chronic low back dysfunction patient has erector spinae muscle activity that differs from the normal when postural and other functional activities are compared (48).

Much clinical debate has also focused on the role of the abdominal musculature in the control of the lumbar spine. Although it is not the role of this volume to discuss the merit of the necessity for large tensions in the abdominal muscles, they would, at least on an empirical basis, appear to be desirable. Certainly one of the advantages of contraction of this muscle group, initiated just prior to the lift, is that the intraabdominal pressure would be increased. Subsequently, "splinting" of the trunk should be aided, thus assisting with the production of an effective extensor moment.

Training may also have to ensue in order to assure that patients perform functional activities and lifting tasks while using the proper mechanics. The lifting techniques and their effect on the lumbar spine have been discussed in previous sections of this chapter. Specific recommendations may need to be made to the patient as to the frequency and duration of the lifting to be performed. The load will also have to be closely monitored.

That the lifting requirements and work postures are of importance can be verified through the literature. One study evaluated the amount of trunk motion during work by dentists, nurses, and warehouse employees. Although the dentists performed mostly in a semiflexed posture and the nurses in the upright position, the dentists performed only eight flexions requiring more than 73° while the nurses completed 70 deep flexions in the same 1-hour time period. The expectation of the warehouse worker was clearly shown in the study. In their case less than one-half the time was spent in the upright position while 153 deep flexions were required that in almost all cases included lifting some object (41). This study points out the importance of recognizing what the work demands for the patient will be. Similar importance may be attached to the sitting or standing posture to be assumed by these patients because prolonged positioning in one posture may have negative effects on the low back.

Great amounts of information need to be gathered not only on the effect of various therapeutic regimens, but also on the torque generating requirements of both the flexor and extensor musculatures. Only after gathering these data, connected with epidemiological studies, will we have a sufficiently clear picture as to the most effective procedures to follow for the successful management of the patient with low back dysfunction. The pathologies, clearly identifiable or nondescript, simply point out the need for the therapist to consider ergonomics in the total rehabilitation of the patient.

SUMMARY

This chapter has discussed relevant portions of the field of ergonomics. Therapists must take into account the various factors presented in this chapter because often the success of treatment, as judged by the patient and by society, will be the abiltiy of the patient to return to work. In this context the last section of this chapter discussed the implications for patients with shoulder, wrist, and low back injuries or dysfunction.

References

1. Addison R, Schultz A: Trunk strength in patients seeking hospitalization for chronic low back disorders. *Spine* 5:539–544, 1980.
2. Andersson GBJ, Murphy RW, Ortengren R, Nachemson AL: The influence of backrest inclination and lumbar support on the lumbar lordosis in sitting. *Spine* 4:52–58, 1979.
3. Andersson GBJ, Ortengren R: Lumbar disc pressure and myoelectric back muscle activity during sitting. III. Studies on a wheelchair. *Scand J Rehabil Med* 6:122–127, 1974.
4. Andersson GBJ, Ortengren R, Nachemson A, Elfstrom G: Lumbar disc pressure and myoelectric back muscle activity during sitting. I. Studies on an experimental chair. *Scand J Rehabil Med* 6:104–114, 1974.
5. Automakes J: Claims cost of back pain. *Best's Review*, September 1981.
6. Bell SA, Koester JA, Wilking BJ, Cook TM: Erector spinae EMG during asymmetric and symmetric lifting. *Phys Ther*, submitted for publication, 1985.
7. Bendix T, Biering-Sorenson F: Posture of the trunk when sitting on forward inclining seats. *Scand J Rehabil Med* 15:197–203, 1983.
8. Blom L, Hauch A: Physiotherapists in ergonomics. *Appl Ergonomics* 13:289–292, 1982.
9. Brunswic M: Seat design in unsupported sitting. Toronto, Ontario, Proceedings of the 1984 International Conference on Occupational Ergonomics, 1984, pp 294–298.
10. Chaffin DB: Localized muscle fatigue—definition and measurement. *J Occup Med* 15:346–354, 1973.
11. Chaffin DB, Andersson GBJ: *Occupational Biomechanics.* New York, John Wiley & Sons, 1984.
12. Drury CG, Francher M: Evaluation of a forward-sloping chair. *Appl Ergonomics* 16:41–47, 1985.
13. Drury CG, Law C, Pawenski CS: A survey of industrial box handling. *Hum Factors* 24:553–565, 1982.

14. Eastman MC, Kamon E: Posture and subjective evaluation at flat and slanted desks. *Hum Factors* 18:15–26, 1976.
15. Eggleton EM (ed): *Ergonomic Design for People at Work.* Belmont, CA, Lifetime Learning Publications, 1983, vol 1.
16. Farfan HF: Muscular mechanisms of the lumbar spine and the position of power and efficiency. *Orthop Clin North Am* 6:135–144, 1975.
17. Farfan HF: The torsional injury of the lumbar spine. *Spine* 9:53, 1984.
18. Fountain FP, Minear WL, Allison RD: Function of longus colli and longissimus cervicis muscles in man. *Arch Phys Med Rehabil* 47:665–669, 1966.
19. Frievalds A, Chaffin DB, Garg A, Lee KS: A dynamic biomechanical evaluation of lifting maximum acceptable loads. *J Biomech* 17:251–262, 1984.
20. Garg A: Lifting and back injuries. *Plant Engineering* 36:89–93, 1982.
21. Gracovetsky S, Farfan HF, Lamy C: The mechanism of the lumbar spine. *Spine* 6:249–262, 1981.
22. Grandjean E: *Fitting the Task to the Man: An Ergonomic Approach.* London, Taylor & Francis Ltd., 1982.
23. Grew ND: Intraabdominal pressure response to loads applied to the torso in normal subjects. *Spine* 5:149–154, 1980.
24. Hemborg B, Moritz U, Hamberg J, et al: Intraabdominal pressure and trunk muscle activity during lifting—effect of abdominal muscle training in healthy subjects. *Scand J Rehabil Med* 15:183, 183, 1983.
25. Hurberts P, Kamh hus K, Andersson G, Peterson I. Shoulder pain in industry: an epidemiological study on welders. *Acta Orthop Scand* 52:299–306, 1981.
26. Herrin G, Chaffin D, Mach R: Criteria for research on the hazards of manual materials handling. Cincinnati, OH, NIOSH Contract Report CDC 99-74-118, 1974.
27. Jokl MV: The effect of the environment on human performance. *Appl Ergonomics* 13:269–280, 1982.
28. Jorgensen K: Back muscle strength and body weight as limiting factors for work in standing slightly-stooped position. *Scand J Rehabil Med* 2:149–153, 1970.
29. Keegan JJ: Alterations to the lumbar curve related to posture and seating. *J Bone Joint Surg [Am]* 35:589–603, 1953.
30. Knutsson B, Lindh K, Telhag H: Sitting—an electromyographic and mechanical study. *Acta Orthop Scand* 37:415–428, 1966.
31. Kroemer KHE: Seating in plant and office. *Am Ind Hygiene Assoc J* 32:633–652, 1971.
32. Leskinen TPJ, Stalhammar HR, Kuorinka IAA: A dynamic analysis of spinal compression with different lifting techniques. *Ergonomics* 26:595–604, 1983.
33. Lindh M: Biomechanics of the lumbar spine. In Frankel FH, Nordin M: *Basic Biomechanics of the Skeletal Spine.* Philadelphia, Lea & Febiger, 1980.
34. Lundervold A: Electromyographic investigations during sedentary work, especially typewriting. *Br J Phys Med* 14:32–36, 1951.
35. Majeske C, Buchanan C: Quantitative description of two sitting postures: with and without a lumbar support pillow. *Phys Ther* 64:1531–1533, 1984.
36. Mandal AC: The seated man (Homo sedens): the seated work position: theory and practice. *Appl Ergonomics* 12:19–26, 1981.
37. Marras WS, King AI, Joynt RL: Measurements of loads on the lumbar spine under isometric and isokinetic conditions. *Spine* 9:176–187, 1984.
38. Meister D: The present and future of human factors. *Appl Ergonomics* 13:281–287, 1982.
39. Nachemson AL: Lumbar interdiscal pressure. In Jayson MIV (ed): *The Lumbar Spine and Back Pain.* Kent, England, Pitman Medical, 1980.
40. Nachemson AL: The lumbar spine: an orthopaedic challenge. *Spine* 1:59–71, 1976.
41. Nordin M, Ortengren R, Andersson GBJ: Measurements of trunk movements during work. *Spine* 9:465–469, 1984.
42. Ortengren R, Andersson GBJ, Nachemson AL: Studies of relationships between lumbar disc pressure, myoelectric back muscle activity, and intraabdominal (intragastric) pressure. *Spine* 6:98–103, 1981.
43. Poulsen E: Back muscle strength and weight limits in lifting burdens. *Spine* 6:73–75, 1981.
44. Rab GT, Chao EYS, Stauffer RN: Muscle force analysis of the lumbar spine. *Orthop Clin North Am* 8:193–199, 1977.

45. Schultz AB, Andersson GBJ: Analysis of loads on the lumbar spine. *Spine* 6:76–82, 1981.
46. Schultz AB, Andersson GBJ, Haderspeck K, Ortengren R, Nordin M, Bjork R: Analysis and measurement of lumbar trunk loads in tasks involving bends and twists. *J Biomech* 15:669–675, 1982.
47. Smidt G, Herring T, Amundsen L, Rogers M, Russell A, Lehmann T: Assessment of abdominal and back extensor function: a quantitative approach and results for chronic low-back patients. *Spine* 8:211–219, 1983.
48. Soderberg GL, Barr JO: Muscular function in chronic low-back dysfunction. *Spine* 8:79–85, 1983.
49. Soderberg GL, Blanco MK, Cosentino TL, Kurdelmeier KA: An EMG analysis of posterior trunk musculature during flat and anteriorly inclined sitting. *Hum Factors*, submitted for publication, 1985.
50. Tichauer ER: *The Biomechanical Basis of Ergonomics*. New York, Wiley-Interscience, 1978.
51. Webb RDG: *Industrial Ergonomics*. Ontario, The Industrial Accident Prevention Association, 1982.
52. *Work Practices Guide for Manual Lifting*. Cincinnati, OH, DHHS (NIOSH) Publ. No. 81–122, 1981.

APPENDIX A

Trigonometry Review

It is possible to solve many force and velocity problems by use of vector diagrams. However, the degree of accuracy is dependent upon the exactness of the person doing the drawing and measuring. In addition, this approach is time consuming when compared to the quicker more accurate method using trigonometry. The word trigonometry means literally, the measurement of triangles. Most problems in motion analysis involve the use of right triangles. A right triangle is one containing an internal right angle (90°). Recall that the sum of the three internal angles of a triangle always equal 180°. Also, an angle less than 90° is called an acute angle and greater than 90° an obtuse angle. Two angles are said to be *complementary* if their sum equals 90°. Thus, in a right triangle it is apparent that the two acute angles are complementary. If the sum of two angles equals 180°, they are said to be *supplementary*.

In order to understand the trigonometry functions, one must first be able to identify the parts of a right triangle. The following diagram (Fig. A.1) of a right triangle will be used for the purpose of explanation.

The six component parts of the triangle consist of three angles and three sides. (The symbol "∠" is used to denote the word angle.) It should be noted that the longest of the three sides (c) is opposite the right angle (C). This longest side is called the *hypotenuse*. Because the hypotenuse is always opposite the right angle, it is very easy to identify. The other two sides are referred to as the legs of the right triangle. The second notation used for the sides is called the side *opposite*. Which side this is depends upon the angle in question. Referring to the diagram, the side opposite angle A (∠A) is side "a," On the other hand, the side opposite ∠B is side "b." The *adjacent* side is the third term used in identifying the sides. The side adjacent (or next to) refers to the side which along with the hypotenuse forms the given angle. Thus, the side adjacent to ∠A would be side b. Likewise, the side adjacent ∠B is side a. Thus, understand that the sides opposite and adjacent depend upon which of the two angles is being considered, whereas the hypotenuse is fixed.

Now that each of the parts of the triangle has been named, the trig functions can be introduced. Although there are six functions, only four will be included. These functions are based upon the relationship that exists between the angles and sides of the triangle.

The first of these is called the sine, abbreviated "sin." The sine of an angle is defined as the ratio (one number divided by another) of the side opposite over the hypotenuse. Thus, the sine of angle A (sin A) = a/c, that is, the length of side a is divided by the length of the hypotenuse. Note that the sine of angle B = b/c.

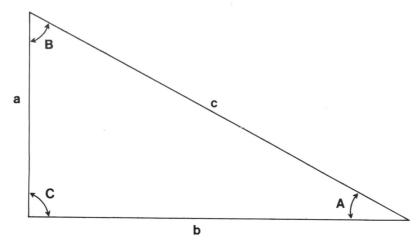

Figure A.1.   The right triangle and descriptors of sides and angles.

The second trig function is called the cosine, abbreviated *cos*, and is defined as the ratio of the side adjacent over the hypotenuse. For angle A the cosine is b/c, and for angle B it is a/c.

The third function is called the tangent (tan) and is defined as the ratio of the side *opposite* over the side adjacent. Thus, the tangent of angle A (tan A) = a/b while the tan B = b/a.

The last function is termed the cotangent (cot) and is defined as the ratio of the side adjacent over the side opposite; hence, the cotangent of angle A (cot A) = b/a and the cot B = a/b.

Now that the trig functions have been defined, their use will be discussed. It has been shown that the trig functions have a specific value for a given angle, regardless of the size of the triangle. Since the trig functions are constants for any given angle, it is possible to include these functions in table form for the various angles. This type of table has been included for reference.

Since the one angle is fixed (90°) in a right triangle, only five parts can vary (three sides and two angles). If either one angle and the length of one side or the length of two sides are known, the remaining parts can be determined. The sides can be used to represent distance, magnitude of force, velocity, or some other physical property.

EXAMPLE

Referring to the diagram, assume that the hypotenuse is 6 inches in length and angle A = 40°. Find the following: (1) angle B; (2) side a; (3) side b.

Angle B can be determined very readily since it is complementary to angle A (40°). So, angle B is found by 90° − 40° = 50°.

To find side a, we must select the trig function that involves side a (which is unknown) and side c, the hypotenuse (which is known). It can be seen that sin A equals side a (opposite) over c (hypotenuse).

In equation form:

$$\sin A = a/c$$

Since c is known to be 6 inches and the sin A (40°) can be secured from the table, the only unknown is side a. Thus, the formula appears as follows:

$$\sin 40° = a/6 \text{ inches}$$

Multiplying both sides of the equation by 6 yields: $6 \times 0.6428 = a$, $a = 3.84$ inches.

The same procedure is followed in solving for side b.

The following problems are included as practice exercises. Answers are at the end of the review.

1. 20 feet = 80 units   1 foot = _____ units   1 unit = _____ feet

2. sine 25 = _____   3. cos 57 = _____   4. tan 80 = _____

5.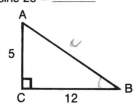

B = _____ degrees

side c = _____

6.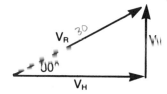

$V_R = 30$ ft/sec

$V_H =$ _____

$V_V =$ _____

7.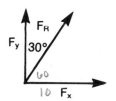

$F_x = 10\#$

$F_y =$ _____

$F_R =$ _____

8. Using a ruler and protractor, devise an appropriate scale factor and sketch the path of a hiker who walks 1 mile at 30°, 3 miles at 120°, 5 miles at 230° and 2 miles at 340°. Measure the resultant displacement of the hiker (magnitude and direction). Use the following coordinate reference system:

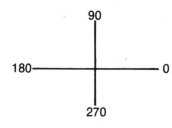

Answers

1. 4 units, .25 feet   5. 22.5°, 13

2. .4226   6. 25.98, 15

3. .5446   7. 17.32, 20

4. 5.6713

CIRCULAR (TRIGONOMETRIC) FUNCTIONS

Degrees	Sines	Cosines	Tangets	Cotangents	
0°00′	.0000	1.0000	.0000		90°00′
1°00′	.0175	.9998	.0175	57.290	89°00′
2°00′	.0349	.9994	.0349	28.636	88°00′
3°00′	.0523	.9986	.0524	19.081	87°00′
4°00′	.0698	.9976	.0699	14.301	86°00′
5°00′	.0872	.9962	.0875	11.430	85°00′
6°00′	.1045	.9945	.1051	9.5144	84°00′
7°00′	.1219	.9925	.1228	8.1443	83°00′
8°00′	.1392	.9903	.1405	7.1154	82°00′
9°00′	.1564	.9877	.1584	6.3138	81°00′
10°00′	.1736	.9848	.1763	5.6713	80°00′
11°00′	.1908	.9816	.1944	5.1446	79°00′
12°00′	.2079	.9781	.2126	4.7046	78°00′
13°00′	.2250	.9744	.2309	4.3315	77°00′
14°00′	.2419	.9703	.2493	4.0108	76°00′
15°00′	.2588	.9659	.2679	3.7321	75°00′
16°00′	.2756	.9613	.2867	3.4874	74°00′
17°00′	.2924	.9563	.3057	3.2709	73°00′
18°00′	.3090	.9511	.3249	3.0777	72°00′
19°00′	.3256	.9455	.3443	2.9042	71°00′
20°00′	.3420	.9397	.3640	2.7475	70°00′
21°00′	.3584	.9336	.3839	2.6051	69°00′
22°00′	.3746	.9272	.4040	2.4751	68°00′
23°00′	.3907	.9205	.4245	2.3559	67°00′
24°00′	.4067	.9135	.4452	2.2460	66°00′
25°00′	.4226	.9063	.4663	2.1445	65°00′
26°00′	.4384	.8988	.4877	2.0503	64°00′
27°00′	.4540	.8910	.5095	1.9626	63°00′
28°00′	.4695	.8829	.5317	1.8807	62°00′
29°00′	.4848	.8746	.5543	1.8040	61°00′
30°00′	.5000	.8660	.5774	1.7321	60°00′
31°00′	.5150	.8572	.6009	1.6643	59°00′
32°00′	.5299	.8480	.6249	1.6003	58°00′
33°00′	.5446	.8387	.6494	1.5399	57°00′
34°00′	.5592	.8290	.6745	1.4826	56°00′
35°00′	.5736	.8192	.7002	1.4281	55°00′
36°00′	.5878	.8090	.7265	1.3764	54°00′
37°00′	.6018	.7986	.7536	1.3270	53°00′
38°00′	.6157	.7880	.7813	1.2799	52°00′
39°00′	.6293	.7771	.8098	1.2349	51°00′
40°00′	.6428	.7660	.8391	1.1918	50°00′
41°00′	.6561	.7547	.8693	1.1504	49°00′
42°00′	.6691	.7431	.9004	1.1106	48°00′
43°00′	.6820	.7314	.9325	1.0724	47°00′
44°00′	.6947	.7193	.9657	1.0355	46°00′
45°00′	.7071	.7071	1.0000	1.0000	45°00′
	Cosines	Sines	Cotangents	Tangents	Degrees

APPENDIX B

*Elements of Vector Algebra**

Detailed analysis of noncoplanar biomechanical systems requires a basic understanding of the elements of vector algebra.

RIGHT HAND RULE

It is customary to use a right handed coordinate system in most mechanical analyses (Fig. B.1). If the fingers of the right hand are curled in the direction necessary to rotate the positive X axis toward the positive Y axis through the 90° angle between them, the thumb will point in the direction of the positive Z axis. Such a coordinate reference frame is termed right-handed.

UNIT VECTORS

Vectors, one unit in length, are utilized to indicate specific directions. The notations **i, j,** and **k** indicate unit vectors directed along the positive X, Y, and Z axes, respectively (Fig. B.2).

VECTOR NOTATION

A vector is often specified in terms of unit vectors **i, j,** and **k,** with each being multiplied by the appropriate magnitude. The vector notation for a line directed from M(Mx,My,Mz) to N(Nx,Ny,Nz) is:

$$\mathbf{MN} = (Nx - Mx)\mathbf{i} + (Ny - My)\mathbf{j} + (Nz - Mz)\mathbf{k}$$

If the vector were directed from N to M, then it would be designated:

$$\mathbf{NM} = (Mx - Nx)\mathbf{i} + (My - Ny)\mathbf{j} + (Mz - Nz)\mathbf{k}$$

Assuming that the coordinates of M and N were (2,1,−2) and (5,−3,10), respectively, the vector directed from M to N would be:

$$\mathbf{MN} = (5 - 2)\mathbf{i} + (-3 - 1)\mathbf{j} + (10 + 2)\mathbf{k}$$
$$= 3\mathbf{i} - 4\mathbf{j} + 12\mathbf{k}$$

The magnitude of **MN** can be calculated using the three dimensional version of the Pythagorean theorem:

$$MN = \sqrt{3^2 + 4^2 + 12^2} = \sqrt{169} = 13$$

---

* Modified from Miller DI, Nelson RC: *Biomechanics of Sport*. Philadelphia, Lea & Febiger, 1973, pp 241–242.

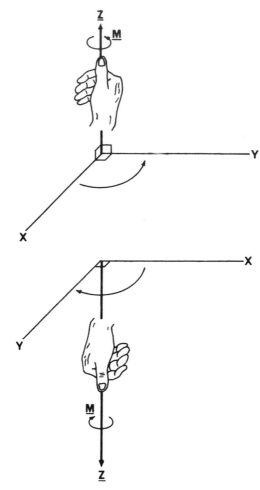

Figure B.1.   Right-handed coordinate reference frames.

MN can be expressed as a unit vector, **u,** by dividing each of its components by the magnitude of the vector. Thus,

$$\mathbf{u} = \frac{\mathbf{MN}}{MN} = \frac{3\mathbf{i} - 4\mathbf{j} + 12\mathbf{k}}{13}.$$

ADDITION AND SUBTRACTION

Vectors can be combined by the addition or subtraction of each of the three orthogonal components. For example, if

$$\mathbf{F} = Fx\mathbf{i} + Fy\mathbf{j} + Fz\mathbf{k} \qquad \text{and}$$
$$\mathbf{G} = Gx\mathbf{i} + Gy\mathbf{j} + Gz\mathbf{k}$$

then $\mathbf{F} + \mathbf{G} = (Fx + Gx)\mathbf{i} + (Fy + Gy)\mathbf{j} + (Fz + Gz)\mathbf{k}.$

DOT OR SCALAR PRODUCT

The dot product of two vectors is, by definition, a scalar equal to the product of the magnitudes of the two vectors multiplied by the cosine of the smaller angle between them. Thus,

$$\mathbf{M} \cdot \mathbf{N} = MN \cos \theta \text{ (Fig. B.3)}.$$

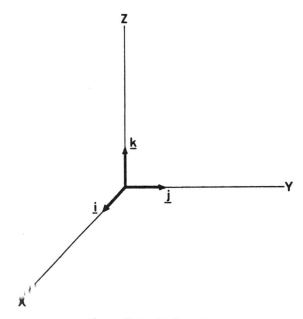

Figure B.2. Unit vectors.

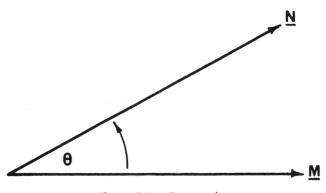

Figure B.3. Dot product.

This gives the component of **M** directed along **N** multiplied by the magnitude of N. It is therefore a suitable vector operation for determining work which is equal to the component of force in the direction of the displacement multiplied by the displacement.

The dot products of unit vectors **i, j,** and **k** are:

$$\mathbf{i} \cdot \mathbf{i} = (1)(1)\cos 0 = 1$$

Similarly, $\mathbf{j} \cdot \mathbf{j} = \mathbf{k} \cdot \mathbf{k} = 1$.

Then, $\mathbf{j} \cdot \mathbf{k} = (1)(1)\cos 90 = 0$ and likewise

$$\mathbf{i} \cdot \mathbf{j} = \mathbf{k} \cdot \mathbf{i} = \mathbf{j} \cdot \mathbf{i} = \mathbf{i} \cdot \mathbf{k} = \mathbf{k} \cdot \mathbf{j} = 0.$$

Using these identities to expand **M·N,**

$$\mathbf{M} \cdot \mathbf{N} = (M_x\mathbf{i} + M_y\mathbf{j} + M_z\mathbf{k}) \cdot (N_x\mathbf{i} + N_y\mathbf{j} + N_z\mathbf{k})$$
$$= M_xN_x + M_yN_y + M_zN_z.$$

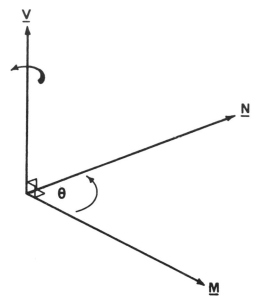

Figure B.4. Cross product.

VECTOR OR CROSS PRODUCT

By definition, the cross product of two vectors **M** and **N** is a vector **V** acting in a direction perpendicular to the plane of the two original vectors in accordance with the right hand rule (Fig. B.4). The magnitude of **V** is equal to the product of the magnitudes of **M** and **N** multiplied by the sine of the smaller angle between them. The cross products of the unit vectors **i, j,** and **k** are:

$$\mathbf{i} \times \mathbf{i} = (1)(1)\sin 0 = 0 \quad \mathbf{j} \times \mathbf{j} = 0 \quad \mathbf{k} \times \mathbf{k} = 0$$
$$\mathbf{i} \times \mathbf{j} = \mathbf{k} \qquad\qquad\quad \mathbf{j} \times \mathbf{k} = \mathbf{i} \quad \mathbf{k} \times \mathbf{i} = \mathbf{j}$$
$$\mathbf{j} \times \mathbf{i} = -\mathbf{k} \qquad\qquad\quad \mathbf{k} \times \mathbf{j} = -\mathbf{i} \quad \mathbf{i} \times \mathbf{k} = -\mathbf{j}.$$

Using these identities, the cross product **M** × **N** can be expanded:

$$\mathbf{M} \times \mathbf{N} = (Mx\mathbf{i} + My\mathbf{j} + Mz\mathbf{k}) \times (Nx\mathbf{i} + Ny\mathbf{j} + Nz\mathbf{k})$$
$$= MxNy\mathbf{k} - MxNz\mathbf{j} - MyNx\mathbf{k} + MyNz\mathbf{i} + MzNx\mathbf{j} - MzNy\mathbf{i}$$
$$= (MyNz - MzNy)\mathbf{i} + (MzNx - MxNz)\mathbf{j} + (MxNy - MyNx)\mathbf{k}$$

This relationship can be more easily expressed in the form of a 3 × 3 determinant:

$$\mathbf{M} \times \mathbf{N} = \begin{vmatrix} \mathbf{i} & \mathbf{j} & \mathbf{k} \\ Mx & My & Mz \\ Nx & Ny & Nz \end{vmatrix}$$

MOMENT OF A FORCE ABOUT A POINT

The vector product **r** × **F** represents the moment of force **F** about a point, where **r** is any position vector directed from the point to the line of action of **F**. Both magnitude and direction of the moment can be obtained by expanding the determinant:

$$\mathbf{r} \times \mathbf{F} = \begin{vmatrix} \mathbf{i} & \mathbf{j} & \mathbf{k} \\ r_x & r_y & r_z \\ F_x & F_y & F_z \end{vmatrix}$$

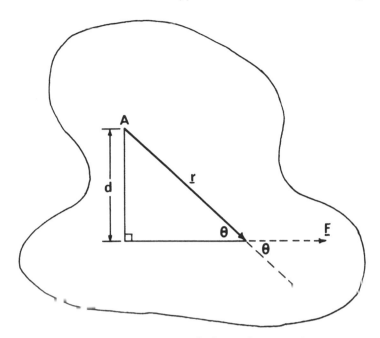

Figure B.5. Moment of a force about a point.

In the planar example shown in Figure B.5, the magnitude of the moment of **F** about point A is equal to the magnitude of the force multiplied by the perpendicular distance d. By trigonometry, it can be seen that

$$d = r \sin \theta$$

It will be recalled that the magnitude of $\mathbf{r} \times \mathbf{F} = rF \sin \theta = Fr \sin \theta$.

MOMENT OF A FORCE ABOUT AN AXIS

The triple scalar product is utilized to determine the moment of force (**F**) about a particular axis (**N**). The axis must first be expressed in unit vector form. Then, the moment of force **F** about axis **N** is $\mathbf{r} \times \mathbf{F} \cdot \mathbf{N}$, where **r** is any position vector joining **N** and **F**, directed toward **F**. In determinant form, the triple scalar product is

$$\mathbf{r} \times \mathbf{F} \cdot \mathbf{N} = \begin{vmatrix} r_x & r_y & r_z \\ F_x & F_y & F_z \\ N_x & N_y & N_z \end{vmatrix}$$

The triple scalar product is the dot product of two vectors, one of which is the cross product of two other vectors. In computing the moment of force about an axis, the triple scalar product gives the component of rotation in the direction of the specified axis.

Example

The following example illustrates some of the basic concepts of vector algebra which are required in biomechanical analysis.

Given

A 20-N force passes through points D(1,3,5) and E(10,10,12), and is directed from D to E. The coordinates are specified in meters.

Find

The moment of the force with respect to an axis through G(−1,−6,−12) and H(−3,−10,−20). The axis is directed from G to H.

Solution

(1) Express the force in vector form.
  (a) Direction of the force

$$\mathbf{DE} = (10 - 1)\mathbf{i} + (10 - 3)\mathbf{j} + (12 - 5)\mathbf{k}$$
$$= 9\mathbf{i} + 7\mathbf{j} + 7\mathbf{k}$$

  (b) Express the direction as a unit vector.

$$\mathbf{U} = \frac{9\mathbf{i} + 7\mathbf{j} + 7\mathbf{k}}{\sqrt{9^2 + 7^2 + 7^2}}$$
$$= \frac{1}{\sqrt{179}} (9\mathbf{i} + 7\mathbf{j} = 7\mathbf{k})$$

  (c) Multiply the unit vector by the magnitude of the force to determine the force vector.

$$\mathbf{F} = (20) \frac{1}{\sqrt{179}} (9\mathbf{i} + 7\mathbf{j} + 7\mathbf{k}) \text{ Newtons}$$

Thus the components of force in the three orthogonal directions are:

$$\mathbf{F}_x = \frac{180}{\sqrt{179}} \quad \mathbf{F}_y = \frac{140}{\sqrt{179}} \quad \mathbf{F}_z = \frac{140}{\sqrt{179}} \text{ Newtons}$$

(2) Calculate a position vector, **r**, joining the axis to the line of action, **F.**
  (a) Of the several possibilities available, namely, **GD, GE, HD,** and **HE,** vector **GD** is arbitrarily chosen:

$$\mathbf{r} = [(1) - (-1)]\mathbf{i} + [(3) - (-6)]\mathbf{j} + [(5) - (-12)]\mathbf{k}$$
$$= 2\mathbf{i} + 9\mathbf{j} + 17\mathbf{k}$$

(3) Express the axis in unit vector form.
  (a) $\mathbf{GH} = [(-3) - (-1)]\mathbf{i} + [(-10) - (-6)]\mathbf{j} + [(-20) - (-12)]\mathbf{k}$
$$= -2\mathbf{i} - 4\mathbf{j} - 8\mathbf{k}$$

  (b) As a unit vector **N,**

$$\mathbf{N} = \frac{-2\mathbf{i} - 4\mathbf{j} - 8\mathbf{k}}{\sqrt{2^2 + 4^2 + 8^2}}$$
$$= \frac{1}{\sqrt{84}} (-2\mathbf{i} - 4\mathbf{j} - 8\mathbf{k}).$$

(4) Use the triple scalar product to determine the moment of the force about the axis.

$$M = \mathbf{r} \times \mathbf{F} \cdot \mathbf{N}$$
$$= [(\mathbf{r} \times \mathbf{F}) \cdot \mathbf{N}]$$
$$= [\mathbf{r} \cdot (\mathbf{F} \times \mathbf{N})]$$
$$= \frac{1}{\sqrt{84}} \cdot \frac{20}{\sqrt{179}} \begin{vmatrix} 2 & 9 & 17 \\ 9 & 7 & 7 \\ -2 & -4 & -8 \end{vmatrix}$$
$$= \frac{20}{\sqrt{84}\sqrt{179}} 2[(7)(-8) - (7)(-4)]$$
$$\qquad - 9[(9)(-8) - (7)(-2)] + 17[(9)(-4) - (7)(-2)]$$
$$= \frac{20}{(9.165)(13.379)} (2)(-28) - (9)(-58) + (17)(-22)$$
$$= \frac{1840}{122.62}$$
$$= 15.01 \text{N} \cdot \text{m}$$

Index